THE THEORETICAL FOUN
DENDRITIC FUNCTION

Computational Neuroscience
Terrence J. Sejnowski and Tomaso A. Poggio, editors

THE THEORETICAL FOUNDATION OF DENDRITIC FUNCTION

Selected Papers of Wilfrid Rall with Commentaries

edited by Idan Segev, John Rinzel, and Gordon M. Shepherd

A Bradford Book
The MIT Press
Cambridge, Massachusetts
London, England

This book was published with the assistance of the Office of Naval Research and the National Institute of Diabetes and Digestive and Kidney Diseases, National Institutes of Health.

This book was printed and bound in the United States of America.

Library of Congress Cataloging-in-Publication Data

Rall, Wilfrid.
  The theoretical foundation of dendritic function : selected papers
  of Wilfrid Rall with commentaries / edited by Idan Segev, John Rinzel, and
  Gordon M. Shepherd.
      p.   cm. — (Computational neuroscience)
  "A Bradford book."
  Includes bibliographical references.
  ISBN 978-0-262-51546-7 (pb.:alk.paper)
  1. Dendrites—Mathematical models. I. Segev, Idan. II. Rinzel, John. III. Shepherd,
Gordon M., 1933–   . IV. Title. V. Series.
QP361.R33   1995
612.8—dc20   94-13538
                                                                        CIP

Contents

Computational neuroscience is an approach to understanding the information content of neural signals by modeling the nervous system at many different structural scales, including the biophysical, the circuit, and the systems levels. Computer simulations of neurons and neural networks are complementary to traditional techniques in neuroscience. This book series welcomes contributions that link theoretical studies with experimental approaches to understanding information processing in the nervous system. Areas and topics of particular interest include biophysical mechanisms for computation in neurons, computer simulations of neural circuits, models of learning, representation of sensory information in neural networks, systems models of sensory-motor integration, and computational analysis of problems in biological sensing, motor control, and perception.

Terrence J. Sejnowski
Tomaso A. Poggio

Foreword by Terrence J. Sejnowski

The exploration of the electrical properties of dendrites pioneered by Wilfrid Rall provided many key insights into the computational resources of neurons. Many of the papers in this collection are classics: dendrodendritic interactions in the olfactory bulb; nonlinear synaptic integration in motoneuron dendrites; active currents in pyramidal neuron apical dendrites. In each of these studies, insights arose from a conceptual leap, astute simplifying assumptions, and rigorous analysis. Looking back, one is impressed with the foresight shown by Rall in his choice of problems, with the elegance of his methods in attacking them, and with the impact that his conclusions have had for our current thinking. These papers deserve careful reading and rereading, for there are additional lessons in each of them that will reward the careful reader.

New techniques have recently allowed direct experimental exploration of mechanisms, such as active membrane currents within dendrites, that previously were only accessible through somatic recordings. The distribution of sodium and calcium currents extends quite widely in the dendritic trees of neocortical and hippocampal neurons. There are still uncertainties in the densities of these ionic currents, and the diversity of their biophysical properties, but it is now clear that the computational repertoire of cortical neurons is far richer than anyone had previously imagined, except perhaps for Rall.

The current work in computational neuroscience has built upon the solid foundations provided by Rall's legacy. Exploring the interplay between the wide range of voltage-sensitive conductances that have been identified, and the spatial interactions within dendrites and between networks of neurons, is now within our grasp. This includes issues such as homeostatic mechanisms for regulating ionic currents in dendrites, the effects of spontaneous activity on dendritic processing, the source of the stochastic variability observed in the spike trains of cortical neurons and role of inhibitory interneurons in synchronizing spike trains in cerebral cortex, and the implications of Hebbian mechanisms for synaptic plasticity. Hidden within dendrites are the answers to many of the mysteries of how brains represent the world, keep records of past experiences, and make us aware of the world.

It would be difficult to imagine the field of computational neuroscience today without the conceptual framework established over the last thirty years by Wil Rall, and for this we all owe him a great debt of gratitude.

1   INTRODUCTION

Overview of Wilfrid Rall's Contributions to Understanding Dendritic Function by Idan Segev, John Rinzel, and Gordon M. Shepherd

The branching structures called dendrites are among the most striking and characteristic features of nerve cells, and understanding their contributions to nerve function has been a supreme challenge to neuroscience. More than thirty years have passed since the three key papers of Wilfrid Rall on the biophysical properties of branching dendritic trees appeared (Rall 1957, 1959, 1960). These papers were revolutionary in several ways. They showed first that dendrites could be analyzed by a rigorous mathematical and biophysical approach, so that studies of the functional properties underlying impulse generation and synaptic responses could be carried out on a par with studies of similar properties in cell bodies and axons. They introduced a new theoretical framework for modeling these complex structures so that their integrative properties could be studied and, through this, their contributions to signal processing in the nervous system. Finally, these studies challenged the dominant hypothesis of contemporary neurobiologists and modelers that neurons are essentially *isopotential* units.

For neural modelers, the assumption of isopotentiality of neurons was very convenient because it allowed them to neglect the daunting spatial properties of dendrites and focus only on temporal aspects of the input-output properties at the cell body (an assumption that continues to this day in most neural network models). This had been the basic premise underlying all theoretical models since the pioneering study of McCulloch and Pitts (1943), in which the neuron was represented as a "point unit" that implements simple binary ("on-off") computation. However, Rall showed that the interrelations between the unique morphology and the specific electrical properties of neurons can be critical for their input-output functions, and that by combining the different kinds of "neuronware" (dendrites, spines, axon, membrane channels, synapses) into complex structures, the neuron can be a computationally powerful unit.

In retrospect it is difficult to understand why dendrites were ignored, functionally, until Rall's pioneering work. They had been the focus of intense anatomical studies for many years since the classical studies of Ramón y Cajal and his contemporaries in the 1890s, and their extended and complex morphology was well appreciated (reviewed in Shepherd 1991). A glance at the drawings of Ramón y Cajal makes it clear that the majority of the surface area of most neurons is in the dendrites and that, most significantly, abundant inputs seem to converge onto the dendritic trees. The electrically distributed nature of dendrites was actually known for many years, simply from the fact that extracellular electrical field potentials, such as the electroencephalogram, can be recorded in the brain; a tissue composed of isopotential units would not give detectable summed extracellular currents. Studies of field potentials in the cortex had further suggested that "decrementing conduction" occurs in dendrites. But these considerations were overridden by the need for simplifying assumptions in facing the complexity of the nervous system, and once they were established, it was difficult to abandon them in favor of new ones.

Reflecting Rall's methodical approach and modest personality, his theory for dendrites penetrated the scientific community slowly and then deeply. It spread among cellular neuroanatomists and neurophysiologists, and, with time, the functional consequences of dendrites began to attract serious attention. Old experimental results were reinterpreted, and new experimental and theoretical studies were designed to explore the input-output function of dendrites (e.g., Rall et al. 1967; Rall 1967; see reviews in Jack et al. 1975; Rall 1977, Rall et al. 1992, and Mel 1994). We know now that most of the synaptic information transmitted between nerve cells is indeed processed in the dendrites, and that it is there that many of the plastic changes underlying learning and memory take place. It is now generally agreed that the specific aspects of dendritic morphology characteristic of different types of nerve cells must be considered when the computational and plastic functions of the brain are to be understood. Thus, we speak naturally today about "dendritic integration," "spatiotemporal summation of synaptic inputs," "dendritic nonlinearities," "dendritic plasticity," "chemical compartmentalization," and ion diffusion along dendritic segments. Much of this new vocabulary has emerged from the work of Wilfrid Rall.

In pursuing these early studies, Rall was one of the first to realize the potential of digital computers for biology (Rall 1964). He was a pioneer not only in constructing the first computer-based models of the neuron complete with its dendrites but also in drawing attention to the dendrites as the main computational substrate for signal integration in the nervous system. Most neurobiologists entering the field now are unaware of Rall's seminal 1964 paper on compartmental modeling and the foundations he laid in it and his subsequent papers for the present methods and concepts that are now taken for granted in the computer modeling of neurons. Through this work Rall may, in fact, be regarded as a founding father of computational neuroscience.

This book is a manifestation of the bulk of Rall's theoretical thinking applied to the nervous system. It brings together his major articles that established many of our present concepts and insights regarding the information-processing functions of nerve cells. Each article is accompanied by an introduction that highlights the main insights gained from the paper and puts the work in the appropriate historical perspective. These introductions are written by co-workers who collaborated with Rall in these studies or were his colleagues in the field. They have tried to convey a sense of the context within which the studies were carried out, and of their unique perspective from working with Rall on these problems and being inspired by him. The introductions also point toward the impact of specific papers on the present state of the art of single neuron modeling. Appropriate commentaries are also provided for several important papers that could not be included because of space limitations.

One may wonder why this book is assembled now. There are several reasons. First, in this "Decade of the Brain," when the field of computational neuroscience is becoming so active, it seems timely to group together the work of a major creator of the field. Second, a source book such as this, with appropriate perspectives, should help the newcomer to appreciate where things started and where they may lead. Third, some of Rall's papers are not easily accessible. Fourth, with the passage of time, many fundamental contributions of Rall have been forgotten or have been misinterpreted. For example, many erroneously believe that Rall considered only passive membrane properties, thereby neglecting the functional consequences of synaptic- and voltage-gated nonlinearities in dendritic trees. Nothing could be further from the truth, and this book provides the evidence in his papers and the commentaries. Finally, in keeping with his modest personality, Rall has never received the recognition one would expect of a major creator of modern neuroscience. As he enters retirement and devotes more time to his artistic pursuits, this book serves as an appreciation from all of us who have been influenced by his scientific thinking and personality.

In the remainder of this introduction we highlight for the general reader the major insights that were gained from the main studies of Rall and his collaborators and followers. We do so by emphasizing the leading questions that he posed along the path of his scientific career, and their answers. A fascinating account of the development of his ideas can be found in his recent brief memoir (Rall 1992). More on the general background for the development of his ideas can be found in Rall 1977, Shepherd 1992, and Segev 1992. This background is amplified in the various introductions and commentaries in this book, together with more personal comments by colleagues and co-workers that are not available elsewhere. Theoretical elaboration and extension of Rall's theory can be found in Jack et al. 1975, Butz and Cowan 1974, Horwitz 1981, Poggio and Torre 1978, Koch et al. 1982, Holmes 1986, Abbott et al. 1991, and

Major et al. 1993. The impact of Rall's ideas on computational neuro-science can be found in Sejnowski et al. 1988. The epilogue of this introduction discusses possible future directions for the theoretical and experimental studies on the computational functions of single neurons.

Early Training: From Physics to Neurophysiology

Wilfrid Rall received his early training in physics, graduating from Yale University with highest honors in 1943. The Second World War was in progress, and, like many other young physicists, he became part of the Manhattan Project. A glimpse of his role in that effort as a mass spectro-grapher at the University of Chicago can be gained from his memoir in Rall 1992. At the end of the war he became interested in applying physics to biology. As it happened, the first graduate program in biophysics was being formed at Chicago by K. S. Cole, and Rall enrolled as one of the first students in 1946. Over the next two years, his summers were spent at the Marine Biological Laboratory in Woods Hole as a research assistant to Cole and George Marmont, helping to develop and introduce the new space clamp and voltage clamp methods for the squid axon. At Chicago, in addition to courses in experimental biology, he took courses taught by Rashevsky, Carnap, Fermi, and Sewall Wright. All in all, not a bad way to start a career in biophysics!

While completing requirements for a master's degree in 1948, Rall had corresponded with John C. Eccles at the University of Otago Medical School in New Zealand about Eccles's new theory of synaptic inhibition. This resulted in an offer to come to Dunedin to carry out his doctoral work. There he was immediately plunged into the intensive studies of the neural basis of spinal reflexes that soon led to the pioneering intracellular studies of motoneurons by Brock, Coombs, and Eccles in 1951–1952. At that point Rall turned to a more independent project for his dissertation, a study of the monosynaptic activation of a motoneuron pool and the construction of a probabilistic model for the input-output relations. In this work Rall gained much from the wise counsel of A. K. (Archie) McIntyre, who became Professor when Eccles left for Australia in 1952. Among the students at Dunedin was Julian Jack, one of the contributors to this volume.

One should not think that this life in New Zealand was lived far off the beaten path, certainly not in neurophysiology. Eccles was always on the move. His intracellular studies made Dunedin the center of the world in the 1950s for the new neurophysiology of the central nervous system. McIntyre himself had recently studied at Cambridge, London, and the

Rockefeller Institute; in fact, the new instrumentation he brought back to Dunedin played a critical role in the pioneering intracellular studies. Rall was therefore ideally placed to experience the best in experimental neurophysiology and to be stimulated by the dynamic Eccles and the reflective McIntyre into constructing models that could give insight into experimental findings. Few have brought such a deep understanding of experimental biology, gained from first-hand experience, to the task of theoretical modeling.

After receiving the Ph.D. in 1953, Rall obtained a Rockefeller Foundation postdoctoral fellowship, which enabled him to gain further experience with the leading neurophysiologists of the time. In London in early 1954 he studied in the laboratory of Bernard Katz; during this period Katz and his students were laying the foundations of our modern concepts of the synapse by their work on the physiology of the neuromuscular junction. Rall also had the opportunity to discuss his approach to modeling the membrane properties of the nerve cell body (soma) with Alan Hodgkin in Cambridge, who provided him valuable encouragement (Rall 1992). In New York he worked at the Rockefeller Institute (now Rockefeller University) in the laboratory of David Lloyd, who was responsible for many of the classic experiments in spinal cord reflex physiology. He collaborated mainly with Carlton Hunt, who, with Stephen Kuffler, had established much of the basic physiology of muscle spindles and their contributions to spinal reflexes.

After a final year in Dunedin, Rall returned to the United States to head the laboratory of biophysics at the Naval Medical Research Institute in Bethesda, Maryland, under K. S. Cole. Cole soon left for the National Institutes of Health, along with several others, including J. Z. Hearon, who was asked to set up a new Office of Mathematical Research (OMR). Rall joined that group in 1957, and spent the rest of his career there. The congenial atmosphere established by Hearon, the institutional home for the OMR provided by DeWitt Stetten in the National Institute of Arthritis and Metabolic Diseases, and the overall support provided by the National Institutes of Health for the OMR deserve special mention and recognition. Mention should also be made of the Laboratory of Neurophysiology (LNP), with Wade Marshall, Kay Frank, Mike Fuortes, Phil Nelson, Tom Smith, and Bob Burke, where Rall established close friendships and collaborations with experimenters on the forefront of work on the motoneuron and spinal reflexes. In retrospect it may be seen that here OMR and LNP established one of the first working groups combining experimental and theoretical neuroscience. With this support and in this environment, Rall could concentrate his unique gifts on long-term projects uniting experimental data with theoretical models.

Insights Gained from Models of Motoneuron Populations

Rall's first study, for his doctoral thesis, involved an analysis of the input-output relations of motoneuron populations. This study linked the concept of the motoneuron pool of Sherrington, with whom Eccles had studied in the 1920s, with the modern analysis of activation of the pool by different intensities of afferent nerve stimulation, by Lloyd. Rall was interested in characterizing in a quantitative fashion the fractional activation of a pool at different levels of motoneuron excitability. He constructed a model based on several assumptions: each motoneuron has the same number of synaptic sites (e.g., 5,000); each site has the same probability of being occupied by a monosynaptic connection; each motoneuron fires an impulse when the number of activated monosynaptic connections exceeds a threshold value, which has an inherent variability. A model based on these assumptions gave a close fit to the experimental data (see Rall 1955a,b). Fuller discussion of these papers is to be found in the appendix to this volume, where Julian Jack notes that "this work has yet to be emulated for any other neuronal population" and remains a valuable example for those who may wish to construct models of neurons with a distribution of properties and models of populations of those neurons that perform a range of functions.

Although not directly involved with dendrites, which is the main theme of the present book, this early study was significant for Rall's later work in several ways. First, he brought to it a perspective on the function of a neuronal population in mediating a particular behavior, in this case a spinal reflex; similarly, in his later studies his interpretations went beyond the immediate biophysical properties to *implications for system functions and behavior*. Second, it focused on properties of individual neurons (numbers of synaptic sites; threshold for impulse generation) as being critical for the function of the neuron population; that is, *systems behavior arises out of the properties of realistic neuron models*. And third, it raised for him the question of how the *biophysical properties of the neuronal membrane contribute to the integrative actions of the neuron*, which came to lie at the core of his thinking.

Do Only Adjacent Somatic Synaptic Inputs Sum Successfully?

In thinking about the biophysical properties underlying neuronal integration, Rall became aware of a widely accepted assertion by Lorente de Nó (1938) that spatial summation between several synaptic inputs on the soma membrane is very local, and that successful summation occurs only when activated synapses are close to each other. This was in conflict with Rall's physical intuition, and in 1953 he addressed this question in a short abstract entitled "Electrotonic theory for spherical soma." Modifying the well-established passive cable equations (Hodgkin and Rushton 1946) to the case of a spherical membrane surface, he showed theoretically that the transient voltage in the soma membrane following focal depolarization equalizes very rapidly over the spherical surface. The implication is that, contrary to Lorente de Nó's assertion, synaptic potentials will sum effectively, independently of where they are located on the soma surface. In other words, Rall demonstrated that, functionally, *the soma can be treated as an isopotential unit.*

Can One Neglect the Cable Properties of Dendrites When the Input Is Applied to the Soma?

The next step was to examine the electrical consequences of the dendrites when the input is applied to the soma. By that time, Eccles and his collaborators in Dunedin had obtained their first pioneering results in recording and stimulating cat spinal motoneurons with an intracellular electrode in the soma. In interpreting the voltage transients recorded from the soma, they assumed that the current was confined mostly to the soma. Rall questioned whether it is valid to neglect the cable properties of the dendrites. In a letter to *Science*, Rall (1957) showed that when dendrites are coupled to the soma, a significant portion of the current spreads electrotonically from the soma to the dendrites. Thus, dendrites affect the charging (and discharging) rate of the soma membrane following an input to the soma. Indeed, the resultant voltage transients will build up (and decay) *faster* when dendrites are present compared to the case of a soma without dendrites (i.e., faster when the transient is normalized relative to the steady-state amplitude). In the limiting hypothetical case of a soma without dendrites, one has the case of an isopotential unit consisting of the membrane resistance and capacitance in parallel, and the voltage rise time (and its decay) in response to a step current input is governed by a single exponent having the membrane time constant, τ_m. When dendrites are present, the decay is faster than τ_m; thus, fitting a single exponent to the experimental voltage transient recorded at the motoneuron soma underestimates the actual τ_m (by a factor of about 2 in the case considered by Rall). Rall showed that when the somatic transients were analyzed using the correct value of τ_m, there was no need to invoke a "residual synaptic current" in shaping the decay of the somatic EPSPs, as was assumed by Eccles and his co-workers. Thus, Rall provided the theoretical basis for recognizing that *dendritic neurons are not isopotential units.*

What Is the Effect of Dendritic Inputs on the Soma Depolarization?

Having shown that signals at the soma are affected by the presence of dendrites, Rall turned his attention to the question of how inputs to the dendrites are integrated at the soma. This question inspired the majority of Rall's studies. The working hypothesis during the 1950s was that synapses on the dendrites, in particular on distal branches, are essentially ineffective, and that only the synapses at the soma and the proximal dendrites contribute to a neuron's output. The complex patterns of dendritic branching made this problem seem intractable to most approaches. In order to deal with it, Rall developed first an analytical cable theory for dendrites (Rall 1959, 1960), followed by a numerical approach utilizing compartmental models (Rall 1964); these form the theoretical foundation for exploring the input-output functions of dendrites.

In order to make his methods as accessible as possible to experimentalists, Rall drew attention to certain simplifying approaches among the broader theoretical framework he constructed. Although this had the virtue of facilitating use of the methods, it meant that many workers have been unaware of the full power of the comprehensive theory. For example, there is a misunderstanding that Rall's cable theory for dendrites can treat only passive trees with uniform membrane resistance, unvarying branch diameters, and a rigid branching pattern. In fact, the methods specifically embrace *arbitrary branching geometries* and *branching patterns* and in which the branches may have *nonuniform membrane properties* (for example, simulating steady background synaptic conductance input to the tree: see Rall 1959, 1962a). For simplicity Rall first applied his analytical theory assuming that the dendritic tree belongs to a class of trees that are electrically *equivalent to a single cylinder*.

It is difficult for a person coming into the field today to appreciate how this simple "equivalent cylinder" model provided for a new world of understanding of dendritic functions. The major insights regarding voltage spread in passive trees came from the analysis of such trees (Rall and Rinzel 1973; Rinzel and Rall 1974). Here we briefly summarize these insights.

1. The degree of branching and the extremely thin diameters of dendritic branches at distal locations, together with the small dimensions of dendritic spines, imply large input resistances (and input impedances) at these locations (on the order of a few hundred megohms and more). Thus, a small excitatory synaptic conductance change (of less than 1 nS) is sufficient to produce a large local dendritic depolarization of a few tens of mV

(Rall and Rinzel 1973; Rinzel and Rall 1974; Rall 1977). In brief, small processes generate large local responses.

2. The local dendritic depolarization is expected to attenuate severely in the central (dendrites-to-soma) direction. Steady voltage is expected to attenuate about 10-fold whereas fast transients may attenuate 100-fold or more when spreading from distal dendritic tips to the soma. The attenuation within the tree is asymmetrical; a much less severe attenuation is expected in the peripheral (soma-to-dendrites) direction. This asymmetry in peripheral versus central directions implies that from the *soma viewpoint*, dendrites are electrically rather compact (average electrotonic length of 0.3–2), whereas from the *dendrites (synaptic) viewpoint* the tree is electrically far from being compact (Rall and Rinzel 1973; Rinzel and Rall 1974).

3. The large voltage attenuation from dendrites to soma for transient synaptic inputs implies that many (several tens) excitatory inputs should be activated within the integration time window, τ_m, in order to sum and produce sufficient (10–20 mV) somatic depolarization that can reach threshold for impulse initiation at the axon hillock.

4. Although severely attenuated in *peak* values, the degree of attenuation of the *area* of transient potentials is relatively small because of the more prolonged time course of the response. Thus, the "cost" (in term of voltage area as well as the charge) of placing the synapse at the dendrites rather than at the soma is quite small. Hence, even in completely passive trees, distal dendritic synapses contribute to the somatic depolarization and can modify the output discharge of the neuron (Rall 1964).

5. Synaptic potentials are delayed, and they become significantly broader, as they spread away from the input site (Rall 1964; Rall 1967; Rall et al. 1967; Rinzel and Rall 1974). The input response at a distal branch (see figure 2 of Rinzel and Rall 1974) implies that, locally, synaptic potentials are very brief. At the soma level the time course of the synaptic potentials is primarily governed by τ_m. This range in width (duration) of the synaptic potential implies multiple time windows for synaptic integration in the tree (Agmon-Snir and Segev 1993, and see also Stratford et al. 1989).

These results demonstrated that the distributed structure of dendrites and their morphological complexity have the functional consequence that dendritic synaptic inputs should give large local responses that undergo marked attenuation within the tree. This implies that, in principle, the tree can be functionally fractionated into many *semi-independent functional subunits,* each of which can perform its computational task locally. The result of this local computation can have a global effect on the input-output (dendrites-to-soma) function of the neuron under appropriate conditions of synchronous activation of critical numbers of inputs with critical spatial relations. There can also be very local effects controlling local input-output dendritic processing through dendrodendritic synapses. And there can be local activity-dependent plasticity, as in dendritic spines (see Rall et al. 1966; Rall 1974; see also Koch et al. 1982; Shepherd and Brayton 1987; Rall and Segev 1987; Rinzel 1982; Woolf et al. 1991; and a recent review by Mel [1994]).

What Can We Learn about the Dendrites from Intracellular Recording at the Soma?

Being both theoretician and experimentalist, Rall felt it was important that his theoretical models would help experimentalists to learn more about the electrical properties of neurons. Indeed, Rall's theory is based on biophysical parameters that, in principle, can be measured experimentally. Furthermore, in many of his studies Rall suggested critical experiments that allow one to extract these biophysical parameters (e.g., the "shape index" to characterize and compare synaptic potentials in Rall et al. 1967, and the "peeling method" for estimating the membrane time constant and the time constants for equalization of transient potentials in Rall 1969).

The challenge was to get these biophysical estimations from recordings made with an intracellular electrode at only one point, the soma. At first, it may seem quite impossible to gain information about a large treelike structure from a local (somatic) recording at its origin. Yet Rall showed that many of the important electrical properties of dendrites can be estimated rather faithfully from such recordings. He showed how one can estimate the cable length of the dendrites (L), the specific properties of the membrane (R_m, C_m) and of the cytoplasm (R_i), the time constant of the dendritic tree (τ_m), the dendrite-to-soma conductance ratio (ρ), and, surprisingly, the properties of the synaptic input (i.e., its electrical distance from the soma ($X = x/\lambda$), its time course ($\alpha = 1/T_{peak}$), and its amplitude).

From the application of Rall's experimental suggestions and from their extensions by Jack and his collaborators (Jack et al. 1975) we know that, depending on the neuron type and experimental condition, R_m ranges between 5,000 and 50,000 ohm cm^2. Present-day researchers may be surprised to learn that the earliest suggestions for the specific membrane resistance, based on assumptions of current flow only across soma membrane, were less than 1,000 ohm cm^2; when Rall first suggested, based on his analysis of current flow into the dendrites in 1959, that it should be at least 2,000 ohm cm^2 and probably 4000, or even higher, his was a lone voice in the wilderness. The specific capacitance (C_m) is assumed to be constant at $1-2$ $\mu F/cm^2$, and R_i is estimated to range between 70 and 250 ohm cm. The time constant of dendritic membrane is, thus, 5–50 msec. The cable length of dendrites (from the soma viewpoint) was estimated to be rather small $(0.3-2)\lambda$; this implied that, for steady input to the soma, dendrites are electrically compact. The dendrite-to-soma conductance ratio (ρ) was estimated to be between 4 and 25 (and maybe more), and, this implied that most of the membrane conductance is in the dendrites.

Regarding the properties of the synaptic input, Rall showed that the variable time courses of EPSPs recorded at the soma are indicative of a wide distribution of the excitatory inputs over the dendritic surface. Thus, the electrotonic distance to the soma (X) may range from 0 (a somatic input) to 1.5 or 2 (distal dendritic inputs). The theory (Rall 1967) allowed estimations of X for individual synaptic inputs. Dramatic confirmation was obtained in the study of Redman and Walmsley (1983) who showed that the value for X that was estimated from Rall's theory agrees extremely well with the actual anatomical location of the synapse as found by labeling and reconstructing both the presynaptic (Ia) axon and the postsynaptic dendrites of the spinal alpha motoneuron.

Current experimental work on synaptic integration is concerned with discriminating between different subtypes of excitatory and inhibitory synapses. A summary of this work is beyond the scope of this introduction. Suffice it to say that synaptic inputs can be generally divided into at least two types of excitatory inputs, one with a fast (AMPA) time course (rise time of smaller than 1 msec) and the other with 10-fold slower kinetics (NMDA), and at least two types of inhibitory inputs, a fast one $(GABA_A)$ and a slow one $(GABA_B)$. Rall's theory of dendritic function will continue to be a critical tool in analyzing the contributions of each type of synaptic response to the integrative functions of the neuron.

What Can We Learn about Neuronal Organization from Extracellular Potentials?

Thus far we have considered analysis of the functional organization of the neuron based only on recordings of intracellular potentials. However, the extracellular potentials due to extracellular current also provide important information. At the time that Rall became interested in these potentials in relation to dendritic function, nearly a century of research had been carried out on the extracellular currents generated by the impulse in peripheral nerves. From this had emerged generally accepted concepts for interpreting the compound extracellular potentials recorded by two different methods: between a focal electrode and a distant ground when the nerve is placed in a volume conductor, and between two electrodes on the nerve when it is surrounded by a nonconducting medium (i.e., mineral oil) (see Fulton 1955).

Unitary Extracellular Potentials

When the first unitary extracellular potentials were recorded routinely from neurons in the 1950s, it was presumed that the volume conductor interpretation was applicable, and it was expected that the potentials, interpreted in this way, could be used to answer such critical questions as whether impulses spread actively or passively into the dendrites. The biphasic nature of the spikes recorded from near the soma seemed to support the idea of active impulse invasion into the dendrites; that is, the second phase of positivity of the soma recording was assumed to reflect active current sinks associated with the spike in the dendrites (see Fatt 1957). However, Rall's earliest studies of intracellular current indicated to him that the biphasic nature of the extracellular spikes was more likely due to a reversal of longitudinal current between an active soma and largely passive dendrites. Building on his analysis of intracellular currents, he carried out laborious and detailed calculations of the associated currents along the dendrites, and he showed that the second positive phase of the soma spike could be due to the rapid repolarization of the soma rather than to active impulse invasion of the dendrites (Rall 1962b).

Although the interpretation of extracellular unitary spikes now seems a somewhat arcane subject, it was a hotly debated topic at the time because of the possible insights it could give into the question of active dendrites. Excerpts from Rall's paper are published here, together with commentaries that explain the significance of this study for the interpretation of extracellular unit potentials recorded from motoneurons in the spinal cord (Nelson and Frank 1964). This work was of further importance as one of the foundations for the study that led to the identification of dendrodendritic synaptic interactions in the olfactory bulb.

Extracellular Field Potentials

In contrast to extracellular unitary potentials, extracellular field potentials are due to the summed activity of populations of synchronously active neurons. Building on his insight into the longitudinal currents in dendrites set up by impulses or synaptic potentials, Rall inferred that field potentials are due to summed extracellular currents outside dendrites arranged in parallel. This meant that the situation contains elements of recording both from peripheral nerves in oil and from a nerve in a volume conductor: within the active region the current paths are constrained in parallel, but outside the region the current returns within a volume conductor. This gives rise to a "potential divider" effect of the recording electrodes along these current paths.

The utility of this concept was demonstrated in reconstructing evoked potentials in the olfactory bulb in the study of Rall and Shepherd (1968). The concept provided the key to understanding the way that different phases of the extracellular field potentials could be correlated with the sequence of intracellular potential changes associated with impulse generation. This was a break with a long tradition in electrophysiology (unfortunately still surviving) of assigning labels to different parts of an extracellular transient and assuming that each is a direct reflection of a propagating intracellular impulse or spreading synaptic potential. With the increased accuracy of the model, it was possible to use the field potentials to localize sites of synaptic interactions, which led to the prediction of dendrodendritic synapses between mitral and granule cells in the olfactory bulb. The generality of the potential divider model in reconstructing evoked potentials for different extents of activated neuronal populations in the cerebral cortex was subsequently demonstrated by Klee and Rall (1977).

Output Functions of Dendrites: Dendrodendritic Synaptic Interactions

The new approaches that Wilfrid Rall developed during the late 1950s and early 1960s came together during the 1960s in a study of the functional organization of neurons in the olfactory bulb. Up to that time Rall had worked mainly with the group of Kay Frank, Michael Fuortes, and their colleagues at NIH on the motoneuron model. His motivation for becoming interested in the olfactory bulb came first from the realization that the field potentials elicited in the bulb by antidromic activation of the output neurons come very close to meeting criteria of synchrony and symmetry, and that the bulb would therefore be an attractive model in which the "potential divider" approach could be used to analyze the relation between field potentials and underlying intracellular activity.

The study of mitral and granule cells in the olfactory bulb brought together most of the methods that Rall had developed in his classical work and added several new ones. Thus, the compartmental approach, developed initially for the motoneuron, was used to construct a model of the output neuron, the mitral cell, and the main interneuron, the granule cell, in the olfactory bulb. Excitatory and inhibitory synaptic potentials were simulated as in the motoneuron model. A new action-potential model, approximating the conductances of the Hodgkin-Huxley model, was developed specifically for this study. The extracellular currents were derived from the intracellular potential distributions, and the extracellular potentials were calculated according to the "potential divider" model. It was the first study to combine all of these experimental and theoretical approaches.

The hypothesis tested in this work was that the Renshaw circuit for recurrent inhibition in the spinal cord, by means of axon collaterals through an inhibitory neuron, could be extended to the olfactory bulb in the form of a recurrent inhibitory circuit from mitral cell axon collaterals through the granule cells. The unexpected result from the study, however, was that this feedback is mediated primarily not by an axon collateral pathway but by a reciprocal synaptic interaction between the mitral dendrites and the granule cell dendrites. The morphological evidence subsequently supported this interpretation, and the combined electrophysiological, biophysical, computational, and morphological study was published in Rall et al. 1966 and Rall and Shepherd 1968.

If Rall's previous studies had given a new picture of the functions of dendrites in receiving and integrating synaptic *inputs*, the olfactory bulb study opened up new ideas concerning the *output* functions of neurons in general and the dendrites in particular. The classical idea, dating back to the doctrine of the "dynamic polarization of the neuron" of Cajal and van Gehuchten (see Ramón y Cajal 1989), was of the dendrites as exclusively receptive parts of the neuron and the axon as the exclusively output part. The olfactory bulb study showed that this classical idea needed to be replaced by an enlarged view, in which dendrites are also potential output sites. The fact that outputs from granule cell spines can be activated by the mitral cell dendritic inputs indicated that neuronal outputs can be activated locally, so that parts of a neuron can mediate semiindependent input-output functions. The computational complexity of a neuron and its interactions was thus greatly increased over the classical model.

This was the first evidence for the possible output functions of dendrites, which subsequently has become a rich field of study, embracing not only synaptic outputs from many kinds of dendrites but also nonsynaptic transmitter release from dendrites (cf. Glowinski et al. 1984), and currently the implication of gaseous messengers such as NO and CO in feedback from dendritic spines onto axon terminals (Garthwaite 1991) and onto other dendrites (Breer and Shepherd 1993). The dendrodendritic circuit was subsequently modeled as a functional unit mediating reciprocal and lateral inhibition of mitral cells (Shepherd and Brayton 1979), an early example of a specific "microcircuit" in the nervous system (Shepherd 1978).

What Are the Consequences of Synaptic Nonlinearities in Dendrites?

In his early analytical studies Rall assumed that as a first approximation the synaptic input can be modeled as a transient current input. This allowed analytical solutions for passive trees. Rall was the first to point out that synaptic responses and their interactions are inherently nonlinear— that they characteristically involve a transient conductance change in the membrane that perturbs the electrical properties of the entire tree considered as an interconnected system. One of the great utilities of the compartmental approach introduced by Rall in his classical paper of 1964 was the ability not only to model arbitrarily complex branching geometries but also to incorporate and explore the consequences of dendritic nonlinearities, either synaptic (time-dependent) or excitable (time- and voltage-dependent) membrane channels.

In the 1964 paper Rall started to explore how *synaptic nonlinearities* influence the input-output properties of dendrites. The main results are summarized:

1. Because of the inherent conductance change associated with synaptic inputs, it is a general rule that synaptic potentials summate nonlinearly (less than linearly) with each other. This effect decreases with increasing separation between the synapses. Consequently, in passive trees, spatially distributed excitatory inputs summate more linearly (produce more charge) than do spatially clustered synapses.

2. Inhibitory synapses located on the path between the excitatory input and the "target" point (e.g., soma) can reduce the excitation more effectively than when placed distal to the excitatory input. This basic property has been studied and emphasized in subsequent work (see Jack et al. 1975; Koch et al. 1982). Thus, the strategic placement of inhibition relative to excitation is critical for dendritic integration. Another important rule of dendritic integration is that inhibition near the soma will have a global veto effect whereas inhibition on dendrites will have more localized veto effects on the responses and integration in local subunits.

3. The somatic depolarization, resulting from activation of excitatory inputs at the dendrites, is very sensitive to the temporal sequence of the synaptic activation. It is largest (but most transient) when the excitatory synaptic activation starts at distal dendritic sites and progresses proximally. Activation of the same synapses in the reverse order in time (proceeding from soma to distal dendrites) will produce smaller (but more sustained) somatic depolarization. Thus, the output of neurons with dendrites is inherently *directional selective* (see also Torre and Poggio 1978).

4. Background synaptic inputs effectively alter the cable properties (electrotonic length, input resistance, time constant, etc.) of the postsynaptic cell. Hence, this activity dynamically changes the computational (input-output) capabilities of the neuron (Rall 1962a; Holmes and Woody 1989; Bernander et al. 1991; Rapp et al. 1992).

Finally, at an early stage, Rall pointed out that, in principle, nonlinear dendrites are computationally richer than passive dendrites (see Rall 1970). The electroanatomical properties of the dendritic tree, the functional architecture of synaptic inhibition and excitation on the tree and their precise timing, and the context (background activity) upon which the input acts, combine to determine the integrative capability of the tree. The repertoire of operations within a tree is greatly extended by excitable channels in dendrites (cf. Llinas 1988).

What Are the Functional Properties of Dendritic Spines?

Dendritic spines are very thin and short appendages that terminate with a bulbous head. In spiny neurons, they come in large numbers and cover much of the dendritic surface, and are the major target for excitatory synaptic inputs. But what is their function? To paraphrase the old saying, if dendrites have been a puzzle, their spines have been an enigma wrapped in that puzzle. Rall was led to this enigma by several routes, including the work on the cable properties of thin dendritic branches, the analysis of current spread between granule cell spines in the olfactory bulb, and exposure to new data on the dimensions of dendritic spines in cortical pyramidal neurons.

The Role of Dendritic Spines in Synaptic Plasticity

Rall was particularly intrigued by the finding that, in the apical dendrites of cortical pyramidal neurons, distal dendritic spines tend to have longer and thinner stems than do more proximal spines. This seemed counter-intuitive (always a useful starting point for a theoretical study) because it would appear to add a further disadvantage to the distal location. In the late 1960s and early 1970s, Rall and Rinzel constructed an electrical model of the dendritic spine and explored the consequence of the partial electrical decoupling of the spine head (the synaptic input) from the dendrite (and soma) provided by the thin spine stem (large resistance).

Rall and Rinzel (1971a,b) and Rall (1974) showed that, although the efficacy of spiny synaptic inputs is reduced because of the spine stem resistance, this resistance could be a locus for neural plasticity because changes in the stem (e.g., increased diameter) could change (e.g., increase) the efficacy of spiny synapse in a very specific manner. They showed that small changes in spine neck resistance would have a significant effect on the synaptic efficacy only if the spine stem resistance is matched with the input resistance at the spine base, and that this could explain the observation that distal spines tend to have thinner (larger resistance) stems.

Excitable Spines

These theoretical results led to further exploration of the possible consequences of excitable channels in dendrites as found recently in many neuron types (e.g., Stuart and Sakmann 1994). These studies have demonstrated that excitable channels in dendrites, in particular on dendritic spines, can amplify synaptic efficacy. Furthermore, compared to the case of spines with passive membrane, spines with voltage-gated or voltage-sensitive membrane properties can produce a sharper "operating range" for changes of synaptic efficacy. These changes can be brought about by changes in the spine stem dimensions, or by other modifications (such as changes in internal cytoplasm resistivity or movement of organelles). A "chain reaction" of firing of excitable spines following excitatory synapses to a few spines was conjectured, and the great sensitivity of the spread of this chain reaction on the location and timing of inhibition was theoretically explored (Segev and Rall 1988). The consequences of such chain reactions for synaptic amplification and for the repertoire of possible logical operations in dendrites have been discussed (e.g., Miller et al. 1985; Shepherd et al. 1985; Rall and Segev 1987; Shepherd and Brayton 1987; Baer and Rinzel 1991). A recent review on the electrical and chemical properties of dendritic spines can be found in Koch and Zador 1993.

Epilogue: The Future

Currently there is great excitement in the neurobiological community in the finding of the richness of ion channels in the soma-dendritic membrane, in particular voltage-dependent channels (see Llinas 1988). One challenge for the experimental research on dendrites is to characterize these channels in terms of types, kinetics, and distribution over the dendritic surface. Theoretical explorations of the consequences of these channels (e.g., the NMDA channel) for the computational functions of single neurons as well as for their plastic functions are already underway (e.g., Mel 1993; De Schutter and Bower 1994). Thus it is apparent that, for molecular biologists, the methods of Rall have special relevance. It is well recognized that the cloning of a gene is only the start in understanding its role in nervous function. A critical step is to understand the cellular function of a gene product, such as a synaptic- or voltage-gated membrane channel. Because in a neuron that channel will be expressed in a specific location, the methods of Rall will be necessary for understanding the contribution of that gene product to the overall functioning of the neuron. Research on the consequences of nonlinear channels for the dynamics of neural networks has also started and is expected to flourish in coming years (cf. Traub and Miles 1991).

Novel technologies are proving useful for probing, physically emulating, and finely altering local sites of active neurons within the nervous system. Among these are voltage-dependent dyes that enable one to view, in real time, the electrical activity of neurons when the system carries out specific computations. VLSI technology potentially makes it possible to emulate the electrical (and chemical) activity of synapses, dendrites, and axons and to construct realistic neural networks in chips that operate in real time. These, and molecular biological methods including antibodies against specific ion channels, combined with high-resolution optical probes, may serve as the essential link between the single-neuron level and the system levels. Again, the theoretical basis for this link between single-neuron computations and systems computations will continue to draw on the methods of Rall.

We are presently in an era when the new methods are revealing the complexity of dendritic branching systems in all their glory. An important theoretical endeavor that is likely to develop in the next few years is the search for systematic methods to reduce this complexity in single-neuron models while retaining the essential input-output functions of the full models. Rall has argued eloquently for focusing on such reduced and tightly constrained models as the means to obtain the best insights into principles, rather than building models incorporating more and more complexity without adequate constraints (see Rall 1992). These "canonical" models will not only elucidate the principles that govern the operation of neurons, but they will also be the building blocks of models of large neuronal networks (see Stratford et al. 1989; Shepherd 1992; and Segev 1992).

We are at the dawn of interesting times, when experimental and theoretical tools are developing very rapidly. Many of the mysteries of neurons and dendrites may soon be solved. At the core of these mysteries is the contribution of individual neurons and their dendritic trees to the processing of information in neural systems, as the basis for behavior and cognitive functions. The contributions of Wilfrid Rall gathered in this volume will likely serve as key tools in unlocking the doors to those mysteries.

References

Abbott, L. F., Fahri, E., and Gutmann, S. (1991). The path integral for dendritic trees. *Biol. Cyber.* 66:49–60.

Agmon-Snir, H., and Segev, I. (1993). Signal delay and propagation velocity in passive dendritic trees. *J. Neurophys.* 70(5):2066–2085.

Baer, S. M. and Rinzel, J. (1991). Propagation of dendritic spikes mediated by excitable spines: a continuum theory. *J. Neurophysiol.* 65:874–890.

Bernander, O., Douglas, R. J., Martin, K. A., and Koch, C. (1991). Synaptic background activity influences spatiotemporal integration in single pyramidal cells. *Proc. Natl. Acad. Sci.* 88:11569–11573.

Breer, H., and Shepherd, G. M. (1993). Implications of the NO/cGMP system for olfaction. *Trends Neurosci.* 16:5–9.

Butz, E. G., and Cowan, J. D. (1974). Transient potentials in dendritic systems of arbitrary geometry. *Biophys. J.* 14:661–689.

De Schutter, E., and Bower, J. M. (1994). An active membrane model of the cerebellar Purkinje cells. I. Simulation of current clamps in slice. *J. Neurophys.* 71:375–400.

Douglas, R. J., and Martin, K. A. C. (1990). Neocortex. In *The Synaptic Organization of the Brain*, ed. G. M. Shepherd. New York: Oxford University Press, 389–438.

Fatt, P. (1957). Electric potentials around an antidromically activated motoneurone. *J. Neurophysiol.* 20:27–60.

Fulton, J. F. (1955). *Textbook of Physiology.* 17th Edition. Philadelphia: W. B. Saunders.

Garthwaite, J. (1991). Glutamate, nitric oxide and cell-cell signalling in the nervous system. *Trends Neurosci.* 14:60–67.

Glowinski, J., Tassin, J. P., and Thierry, A. M. (1984). The mesocortico-prefrontal dopaminergic neurons. *Trends Neurosci.* 7:415–418.

Hodgkin, A. L, and Rushton, W. A. H. (1946). The electrical constants of crustacean nerve fiber. *Proc. R. Soc. Lond. B. Biol. Sci.* 133:444–479.

Holmes, W. R. (1986). A continuous cable method for determining the transient potential in passive dendritic trees of known geometry. *Biol. Cyber.* 55:115–124.

Holmes, W. R., and Woody, D. (1989). Effect of uniform and nonuniform synaptic "activation-distribution" on the cable properties of modeled cortical pyramidal cells. *Brain Res.* 505:12–22.

Horwitz, B. (1981). An analytical method for investigating transient potentials in neurons with branching dendritic trees. *Biophys. J.* 36:155–192.

Jack, J. J. B., Noble, D., and Tsien, R. W. (1975). *Electric Current Flow in Excitable Cells.* Oxford: Oxford University Press.

Klee, M., and Rall, W. (1977). Computed potentials of cortically arranged populations of neurons. *J. Neurophysiol.* 40:647–666.

Koch, C., Poggio, T., and Torre, V. (1982). Retinal ganglion cells: A functional interpretation of dendritic morphology. *Phil. Trans. Roy. Soc. Lond. B.* 298:227–264.

Koch, C., Poggio, T., and Torre, V. (1983). Nonlinear interactions in a dendritic tree: Localization, timing and role in information processing. *Proc. Natl. Acad. Sci. USA* 80:2799–2802.

Koch, C., and Zador, A. (1993). The function of dendritic spines: Devices subserving biochemical rather than electrical compartmentalization. *J. Neuroscience.* 13(2):413–422.

Llinas, R. (1988). The intrinsic electrophysiological properties of mammalian neurons: Insights into central nervous system function. *Science* 242:1654–1664.

Lorente de Nó, R. (1938). Synaptic stimulation as a local process. *J. Neurophys.* 1:194–207.

McCulloch, W., and Pitts, W. (1943). A logical calculus of ideas immanent in nervous activity. *Bull. Math. Biophys.* 5:115–133.

Major, G. J., Evans, D., and Jack, J. J. B. (1993). Solutions for transients in arbitrary branching cables: I. Voltage recording with a somatic shunt. *Biophys. J.* 65:423–449.

Mel, B. W. (1993). Synaptic integration in an excitable dendritic tree. *J. Neurophys.* 70:1086–1101.

Mel, B. W. (1994). Information processing in dendritic trees. *Neural Computation* (in press).

Miller, J. P., Rall, W., and Rinzel, J. (1985). Synaptic amplification by active membrane in dendritic spines. *Brain Res.* 325:325–330, 1985.

Nelson, P. G., and Frank, K. (1964). Extracellular potential fields of single spinal motoneurons. *J. Neurophysiol.* 27:913–927.

Poggio, T., and Torre, V. (1978). A new approach to synaptic interaction. In *Theoretical Approaches to Complex Systems*, ed. R. Heim and G. Palm. New York: Springer-Verlag.

Rall, W. (1955a). A statistical theory of monosynaptic input-output relations. *J. Cell. Comp. Physiol.* 46:373–411.

Rall, W. (1955b). Experimental monosynaptic input-output relations in the mammalian spinal cord. *J. Cell. Comp. Physiol.* 46:413–437.

Rall, W. (1957). Membrane time constant of motoneurons. *Science* 126:454.

Rall, W. (1959). Branching dendritic trees and motoneuron membrane resistivity. *Expt. Neurol.* 1:491–527.

Rall, W. (1960). Membrane potential transients and membrane time constant of motoneurons. *Expt. Neurol.* 2:503–532.

Rall, W. (1962a). Theory and physiological properties of dendrites. *Ann. N.Y. Acad. Sci.* 96:1071–1092.

Rall, W. (1962b). Electrophysiology of a dendritic neuron model. *Biophys. J.* 2:145–167.

Rall, W. (1964). Theoretical significance of dendritic trees and motoneuron input-output relations. In *Neural Theory and Modeling*, ed. R. F. Reiss. Stanford: Stanford University Press.

Rall, W. (1967). Distinguishing theoretical synaptic potentials computed for different soma-dendritic distributions of synaptic input. *J. Neurophysiol.* 30:1138–1168.

Rall. W. (1969). Time constants and electrotonic length of membrane cylinders and neurons. *Biophys. J.* 9:1483–1508.

Rall, W. (1970). Cable properties of dendrites and effects of synaptic location. In *Excitatory Synaptic Mechanisms*, ed. P. Anderson, and J. K. S. Jansen. Oslo: Universitetsforlag.

Rall, W. (1974). Dendritic spines, synaptic potency in neuronal plasticity. In *Cellular Mechanisms Subserving Changes in Neuronal Activity*, ed. C. D. Woody, K. A. Brown, T. J. Crow, and J. D. Knispel. Los Angeles: Brain Information Service.

Rall, W. (1977). Core conductor theory and cable properties of neurons. In *The Nervous System*, Vol. I: *Cellular Biology of Neurons*, Part 1, ed. E. R. Kandel. Bethesda: American Physiological Society.

Rall, W. (1992). Path to biophysical insights about dendrites and synaptic function. In *The Neuroscience: Paths to Discoveries*, ed. F. Samson and G. Adelman. Boston: Birkhauser.

Rall, W., Burke, R. E., Smith, T. G., Nelson, P. G., and Frank, K. (1967). Dendritic location of synapses and possible mechanisms for the monosynaptic EPSP in motoneurons. *J. Neurophysiol.* 30:1169–1193.

Rall, W. and Rinzel, J. (1971a). Dendritic spines and synaptic potency explored theoretically. *Proc. I.U.P.S. (XXV Intl. Congress)* IX:466.

Rall, W. and Rinzel, J. (1971b). Dendritic spine function and synaptic attenuation calculations. *Program & Abstracts Soc. Neurosci. First Annual Mtg.* p. 64.

Rall, W., and Rinzel, J. (1973). Branch input resistance and steady attenuation for input to one branch of a dendritic neuron model. *Biophys. J.* 13:648–688.

Rall, W., and Segev, I. (1987). Functional possibilities for synapses on dendrites and on dendritic spines. In *Synaptic Function*, ed. G. M. Edelman, W. F. Gall, and W. M. Cowan. Neurosci. Res. Found. New York: John Wiley, 605–636.

Rall, W., and Shepherd, G. M. (1968). Theoretical reconstruction of field potentials and dendro-dendritic synaptic interactions in olfactory bulb. *J. Neurophysiol.* 31:884–915.

Rall, W., Shepherd, G. M., Reese, T. S., and Brightman, M. W. (1966). Dendrodendritic synaptic pathway for inhibition in the olfactory bulb. *Exp. Neurol.* 14:44–56.

Ramón y Cajal, S. (1911). *Histologie du Système Nerveux de l'Homme et des Vertébrés.* Trans. L. Azoulay. Paris: Maloine, 2 vols.

Ramón y Cajal, S. (1989). *Recollections of My Life.* Cambridge, Mass.: MIT Press.

Rapp, M., Yarom, Y., and Segev, I. (1992). The impact of parallel fiber background activity on the cable properties of cerebellar Purkinje cells. *Neural Computation* 4:518–532.

Redman, S. J., and Walmsley, B. (1983). The time course of synaptic potentials evoked in cat spinal motoneurons at identified group Ia synapses. *J. Physiol.* 343:117–133.

Rinzel, J. (1982). Neuronal plasticity (learning). In *Some Mathematical Questions in Biology-Neurobiology,* ed. R. M. Miura. Lectures on Mathematics in the Live Sciences **15.** Providence, RI: Amer. Math. Soc.

Rinzel, J., and Rall W. (1974). Transient response in a dendritic neuron model for current injected at one branch. *Biophys. J.* 14:759–790.

Segev, I. (1992). Single neurone models: oversimple, complex and reduced. *TINS* 15:414–421.

Segev, I., and Rall, W. (1988). Computational study of an excitable dendritic spine. *J. Neurophysiol.* 60:499–523.

Sejnowski, T. J., Koch, C., and Churchland, P. S. (1988). Computational neuroscience. *Science* 241:1299–1306.

Shepherd, G. M. (1978). Microcircuits in the nervous system. *Sci. Am.* 238:92–103.

Shepherd, G. M. (1991). *Foundations of the Neuron Doctrine.* New York: Oxford University Press.

Shepherd, G. M. (1992). Canonical neurons and their computational organization. In *Single Neuron Computation,* ed. T. Mckenna, J. Davis, and S. E. Zornetzer. Boston: Academic Press.

Shepherd, G. M., and Brayton, R. K. (1979). Computer simulation of a dendrodendritic synaptic circuit for self- and lateral-inhibition in the olfactory bulb. *Brain Res.* 175:377–382.

Shepherd, G. M., and Brayton, R. K. (1987). Logic operations are properties of computer-simulated interactions between excitable dendritic spines. *Neuroscience* 21:151–166.

Shepherd, G. M., Brayton, R. K., Miller, J. F., Segev, I., Rinzel, J., and Rall, W. (1985). Signal enhancement in distal cortical dendrites by means of interactions between active dendritic spines. *Proc. Natl. Acad Sci. USA* 82:2192–2195.

Stratford, K., Mason, A., Larkman, A., Major, G., and Jack, J. J. J. B. (1989). The modeling of pyramidal neurons in the visual cortex. In *The Computing Neuron,* ed. R. Durbin, C. Miall, and G. Mitchison. Reading, MA: Addison-Wesley.

Stuart, G. J., and Sakmann, B. (1994). Active propagation of somatic action potentials into neocortical pyramidal cell dendrites. *Nature* 367:69–72.

Torre, V., and Poggio, T. (1978). A synaptic mechanism possibly underlying directional selectivity to motion. *Proc. R. Soc. Lond. (Biol.).* 202:409–416.

Traub, R. D., and Miles, R. (1991). *Neuronal Networks of the Hippocampus.* Cambridge, UK: Cambridge Univ. Press.

Tuckwell, H. C. (1988). *Introduction to Theoretical Neurobiology: Volume 1: Linear Cable Theory and Dendritic Structure. Volume 2: Nonlinear and Stochastic Theories.* Cambridge: Cambridge University Press.

Woolf, T. B., Shepherd, G. M., and Greer, C. A. (1991). Serial reconstructions of granule cell spines in the mammalian olfactory bulb. *Synapse* 7:181–192.

2 CABLE PROPERTIES OF NEURONS WITH COMPLEX DENDRITIC TREES

2.1 Introduction by Julian Jack and Stephen Redman

Rall, W. (1957). Membrane time constant of motoneurons. *Science* 126:454.

Rall, W. (1959). Branching dendritic trees and motoneuron membrane resistivity. *Exptl. Neurol.* 1:491–527.

Rall, W. (1960). Membrane potential transients and membrane time constant of motoneurons. *Exptl. Neurol.* 2:503–532.

After Wil Rall arrived in Dunedin, New Zealand, in 1949, to study for his Ph.D. under the supervision of John Eccles, significant events in the history of neuroscience took place there. Eccles, with his colleagues Brock and Coombs, made his first intracellular recordings from motoneurones. EPSPs and IPSPs were recorded for the first time. The scientific disputes that subsequently arose between Rall and Eccles (after Rall had returned, in 1956, to the United States) over the correct interpretation of recordings from motoneurones can be traced to the lack of attention that Eccles paid to cable properties of motoneurones. These disputes were over the correct value of the specific membrane resistivity for the motoneurone membrane, the time course of excitatory and inhibitory synaptic currents, and the effectiveness of synapses on dendrites.

Rall began his analysis of the electrotonic characteristics of dendritic trees with very little quantitative morphological material available. One motoneurone had been reconstructed from serial sections by Haggar and Barr (1950). Chu (1954) had obtained motoneurones from human spinal cord by shaking fresh autopsy tissue in a jar containing glass beads. (This was probably the first preparation of dissociated neurones.) The cell bodies and their proximal dendrites remained intact. The branching patterns, dendritic lengths, and diameters obtained from these data formed the basis of Rall's 1959 paper, "Branching dendritic trees and motoneurone resistivity." His aim was to provide a method for reducing the geometrical complexity of a branching dendritic tree, while preserving its electrical properties. The scheme he used was a recursive calculation for the steady-state input conductance of a finite length of a cylindrical dendrite terminating with further branching. Each length of dendrite was terminated by a conductance that was the input conductance of the subsequent branchings. Repeated substitutions for the input conductance at each branch point led to a compact expression for the input conductance of a dendritic trunk. This procedure placed no restrictions on branching rules and did not require the specific resistivities of the membrane and cytoplasm to remain constant throughout the dendrites. Rall made the important observation that if k branches (of diameter d_{jk}) originate at the jth branch in a tree and satisfy the relationship

$$d_{(j-1)}^{3/2} = \sum_k d_{jk}^{3/2}$$

then these k branches could be collapsed into a continuation of the

$(j-1)$th element (diameter $d_{(j-1)}$) with no electrical discontinuity occurring at the jth branch point. If this branching rule (which became known as the 3/2 power law) applied throughout the entire dendrite, the dendritic tree could be collapsed to a continuous extension of the trunk dendrite. (In this treatment, the question of how to terminate the dendritic cylinder was not discussed, although it was implicit in the recursive procedure that the dendritic cylinder would terminate.) The limited morphological material available to Rall at the time suggested that the 3/2 power law might be approximately obeyed, at least at proximal branches. This simplification was enormously important for the subsequent mathematical treatment of transient potentials in dendrites.

Rall's reduction of a dendritic tree to an equivalent dendrite was sometimes criticized in the mistaken belief that it was only valid when the 3/2 power law could be applied at branch points. This misunderstanding may have arisen because much of the subsequent analytical treatment of the neurone model in the 1960s and 1970s assumed an equivalent dendrite of uniform diameter, which does require the 3/2 power law.

Input resistances of motoneurones were measured by Coombs, Eccles, and Fatt (1955); Coombs, Curtis, and Eccles (1959); and Frank and Fuortes (1956). Eccles and his collaborators described a "standard motoneurone," derived from the same morphological data that was available to Rall, as having five dendrites of 5 μm diameter and infinite length attached to a 70 μm diameter soma. Using this model, Coombs et al. (1955) calculated the membrane resistivity (R_m) to be 500 Ωcm^2. Rall went to considerable effort to demonstrate that Eccles had seriously underestimated the size of the dendritic tree, and therefore R_m. Rall's calculations suggested a mean value of 4,000 Ωcm^2. The difference between these two estimates of R_m was to have a profound influence on the opposing positions Rall and Eccles subsequently took on the effectiveness of dendritic synapses. Eccles (1957, 1960) calculated that the dendrites would exceed three space constants in length, and that synapses located at such large electrotonic distances from the soma could not contribute to the somatic membrane potential. Thereafter Eccles attached little significance to synapses on dendrites. In contrast, Rall subsequently calculated that motoneurone dendrites extended to between one and two space constants and that dendritic synapses could make significant alterations to the somatic membrane potential.

Apart from the issue of whether dendritic synapses were effective, a second debate developed about the time course of the synaptic current generating the EPSP in the motoneurone. Both Frank and Fuortes (1956) and Coombs, Curtis, and Eccles (1956) had concluded that the time constant of the motoneurone membrane was much shorter than the time constant of decay of the EPSP; Coombs, Curtis, and Eccles took this further and suggested that the explanation for the difference was that there was a prolonged phase of transmitter action (i.e., a prolonged current injection) lasting throughout the time course of the synaptic potential. At that time, Fatt (1957) offered a different interpretation, suggesting that the slow decay was "passive and involves a spatial factor." Fatt had presented evidence from extracellular recording that he interpreted as indicating that a substantial part of the synaptic input came from the dendrites. Nevertheless, Fatt accepted the measure of the "somatic" membrane time constant provided by the other groups and concluded that there was a difference between somatic and dendritic membrane time constant.

The scene was set for Rall to provide the calculations arising from his soma-dendritic model of the cell. In his brief report in *Science* (1957), he set out the issue with stark clarity and concluded that all the data was compatible with the assumption of a uniform membrane time constant of higher value than the previous estimates. The "somatic" membrane time constant measured by passing a pulse of current through a microelectrode in the soma was underestimated if the time course was assumed to be a simple exponential, by a factor of about two. Thus, in both this debate as well as the one arising from consideration of the input resistance of motoneurones, the issue was the value of the membrane properties.

Eccles and his colleagues resisted this conclusion and in 1959 published two papers (Coombs, Curtis, and Eccles 1959; Curtis and Eccles 1959) reasserting that the membrane time constant was less than the decay time constant of the EPSP, although, as a result of partly acknowledging Rall's criticism, the difference between the two was now judged to be smaller. They insisted that there was clear evidence for a residual phase of synaptic excitatory current and adduced two further pieces of evidence in favor of such residual action: (i) the fact that an antidromic action potential did not abolish the EPSP when timed to coincide with its peak; (ii) the observation that hyperpolarization shortened the time constant of decay of the EPSP. Curtis and Eccles argued that this could not be accounted for other than by the hyperpolarization having a direct action on either the binding or clearance of the transmitter substance. A final, ingenious argument was offered by Curtis and Eccles. Having accepted that there would be some current spread from soma to dendrites, they suggested that it would be much less than Rall calculated, and hence maintained that the membrane time constant was less than the synaptic decay time constant. Using the assumption of a simple spherical model of the nerve cell, they derived the time course of the synaptic current anew and found that between the initial brief phase and a subsequent prolonged residual phase there was a brief reversal of the current. They offered the interpretation that the preponderance of active synapses were on the soma and proximal dendrites and this brief current reversal was attributable to spread of the excitatory current into the distal dendrites, temporarily "hiding" the low residuum of synaptic excitatory current. The fact that they used an isopotential, non-distributed model to derive the time course of synaptic current and then assumed a nonisopotential distributed model to interpret it, seemed to have escaped them!

Rall's response in his 1960 paper was magisterial. In the introduction he reviewed the past history and then started the analysis by introducing a simple procedure for the soma-dendritic model that would allow determination of the membrane time constant; this was to plot $\sqrt{t}$ *times* dV/dt (for response to a current step) versus t, instead of the conventional dV/dt versus t, on a semilogarithmic scale. The negative slope of the resulting line gives the reciprocal of the membrane time constant, providing there is a "dendritic dominance" (i.e., more current spreads into the dendrites than passes across the soma membrane) of the order that he, and Eccles, calculated to be appropriate. He then showed that the experimental data from two cells reported by Coombs, Curtis, and Eccles (1959) gave an estimate of the membrane time constant greater than that deduced by them (of the order of 30 percent).

Rall then went on to draw attention to a technique using sinusoidal applied current, which might have been useful in judging the dendritic dominance. He thus provided a safeguard in terms of the techniques available, so that both dendritic dominance and the membrane time constant could be estimated, with the method for their joint estimation achieved by successive approximation if dendritic dominance was not large.

The final part of the paper (other than the mathematical appendix, presenting the detailed derivation of the equations on which the reasoning in the paper is based) then gave a clear and decisive review of the hypotheses advanced both by Fatt and by Eccles and his colleagues. Rall pointed out that Fatt's suggestion was not in conflict with his conclusion, but that there was no necessity to adopt this more complicated model (different time constants for soma and dendrites). The discussion (pages 519–523) then systematically treated the arguments that Eccles and his colleagues had advanced and showed that there was an alternative explanation for each.

Eccles (1961) subsequently stoutly defended his view that there was a prolonged phase of synaptic current, using new data on the structure of motoneurones provided by Aitken and Bridger (1961) and further electrophysiological measures. It would be inappropriate to give a detailed critique of his arguments, but it was hardly a compelling defense. As Eccles himself pointed out in 1964, the analysis remained unsatisfactory unless the structure were known of the particular neurone from which the experimental results were obtained.

It may seem strange to introduce Rall's classic early papers on nerve cell modeling by describing a controversy. But the controversy, which rumbled on for about a decade, was a decisive influence in shaping the way Rall presented his initial work. Until recently, when specialist journals have become available, it was always a struggle to persuade the editorial boards of physiological journals to accept papers of a purely theoretical nature. Rall was the pioneer of nerve cell modeling—for structures more complicated than the axon—and remained virtually the sole worker in the field for nearly two decades (his first publication, studying the isopotentiality properties of spherical nerve cells, was published in 1953). In that time, he not only laid a complete foundation for the more sophisticated models of today but did so in a period where his work was commonly greeted with indifference or, as in the case of the aforementioned controversy, strong opposition. It may not have escaped the reader's attention that a substantial period elapsed between the preliminary report in *Science* and the subsequent publications two and three years later in the new and then rather obscure journal *Experimental Neurology*. To those of us who developed an interest in the field at this time, it was with a sense of justice finally done that we saw Rall's subsequent work being published in prestigious journals such as *Biophysical Journal* and the *Journal of Neurophysiology*.

We would like to add some even more personal aspects to our commentary. One of us (Julian Jack) was a young premedical student in Dunedin, in the period after Eccles had gone to Canberra but before Wil returned to the United States. Wil presented two seminars to interested students on his cable theory. This work was of such novelty and interest that it inspired J. Jack to attend undergraduate mathematics lectures in his spare time and subsequently (in 1959, long after Rall had left) to persuade his research supervisor, Archie McIntyre, to allow him to take a break from spinal cord reflex studies and make a few intracellular recordings from cat motoneurones. The explicit objective of these experiments was to see whether, with very restricted stimulation of the group Ia fiber excitatory input, it might be possible to detect EPSPs with different rise times; the hope was that individual fiber inputs might be located either near to the soma or further out on the dendrites and thus show different time courses, since this was the possibility that Rall had implied in his seminar. The experiments did indeed confirm Rall's prediction, but they were not pursued further until after J. Jack had completed his medical studies in

England and subsequently linked up with Bob Porter, Simon Miller (Jack, Miller, and Porter 1967), and, finally, S. J. Redman (see Jack, Miller, Porter, and Redman 1971). The long incubation on this occasion was not because of any external opposition but because in order to make as satisfactory as possible a quantitative treatment of the data, we had to develop the theory and make matching computations. By then the similar work from NIH was published (see Rall 1967; Rall et al. 1967). Both of us have the most pleasant memories of first meeting Wil and then visiting him at NIH together. He was extremely encouraging to us and subsequently very generous in his referencing of our work, even before it was published (see Rall 1969a, footnotes 10, 18, 19). He subsequently made very helpful suggestions on drafts of our papers. Since those days, he has remained a good friend and a supportive colleague. We have admired the high standards he has maintained in his publications, and his scholarly attitude and integrity has been an inspiration for us.

References

Aitken, J. T., and J. E. Bridger (1961) Neuron size and neuron population density in the lumbosacral region of the cat's spinal cord. *J. Anat.*, **95**:38–53.

Chu, L. W. (1954) A cytological study of anterior horn cells isolated from human spinal cord. *J. Comp. Neurol.*, **100**:381–414.

Coombs, J. S., D. R. Curtis, and J. C. Eccles (1956) Time courses of motoneuronal responses. *Nature*, **178**: 1049–1050.

Coombs, J. S., D. R. Curtis, and J. C. Eccles (1959) The electrical constants of the motoneurone membrane. *J. Physiol., London*, **145**:505–528.

Coombs, J. S., J. C. Eccles, and P. Fatt (1955) The electrical properties of the motoneurone membrane. *J. Physiol., London*, **130**:291–325.

Curtis, D. R., and J. C. Eccles (1959) Time courses of excitatory and inhibitory synaptic actions. *J. Physiol., London*, **145**:529–546.

Eccles, J. C. (1957) *The Physiology of Nerve Cells.* Baltimore: Johns Hopkins Press.

Eccles, J. C. (1960) The properties of the dendrites. In *Structure and Function of the Cerebral Cortex*, ed. D. B. Tower and J. P. Schade. Amsterdam: Elsevier.

Eccles, J. C. (1961) Membrane time constants of cat motoneurones and time courses of synaptic action. *Exptl. Neurol.*, **4**:1–22.

Eccles, J. C. (1964) *The Physiology of Synapses.* Berlin: Springer-Verlag.

Fatt, P. (1957) Sequence of events in synaptic activation of a motoneurone. *J. Neurophysiol.*, **20**:61–80.

Frank, K., and M. G. F. Fuortes (1956) Stimulation of spinal motoneurones with intracellular electrodes. *J. Physiol., London*, **134**:451–470.

Haggar, R. A., and M. L. Barr (1950) Quantitative data on the size of synaptic end-bulbs in the cat's spinal cord. *J. Comp. Neurol.*, **93**:17–35.

Jack, J. J. B., S. Miller, and R. Porter (1967) The different time courses of minimal EPSPs in spinal motoneurones. *J. Physiol., London*, **191**:112–113.

Jack, J. J. B., S. Miller, R. Porter, and S. J. Redman (1971) The time course of minimal excitatory post-synaptic potentials evoked in spinal motoneurones by group Ia afferent fibres. *Physiol., London*, **215**:353–380.

Rall, W. (1953) Electrotonic theory for a spherical neurone. *Proc. Univ. Otago. Med. School*, **31**:14–15.

Rall, W. (1957) Membrane time constant of motoneurons. *Science*, **126**:454.

Rall, W. (1959) Branching dendritic trees and motoneuron membrane resistivity. *Expt. Neurol.*, **1**:491–527.

Rall, W. (1960) Membrane potential transients and membrane time constant of motoneurons. *Expt. Neurol.* **2**:503–532.

Rall, W. (1967). Distinguishing theoretical synaptic potentials computed for different soma-dendritic distributions of synaptic input. *J. Neurophysiol.* **30**:1138–1168.

Rall, W. (1969a). Time constants and electrotonic length of membrane cylinders and neurons. *Biophys. J.* **9**:1483–1508.

Rall, W., R. E. Burke, T. G. Smith, P. G. Nelson, and K. Frank (1967). Dendritic location of synapses and possible mechanisms for the monosynaptic EPSP in motoneurons. *J. Neurophysiol.* **30**:1169–1193.

Wilfrid Rall

New information about motoneuron membranes has been obtained in recent experiments in which intracellular electrodes were used for both stimulation and recording at the motoneuron soma (*1–6*). Unexpectedly low membrane time-constant values have been inferred from the subthreshold transients of membrane potential observed when constant current was applied across the soma membrane (*2–4*). It is shown in this report, however, that these experimental transients are theoretically consistent with significantly larger membrane time-constant values, provided that the cablelike properties of dendrites are taken into account. This correction removes the apparent discrepancy (*3–5*) between the soma membrane time constant and the time constant of synaptic potential decay and thus removes the need for special explanations, such as a hypothetical prolongation of synaptic depolarizing activity (*4, 6*), or a prolongation of soma synaptic potential by electrotonic spread from a larger and slower synaptic potential postulated to occur in the dendrites (*5*).

The membrane time constant τ is defined as the product of passive membrane resistance and capacitance. The assumption (*2–4, 6*) that the experimentally observed membrane transients may be regarded as exponential curves having this time constant τ would be valid only if constant current were applied uniformly to the entire membrane surface. For the experiments in question, this could be true only for the hypothetical case of a *soma without dendrites*. The lower dashed curve in Fig. 1 illustrates the exponential time course of membrane potential change V, relative to its final steady value V_s for this hypothetical case.

Since the motoneurons are known to possess several large dendrites, a significant portion of the current applied to the soma must spread (electrotonically) along these several dendrites. This will change the time course of soma membrane potential. For example, as the size and number of dendrites is increased relative to soma size, there is a limiting case, *dendrites without soma*. This case is illustrated by the upper dashed curve in Fig. 1, on the assumption that these dendrites have the same membrane time constant τ and that they may be represented as cylinders of infinite length. This time course can be precisely expressed as

$$V/V_s = \mathrm{erf}\sqrt{t/\tau}$$

for the membrane potential at the point (soma) where constant current is applied across the membrane of each dendrite. It is the same as that

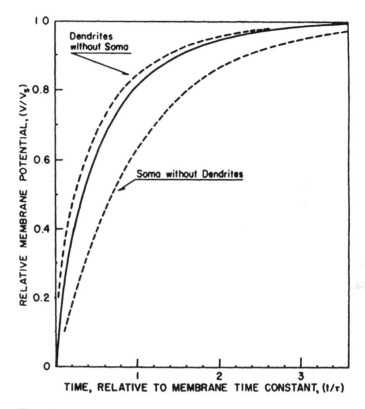

Figure 1
Membrane potential transients at the neuron soma and origins of dendrites, when constant current is applied across the soma membrane.

obtained in the more familiar problem of electrotonic potential beneath an electrode ($x = 0$), when constant current is applied between external electrodes placed far apart on a cylindrical axon (7). This curve is not a simple exponential: the time required to reach half of the steady value V_s is one-third of the time required in the lower dashed curve, while the time required to reach 90 percent of V_s is about three-fifths of that required in the lower dashed curve.

The middle curve in Fig. 1 corresponds to an intermediate relation between dendrites and soma (8). It has been assumed that soma and dendrite membranes have the same membrane time constant and that the membrane potential at any moment is uniform over the soma surface (9), up to and including the origins of the dendrites. The dendrites can be treated either as cylinders of infinite length or as structures which taper and branch exponentially.

This intermediate curve was calculated with a value of 5 for the ratio between the steady-state membrane current drawn by the dendrites and the steady-state current drawn by the soma membrane. This value is theoretically consistent with the specific example of a soma with six cylindrical dendrites (used in *1* and *6*, as well as in *3*), provided that a value of about 2000 ohm cm² is used for the membrane resistivity. Since this example probably underestimates the size and number of dendrites (*1*, p. 322), it is predicted that the time course of soma membrane potential change, when constant current is applied to the soma, will lie *between* the two upper curves in Fig. 1, for many motoneurons.

On the basis of this theoretical prediction, the membrane time constant can be estimated as being the time required for the experimental transients to reach about 82 percent of the final steady value. Since, however, the experimental error permits exponential curves to be fitted to the experimental transients (*2–4*), it should be noted that the time constants of such curves can be expected to be smaller than the actual membrane time constant, by a factor of about 2. It appears, therefore, that these experimental transients do not conflict significantly with the earlier estimate (*10*), of about 4 msec for the membrane time constant of cat motoneurons, which was based on the decay time constant of synaptic potentials (*10*), and of monosynaptic facilitation (*11*).

This is consistent with the simple notion of synaptic potential decay as a purely passive process, having the same characteristics on both soma and dendrites (*12*).

References and Notes

1. J. S. Coombs, J. C. Eccles, P. Fatt, *J. Physiol.* **130**, 291 (1955).

2. T. Araki and T. Otani, *J. Neurophysiol.* **18**, 472 (1955).

3. K. Frank and M. G. F. Fuortes, *J. Physiol.* **134**, 451 (1956).

4. J. S. Coombs, D. R. Curtis, J. C. Eccles, *Nature* **178**, 1049 (1956).

5. P. Fatt, *J. Neurophysiol.* **20**, 61 (1957).

6. J. C. Eccles, *The Physiology of Nerve Cells* (Johns Hopkins Press, Baltimore, Md., 1957).

7. A. L. Hodgkin and W. A. H. Rushton, *Proc. Roy. Soc.* (*London*) **B133**, 444 (1946); L. Davis, Jr., and R. Lorente de Nó, *Studies Rockefeller Inst. Med. Research* **131** 442 (1947).

8. A report of the mathematical treatment of this intermediate problem is in preparation.

9. W. Rall, *Proc. Univ. Otago Med. Sch.* **31**, 14 (1953), and abstract for National Biophysics Conference (1957).

10. L. G. Brock, J. S. Coombs, J. C. Eccles, *J. Physiol.* **117**, 431 (1952).

11. D. P. C. Lloyd, *J. Neurophysiol.* **9**, 421 (1946).

12. The opinions expressed in this note are my own, and are not to be construed as official or as reflecting the views of the U.S. Navy Department or the naval service at large.

Wilfrid Rall

This paper is concerned with both the quantitative information and the theory required for the interpretation of certain experimental results obtained with intracellular microelectrodes. The theory treats the spread of current from a neuron soma into branching dendritic trees. Formulas are derived for the calculation of membrane resistivity from physiological measurements of whole neuron resistance and anatomical measurements of soma and dendritic dimensions. The variability of available anatomical and physiological information is discussed. The numerical result is an estimated range of membrane resistivity values for mammalian motoneurons, and a corresponding set of values for the dendritic to soma conductance ratio. These values are significantly greater than those currently accepted in the literature, mainly because the dendritic dimensions appear to have been underestimated previously. Analysis of the histological evidence also reveals significant quantitative differences between infant, adult, and chromatolytic motoneurons. The theory builds upon the classical theory of axonal membrane electrotonus; all important assumptions are explicitly stated and discussed. The theory is general and can be applied to many types of neurons with many types of dendritic trees; it is also relevant to the diffusion of material in neurons. The 3/2 power of dendritic trunk diameter is shown to be a fundamental index of dendritic size. Another parameter characterizes the extensiveness of dendritic branching.

Introduction

New information about mammalian motoneurons has been obtained recently from experiments using intracellular stimulating and recording

It is a pleasure to acknowledge the stimulation provided by discussions with many colleagues; in particular, I wish to mention J. Z. Hearon, R. J. Podolsky, K. Frank, M. G. F. Fuortes, and G. L. Rasmussen. This work was begun while the author was in the Biophysics Division, Naval Medical Research Institute, National Naval Medical Center, Bethesda, Maryland; the opinions or assertions contained herein are the private ones of the writer and are not to be construed as official or reflecting the views of the Navy Department or the naval service at large.

electrodes (1, 7, 8, 12, 14). Correct interpretation of such experimental results is important because of the following implications: the electric properties of the motoneuron membrane can be estimated; the relative importance of soma and dendrites in both normal and experimental situations can be assessed; and much of accepted motoneuron physiology may require reassessment.

The interpretation of such experiments is complicated by the need to interrelate three different kinds of information: electrophysiological measurements on single motoneurons; morphological measurements of such neurons; a theory of electric current spread from a neuron soma into several branching dendritic trees. The present paper presents such a theory and applies it to the best physiological and morphological information currently available for mammalian motoneurons.

A diagrammatic illustration of the problem is provided by Fig. 1. When an intracellular microelectrode is used to apply electric current between a point inside a nerve cell body and a distant extracellular electrode (not shown in the diagram), some of the current flows directly across the soma membrane, and some of it flows into the dendrites (and axon) for varying distance before crossing the membrane. How much

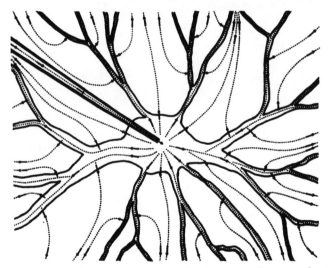

FIG. 1. Diagram illustrating the flow of electric current from a microelectrode whose tip penetrates the cell body (soma) of a neuron. The full extent of the dendrites is not shown. The external electrode to which the current flows is at a distance far beyond the limits of this diagram.

of the total current flows along each of these different paths is determined by a combination of electric and geometric factors. The electric factors, for steady state conditions, are the membrane resistivity and the specific resistivities of the intracellular and extracellular conducting media; the membrane capacity must also be considered during the transient phase of current spread. The geometric factors include the size of the neuron soma, the size and taper of all dendritic trunks, and also some measure of the amount and extent of dendritic branching.

Except for the geometric complications, this theoretical problem resembles the classical problem of passive electrotonic potential spread in axons (5, 9, 20). This fact was used in the first estimate of mammalian motoneuron membrane resistivity (8); it was assumed that the dendritic trees could be represented as cylinders of infinite length. These authors assumed six such cylinders of 5 μ diameter, for cat motoneurons; however, in their discussion (8, p. 322) they suggested that the dendritic processes must contribute rather more than their calculations had allowed. Nevertheless, this first model has become the "standard motoneurone" of Eccles (10), and a large amount of further interpretation has been based upon it. The results of the present paper indicate that this "standard motoneurone" underestimates the dendritic contribution by a significant amount.

The first interpretations of experimental transients of soma membrane potential (in response to the application of a current step across the soma membrane) were also in terms of this "standard motoneurone." Although the transient characteristics of electrotonic potential spread in long cylinders are well established for axons (9, 20), this knowledge was neglected in the estimation of the membrane time constant (6, 10, 14). The need for reinterpretation of these experiments, with suitable allowance for dendritic transient characteristics, was pointed out in preliminary communications (24, 25), and is dealt with more fully in a companion paper (26).

Theory

Assumptions

By means of the following assumptions, the geometric and passive electric properties of a neuron with dendritic trees are idealized to produce a formal theoretical model that is suitable for mathematical treatment. Definitions are introduced as needed; a complete list of all symbols is given in Appendix 1. Assumptions 1–5 are specific to the present model; assumptions 6–8 are equivalent to assumptions already established as basic to the theory of axonal electrotonus (9, 20).

1. A dendritic tree is assumed to consist of a cylindrical trunk and cylindrical branch components. Such a tree is illustrated in Fig. 5. The analysis has been generalized to include taper, but this complication is omitted here.

2. The electric properties of the membrane are assumed to be uniform over the entire soma-dendritic surface, alternative assumptions are possible (12), but this assumption centers attention on the geometric aspects of the problem.

3. The electric potential is assumed to be constant over the entire external surface of the neuron. This is equivalent to assuming infinite conductivity of the external medium; such an assumption is commonly made for axons placed in a large volume of conducting medium. The use of this assumption can be shown to cause negligible error in the results. Briefly, this is because the gradients of electric potential to be expected in an external medium of large volume, and of reasonable conductivity, are very much smaller than the corresponding internal (axial) gradients of potential.[2]

4. The electric potential is assumed to be constant over the internal surface of the soma membrane. Together with assumption 3, this implies a uniform soma membrane potential. In this formal model, therefore, the shape of the soma surface is irrelevant, because the entire soma membrane is effectively a lumped membrane impedance. Thus lumped impedance represents the common point of origin for all dendritic trunks belonging to a single neuron. Strict validity of this assumption, during flow of current into the dendrites from an electrode placed within the soma, would imply infinite conductivity within the soma.[2]

5. The internal potential and current are assumed to be continuous at all dendritic branch points and at the soma-dendritic junction. This is an obvious physical requirement which merits explicit statement because of its importance in the mathematical treatment.

6. The electric current inside any cylindrical component is assumed to flow axially through an ohmic resistance which is inversely proportional to the area of cross section.

7. The electric current across the membrane is assumed to be normal

[2] Further assessment of assumptions 3 and 4 is presented in the discussion portion of this paper, page 521.

to the membrane surface. The uniformly distributed membrane impedance is assumed to consist of an ohmic resistance in parallel with a perfect capacity.

8. A membrane electromotive force, E, is assumed to be in series with the membrane resistance, and is assumed to be constant for all of the membrane. Under steady conditions, and in the absence of current flow, the electric potential difference, V_m, across the membrane has a resting value equal to E.

FUNDAMENTAL EQUATIONS

The derivation of the differential equation for distributions of passive electrotonic potential in uniform cylinders is well established in the theory developed for axons (5, 9, 20). In regions containing no sources or sinks of externally applied current, this differential equation can be expressed

$$\lambda^2 \frac{\partial^2 V}{\partial x^2} = V + \tau \frac{\partial V}{\partial t}, \qquad [1]$$

where $V = V_m - E$ is the electrotonic potential, x represents distance along the axis of the cylinder, $\tau = R_m C_m$ is the membrane time constant, and $\lambda = [(d/4)(R_m/R_i)]^{1/2}$ is the characteristic length constant.[3]

Transient solutions of this differential equation are considered in a companion paper (26). Under steady state conditions, $\partial V/\partial t = 0$, and the general solution of the differential equation can be expressed in terms of exponential or hyperbolic[4] functions, with two arbitrary constants.

---

[3] A more familiar expression for λ would be $[r_m/(r_e + r_i)]^{1/2}$. Here, however, assumption 3 implies $r_e = 0$, and the resistances, r_m and r_i, for unit length, have been expressed in terms of fundamental quantities: R_m = membrane resistance for a unit area (Ωcm^2); R_i = specific resistivity of internal medium (Ωcm); and d is the diameter of the cylinder. Thus $r_m = R_m/\pi d$) and $r_i = 4R_i/(\pi d^2)$. The derivation of Eq. [1] can be indicated briefly as follows: because of assumptions 3 and 6, the axial current, I, is defined by Eq. [8], and (see Fig. 2) the membrane current per unit length of cylinder is $i_m = -\partial I/\partial x = (1/r_i)(\partial^2 V/\partial x^2)$; also, because of assumptions 3, 7, and 8, $i_m = \pi d(C_m \partial V/\partial t + V/R_m)$; equating these two expressions for i_m results in Eq. [1]. Further details can be found in Research Report NM 01 05 00.01.02 of the Naval Medical Research Institute, Bethesda, Maryland.

[4] The hyperbolic sine and cosine are tabulated functions defined as follows: $\sinh u = \frac{1}{2}(e^u - e^{-u})$ and $\cosh u = \frac{1}{2}(e^u + e^{-u})$. The properties relevant to the boundary conditions of the present problem are these: when $u = 0$, $\sinh u = 0$, and $\cosh u = 1$; also, $d/dx (\sinh u) = (\cosh u) du/dx$, and $d/dx (\cosh u) = (\sinh u) du/dx$.

The following form proves to be particularly useful for present purposes

$$V/V_1 = \cosh\left[(x_1 - x)/\lambda_0\right] + B_1 \sinh\left[(x_1 - x)/\lambda_0\right], \qquad [2]$$

where $\lambda = \lambda_0$ refers specifically to the dendritic trunk. The constant, V_1, represents the value of V at $x = x_1$, and the constant, B_1, is related to the amount of axial current flowing at $x = x_1$. For the case of a cylin-

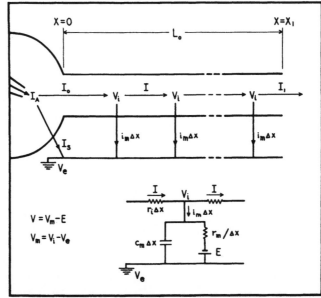

Fig. 2. The upper diagram illustrates electric potentials and current flow for a cylindrical trunk arising from a soma. The lower diagram shows the lumped parameter equivalent circuit for the membrane. Symbols are as given in the text and in Appendix 1, with the addition of Δx, which simply represents the increment in x for which quantities are lumped. The differential equations, of course, imply no lumping (i.e. the limit as $\Delta x \to 0$).

drical trunk, extending from $x = 0$ to $x = x_1$, the soma electrotonic potential, V_0, is related to V_1 by the expression

$$V_0/V_1 = \cosh\left(L_0/\lambda_0\right) + B_1 \sinh\left(L_0/\lambda_0\right), \qquad [3]$$

where $L_0 = x_1$ is the length of the trunk, see Figs. 2 and 4. The value of B_1 is determined by the branches arising at $x = x_1$, as well as by the extensiveness of subsequent branching arising from these primary branches. This dependence of B_1 upon branching is made explicit below, Eq. [16].

For the special case, $B_1 = 1$, Eq. [2] simplifies to the exponential electrotonic decrement,

$$V/V_c = e^{-x/\lambda_0},$$ [4]

already well known for axon cylinders of infinite length. For a dendritic trunk, this solution applies only for the range $0 \leqslant x \leqslant x_1$; it implies that the branches arising at $x = x_1$ provide the same combined input conductance at $x = x_1$ as would an infinite extension of the cylindrical trunk. A value of B_1 greater than unity implies that the dendritic tree is branched more extensively than this, and a value less than unity implies less extensive branching.

Termination of a Cylinder. There are several reasons for briefly considering the special cases, $B_1 = 0$ and $B_1 = \infty$. These special cases represent particular terminal boundary conditions that are relevant, in one case, to a natural "sealed end" of a terminal dendritic branch, and relevant in the other case to experimentally produced "killed end" termination of a dendritic branch or axon. Also, these two special cases result in simplifications of Eq. [2], and they represent two extremes of electrotonic potential decrement with distance along a cylinder; these two cases are compared, in Fig. 3, with the special case, $B_1 = 1$, already considered in Eq. [4].

When $B_1 = 0$, Eq. [2] simplifies to

$$V/V_c = \frac{\cosh\left[(x_1 - x)/\lambda_0\right]}{\cosh\left(L_0/\lambda_0\right)},$$ [5]

which is characterized by a zero slope at $x = x_1$. Curves e, f, and g in Fig. 3 illustrate this solution for the three lengths, $L_0/\lambda_0 = 2$, 1, and 1/2. It is clear that these curves slope less steeply than curve a. This solution would correspond to termination with a "sealed end" that provides a very high resistance between the internal and external media at $x = x_1$. This is a good approximation to the case of a membrane cylinder whose end is sealed with a disk composed of the same membrane; the exact solution for this case is obtained by setting

$$B_1 = \lambda_0 R_i/R_m = [(R_i/R_m)(d_0/4)]^{1/2}$$

in Eq. [2]. Thus, for example, if $R_1 = 50$ Ωcm, $R_m = 1250$ Ωcm^2, and $d_0 = 4$ μ, then $B_1 = 2 \times 10^{-3}$, which differs negligibly from zero.

When $B_1 = \infty$, Eq. [2] simplifies to

$$V/V_0 = \frac{\sinh\,[(x_1 - x)/\lambda_0]}{\sinh\,(L_0/\lambda_0)}, \qquad [6]$$

which is characterized by $V = 0$ at $x = x_1$. Curves b, c, and d in Fig. 3 illustrate this solution for the three lengths, $L_0/\lambda_0 = 2$, 1, and 1/2.

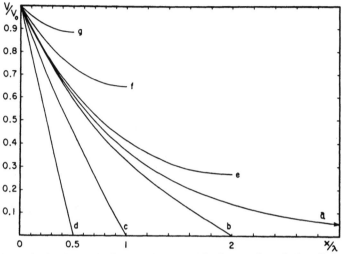

FIG. 3. Distributions of electrotonic potential along unbranched cylinders, for different terminal boundary conditions and different lengths, Eq. [2]. Curve a corresponds to $B_1 = 1$, or to infinite cylindrical extension, Eq. [4]. Curves b, c, and d correspond to $B_1 = \infty$ and $V_1 = 0$, Eq. [6]. Curves e, f, and g correspond to sealed end termination with $B_1 = 0$, Eq. [5].

It is clear that these curves slope more steeply than curve a. This solution represents part of the complete solution for a "killed end" boundary condition at $x = x_1$. When the terminal resistance between the internal and external media is essentially zero, also the terminal membrane potential difference, V_m, must be essentially zero, because the membrane EMF cannot produce an infinite current. Thus, the "killed end" boundary condition is $V = -E$ because the electrotonic potential is defined, $V = V_m - E$; in other words, this boundary condition is equivalent to application of a potential, $-E$, across an uninjured membrane at $x = x_1$. The complete solution which satisfies the two boundary conditions, $V = V_0$ at $x = 0$ and $V = -E$ at $x = x_1$, can be expressed

$$V = \frac{V_0 \sinh\,[(x_1 - x)/\lambda_0] - E \sinh\,(x/\lambda_0)}{\sinh\,(L_0/\lambda_0)}. \qquad [7]$$

INPUT CONDUCTANCE OF A DENDRITIC TREE

Because of assumptions 3 and 6, the axial current at any point, x, can be expressed

$$I = (1/r_i)\left[-\frac{\partial V}{\partial x}\right],\qquad\qquad [8]$$

where r_i represents the axial (core) resistance per unit length of the cylinder. It follows from Eqs. [2] and [8], that for the range $0 \leqslant x \leqslant x_1$,

$$I/V_1 = G_\infty\left\{\sinh\left[(x_1 - x)/\lambda_0\right] + B_1 \cosh\left[(x_1 - x)/\lambda_0\right]\right\}\qquad [9]$$

where

$$G_\infty = (\lambda_0 r_i)^{-1}$$
$$= (\pi/2)(R_m R_i)^{-1/2}(d_0)^{3/2}.\qquad\qquad [10]$$

The dendritic input current, I_0, that flows from the soma into this dendritic trunk at $x = 0$, is obtained by setting $x = 0$ in Eq. [9]. Making use of Eq. [3], the result can be expressed as the dendritic input conductance.

$$G_D = I_0/V_0 = B_0 G_\infty,\qquad\qquad [11]$$

where

$$B_0 = \frac{B_1 + \tanh (L_0/\lambda_0)}{1 + B_1 \tanh (L_0/\lambda_0)}.\qquad\qquad [12]$$

Equations [10], [11], and [12] express a very useful result. The dendritic input conductance, G_D, of any dendritic tree is expressed in terms of the reference conductance, G_∞, corresponding to an infinite extension of the cylindrical trunk, and a factor, B_0, The value of B_0 depends upon the relative trunk length, L_0/λ_0, and upon the value of B_1. The manner in which B_1 depends upon successive branchings, is considered below.

For very short dendritic trunks, B_0 essentially equals B_1, because tanh (L_0/λ_0) is then close to zero. For very long dendritic trunks, B_0 essentially equals unity, regardless of B_1, because tanh (L_0/λ_0) is then close to unity. For intermediate trunk lengths, the value of B_0 always lies between B_1 and unity.

For the special case, $B_1 = 1$, B_0 necessarily equals unity. For the limiting special case, $B_1 = 0$, which is the "sealed end" termination considered with Eq. [5], B_0 assumes its smallest possible value, tanh (L_0/λ_0).

This implies an input conductance, G_D, that is less than or equal to G_∞; it corresponds to the reduced steepness of the initial slopes of curves e, f, and g in Fig. 3. In the other limiting special case, $B_1 = \infty$, which is related to "killed end" termination, cf. Eqs. [6] and [7], B_0 assumes its largest possible value, coth (L_0/λ_0). This implies an input conductance, G_D, that is greater than or equal to G_∞; it corresponds to the increased steepness of the initial slopes of curves b, c, and d in Fig. 3.

Dependence of B_1 *upon Branching.* In order to obtain an expression for B_1 in terms of subsequent branching, it is necessary to satisfy a series of boundary conditions required by assumptions 3 and 5. Continuity of both V and I at every branch point also implies continuity of the ratio, I/V, which has the dimensions of conductance.

At $x = x_1$, Eq. [9] for the dendritic trunk reduces simply to

$$I_1/V_1 = B_1 G_\infty. \qquad [13]$$

For each branch arising at $x = x_1$, there corresponds an equation similar to Eq. [9]; i.e., it is identical except for subscripts (cf. Fig. 4). For the

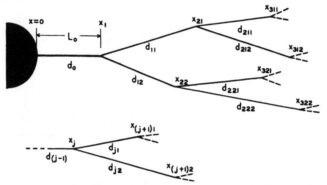

<small>Fig. 4. Dendritic branching diagrams to illustrate the subscript notation used in the text.</small>

kth branch, extending from $x = x_1$ to $x = x_{2k}$, and having a diameter, d_{1k}, a length, L_{1k}, and a characteristic length, λ_{1k}, the I/V value at $x = x_1$ can be expressed

$$I_{1k}/V_1 = B_{1k} G_\infty (d_{1k}/d_0)^{3/2}, \qquad [14]$$

where

$$B_{1k} = \frac{B_{2k} + \tanh (L_{1k}/\lambda_{1k})}{1 + B_{2k} \tanh (L_{1k}/\lambda_{1k})} \qquad [15]$$

and B_{2k} depends similarly upon branching subsequent to $x = x_{2k}$.

Continuity of I/V at $x = x_1$, requires that the sum, composed of one term like Eq. [14] for each branch arising at $x = x_1$, must equal the quantity given in Eq. [13]. This results in the expression

$$B_1 = \sum_k B_{1k}(d_{1k}/d_0)^{3/2}.$$ [16]

For the common case of two unequal branches (cf. Fig. 4), this can be written

$$B_1 = B_{11}(d_{11}/d_0)^{3/2} + B_{12}(d_{12}/d_0)^{3/2}$$ [17]

and for the special case of equal branches, N_1 in number, this can be written

$$B_1 = N_1(d_1/d_0)^{3/2} \left[\frac{B_2 + \tanh{(L_1/\lambda_1)}}{1 + B_2 \tanh{(L_1/\lambda_1)}} \right].$$ [18]

It can be seen that B_1 depends not only on the (primary) branches arising at $x = x_1$, but also (Eq. [15]) on the values of B_{2k}, which depend upon the (secondary) branches arising from the primary branches. This process can be repeated, step by step, until terminal branches are reached.

Generalization to any Branch Point. The results expressed in Eqs. [15] and [16] can be generalized to any branch point, $x = x_j$, of a dendritic tree (cf. Fig. 4). Thus

$$B_j = \sum_k B_{jk}[d_{jk}/d_{(j-1)}]^{3/2},$$ [19]

where

$$B_{jk} = \frac{B_{(j+1)k} + \tanh{(L_{jk}/\lambda_{jk})}}{1 + B_{(j+1)k} \tanh{(L_{jk}/\lambda_{jk})}},$$ [20]

and the subscript, jk, represents the kth branch arising at $x = x_j$; the value of λ_{jk} can be expressed

$$\lambda_{jk} = [(d_{jk}/4)(R_m/R_i)]^{1/2}.$$ [21]

These general results were used to calculate Table 1.

A Hypothetical Dendritic Tree. A specific hypothetical example of an extensively branched dendritic tree is illustrated in Fig. 5. This example contains some symmetry to simplify the illustrative calculations; however, the general method does not require the presence of any symmetry. This example was also intended to be a possible approximation to some of the dendritic trees of mammalian motoneurons, on the assumption that histological preparations usually do not show the full extent of peripheral dendritic branching; how close an approximation it may be is still an open question (see pages 515 and 516).

The trunk and all branch elements are assumed to be cylinders. The trunk is assumed to have a diameter of 15 μ and a length of 50 μ. It bifurcates into two equal branches, 10 μ in diameter and 100 μ in length. All subsequent branches are assumed, for simplicity, to be 200 μ in length; their diameters, in microns, are indicated by the numbers beside

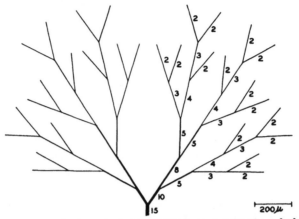

Fig. 5. Diagram of the hypothetical dendritic tree used for the calculations summarized in Table 1. The lengths and largest diameters are drawn to scale. The two halves of the tree are mirror images; the numbers represent dendritic branch diameters in microns. This two-dimensional spread is meant to represent a more compact three-dimensional tree.

them in Fig. 5. The radial extent of this system is approximately one millimeter.

To calculate the dendritic input conductance, G_D, of such a system it is necessary to assume values for the resistivities, R_m and R_i. The calculations in Table 1 have been carried out with two different values for the ratio, R_m/R_i; the larger value, 72 cm, corresponds, for example,

to $R_m = 3600$ Ωcm² and $R_i = 50$ Ωcm; the smaller value is one fourth of the larger. Given the R_m/R_i value, Eq. [21] is used to calculate the λ_{jk} values; then the tanh (L_{jk}/λ_{jk}) values are calculated for each cylindrical component. Beginning with $B_{(j+1)k} = 0$ for the terminal branches, the procedure is to calculate B_{jk} from Eq. [20] and then B_j from Eq. [19]. This provides the $B_{(j+1)k}$ value for a next-to-terminal branch. In this manner, step by step, the calculation approaches the dendritic trunk, where B_0 is defined by Eq. [12] and B_1 is defined by Eq. [16].

Table 1 demonstrates that, with the larger value for R_m, the extensiveness of branching is only just sufficient to make the dendritic input conductance of this tree essentially equal to the input conductance, G_∞, corresponding to an infinite extension of the cylindrical trunk. With the smaller R_m value, the same branching is more than sufficient to satisfy this criterion; in fact, the B value increases from zero to unity in only three steps; in other words, the 8-μ branches could be extended to infinity without changing the input conductance of the dendritic tree. It is clear that for smaller R_m values, less extensive branching is required to make B_0 be close to unity.

For this particular dendritic tree, the result is $G_D = 2 \times 10^{-7}$ reciprocal ohms for $R_m = 3600$ Ωcm², and $G_D = 4.5 \times 10^{-7}$ reciprocal ohms for $R_m = 900$ Ωcm². To obtain the conductance of a whole neuron, several such conductances must be added in parallel with the soma membrane conductance.

Comment. A value of B_0 greater than unity can result only when B_1 is greater than unity. If the B_{2k} values are close to unity, this depends mainly on the sum of the $(d_{1k}/d_0)^{3/2}$ values being greater than unity. The anatomical evidence does include several sets of primary dendritic branches whose diameters approximate this condition.

It is not accidental that any B_{jk} value different from unity always lies between $B_{(j+1)k}$ and unity. This is an algebraic property of Eq. [20]; it is valid for $B_{(j+1)k}$ either less than or greater than unity. Thus, whenever nature keeps the values of

$$\sum_k (d_{jk}/d_{j-1})^{3/2}$$

very close to unity, the values of B_j, as one calculates from the terminal branches to the trunk, must approach stepwise toward unity; once a value close to unity is reached, further steps cannot carry the value away from unity by any significant amount.

WHOLE NEURON CONDUCTANCE

The whole neuron conductance, G_N, can be defined

$$G_N = I_A/V_0 = 1/R_N, \qquad [22]$$

where I_A represents the applied current flowing from an electrode within the neuron soma to an extracellular electrode, and V_0 is the steady value of the electrotonic potential at $x = 0$ (i.e., at the soma and at the origin of every dendrite), that results from this current.

TABLE 1
BRANCHING TREE CALCULATION

d_{j-1} to d_{jk}	$(d_{jk}/d_{j-1})^{3/2}$	$R_m = 3600\ \Omega cm^2$				$R_m = 900\ \Omega cm^2$			
		tanh (L_{jk}/λ_{jk})	$B_{(j+1)k}$	B_{jk}	B_j	tanh (L_{jk}/λ_{jk})	$B_{(j+1)k}$	B_{jk}	B_j
3 μ to { 2 μ	0.54	0.32	0	0.32	0.34	0.58	0	0.58	0.62
{ 2 μ	0.54	0.32	0	0.32		0.58	0	0.58	
4 μ to { 2 μ	0.35	0.32	0	0.32	0.47	0.58	0	0.58	0.75
{ 3 μ	0.65	0.26	0.34	0.55		0.50	0.62	0.85	
5 μ to { 3 μ	0.46	0.26	0.34	0.55	0.70	0.50	0.62	0.85	1.02
{ 4 μ	0.71	0.24	0.47	0.64		0.44	0.75	0.89	
8 μ to { 5 μ	0.49	0.21	0.70	0.80	0.78	0.40	1.02	1.01	0.98
{ 5 μ	0.49	0.21	0.70	0.80		0.40	1.02	1.01	
10 μ to { 5 μ	0.35	0.21	0.70	0.80	0.88	0.40	1.02	1.01	1.05
{ 8 μ	0.71	0.17	0.78	0.84		0.32	0.98	0.99	
15 μ to { 10 μ	0.54	0.08	0.88	0.90	0.98	0.15	1.05	1.03	1.12
{ 10 μ	0.54	0.08	0.88	0.90		0.15	1.05	1.03	
15 μ (at $x = o$)		0.03	0.98	$B_o = 0.98$		0.05	1.12	$B_o = 1.11$	

Physical continuity of current (assumption 5) implies that the applied current, I_A, must equal the sum of the several dendritic input currents plus the current flowing across the soma membrane. Similarly, G_N is the sum of the several dendritic input conductances plus the soma conductance.

Because of assumptions 2–4, the soma conductance can be expressed

$$G_S = S/R_m, \tag{23}$$

where S represents the soma surface area.

Making use of the results obtained for dendritic trees (Eqs. [10]–[12]), the combined dendritic input conductance can be expressed

$$\sum_j G_{Dj} = CD^{3/2}(R_m)^{-1/2} \tag{24}$$

where

$$C = (\pi/2)(R_i)^{-1/2}, \tag{25}$$

and

$$D^{3/2} = \sum_j B_{0j}(d_{0j})^{3/2}. \tag{26}$$

Equation [26] defines a combined dendritic tree parameter. It shows that the combined effect of several dendritic trees is proportional, not to a simple sum or average of the trunk diameters, but to a sum composed of the 3/2 power of each trunk diameter appropriately weighted. The weighting factor, B_{0j}, relates the input conductance, G_{Dj}, of the jth trunk to its infinite cylindrical extension value, see Eqs. [10] to [12]. Because B_{0j} does depend upon R_m/R_i through $\tanh(L_{0j}/\lambda_{0j})$, the parameter, $D^{3/2}$, does not reflect purely geometric characteristics of the dendritic trees. For this reason, it is useful also to define a combined dendritic trunk parameter

$$\sum d_{0j}^{3/2} \tag{27}$$

which does not depend in any way upon the values of R_m and R_i. It is this last parameter that is most easily estimated from histological evidence. If, in addition, study of representative dendritic trees should establish that all the B_{0j} values are close to unity, then the geometric parameter [27] would provide a good approximation to the more general parameter, $D^{3/2}$, defined by Eq. [26]. This approximation has been used in Table 2 below, but its validity is obviously subject to further testing. The following formulas are general, and are not based upon such an approximation.

Making use of Eqs. [23]–[26], the whole neuron conductance can be expressed,

$$G_N = \frac{CD^{3/2}}{\sqrt{R_m}} + \frac{S}{R_m} \qquad [28]$$

where it has been assumed that the same R_m value applies to both soma and dendrites; alternative assumptions would have to be introduced at this point.

Because the practical problem consists of estimating R_m from an experimental measurement of R_N, it is useful to solve Eq. [28] explicitly for R_m. The result is

$$R_m = (1 + \epsilon)C^2D^3R_N^2 \qquad [29]$$

where

$$1 + \epsilon = \frac{1}{4}\left[1 + \sqrt{1 + \frac{4S}{C^2D^3R_N}}\right]^2. \qquad [30]$$

When $C^2D^3R_N$ is greater than $4S$, expansion of [30] yields

$$\epsilon \approx \frac{2S}{C^2D^3R_N}.$$

For a numerical illustration relevant to mammalian motoneurons (see Table 2), consider $S = 1.25 \times 10^{-4}$ cm^2, $D^{3/2} = 2.5 \times 10^{-4}$ cm$^{3/2}$, $C = 0.2$ $(\Omega\text{cm})^{-1/2}$ and $R_N = 1.2$ megohms (7). Then $R_m = 3900$ Ωcm^2; a value of 0.083 is found for ϵ. Increase of R_N to 1.65 megohms (14) increases R_m to 7200 Ωcm^2. These values are shown in Fig. 6, which displays the theoretical relation between R_N and R_m (log-log scaling) for nine different values of the combined dendritic tree parameter, $D^{3/2}$; for this figure, it was assumed that $C = 0.2$ $(\Omega\text{cm})^{-1/2}$, which correponds to R_i between 50 and 75 Ωcm, and that $D^{3/2}/S = 2$ cm$^{-1/2}$, which corresponds to the average in Table 2.

DENDRITIC TO SOMA CONDUCTANCE RATIO

The ratio of combined dendritic input conductance to the soma membrane conductance is simply the quotient of Eqs. [24] and [23]. This ratio is important in the consideration of transients (24, 26). It can be expressed

$$\rho = C[D^{3/2}/S]\sqrt{R_m}. \qquad [31]$$

Clearly, the value of ρ depends upon both geometric and electric quantities. However, when dendritic trees are such that the parameter, $D^{3/2}$, is equal to the purely geometric combined dendritic trunk parameter (compare Eq. [26] with expression [27]), then

$$D^{3/2}/S = \sum_j d_{0j}^{3/2}/S,$$ [32]

and this ratio can then be regarded as purely geometric.

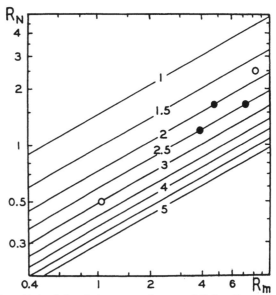

FIG. 6. Theoretical relation between membrane resistivity, R_m, and whole neuron resistance, R_N, for several values of $D^{3/2}$; note log-log scaling. R_m is in 10^3 ohm cm² and R_N is in megohms; the numbers in the middle represent the $D^{3/2}$ values in 10^{-4} cm³/². Filled circles represent specific intermediate values mentioned in the text; open circles represent extreme values of the range presented in the Results section. Because of the log-log scaling, these theoretical curves are almost, but not quite, straight lines. The calculations shared the assumptions of Eq. [33], and were based upon Eqs. [28] and [34].

For the motoneurons of Table 2, this geometric ratio has an average value of about 2 cm⁻¹/²; using also $C = 0.2$ (Ωcm)⁻¹/², Eq. [31] yields the particular numerical formula

$$\rho = 0.4\sqrt{R_m}$$ [33]

where R_m must be expressed in Ωcm². This implies, for example, that values of 400, 1600, 3600, and 6400 Ωcm² for R_m, would correspond to values of 8, 16, 24, and 36 for the ratio, ρ.

For the interpretation of experimental evidence, it should be emphasized that ρ depends upon R_m as well as upon geometry, and that the determination of R_m from the data cannot depend upon the value of ρ (unless a trial and error procedure is employed). The direct procedure for calculation of R_m makes use of Eq. [29]. However, in calculations where a value of R_m is assumed (e.g., Table 2), it is efficient to calculate ρ from Eq. [31], or from formula [33] when applicable, and then to calculate R_N from the relation

$$R_N = \frac{R_m}{(\rho + 1)S} \qquad [34]$$

which follows from the definitions (or from Eqs. [28] and [31]).

Anatomical Information

Ideally, for present purposes, the soma and dendritic dimensions should be those of the same neuron upon which the electrophysiological measurements have been made, and the dimensions should be those of the living neuron. Instead, it is necessary, at present, to use the morphological dimensions of one sample of dead cells in combination with physiological results obtained from a different sample of living, but not completely normal cells. Because of uncertainty in how well these two samples are matched, there is also uncertainty in the interpretations. It is therefore important to consider the variability of the data and the possibilities for systematic error.

The information summarized in Table 2 was obtained by measurement of published histological material, which is identified in the footnotes. These neurons were all large ventral horn cells from the lumbar region of mammalian spinal cord. Although the motor axon was not identifiable in every case, it is generally assumed that such cells are the same as the motoneurons which neurophysiologists have been studying with intracellular microelectrodes.

This quantitative sample is small and is based upon histological illustrations that were not specifically intended for such measurements. I hope that this study will stimulate neurohistologists to provide more extensive measurements from the best possible original material.

Other Anatomical Sources. Ramón y Cajal presented a wealth of material relevant to the present study. There are, however, two disadvantages: Most of his illustrations are from fetal material, and the scale is not given in his figure legends. For the present study, such illustrations as his Figs. 129–131 (27) are especially interesting for the extensiveness of branching that they reveal.

Balthasar (2) has presented a histological study of normal and chromatolytic motoneurons in young cats (ages up to 6 months). Although this study contains considerable information on the dendrites, the published figures are of limited value for present purposes, because the sections were 12 to 20 μ in thickness, and no reconstruction from serial sections was presented. In any single section, some dendritic trunks are likely to be missed completely, and even those which do appear may not display their full diameters. However, even with these disadvantages, measurements of Balthasar's figures reveal general agreement with the results presented in Table 2. Balthasar has been cited by Eccles in support of his "standard motoneurone" (10, p. 6; 7, p. 514). In fact, Balthasar emphasizes the differences between several types of cells with different dendritic complement (2, pp. 356–358, 362–364, 377). Balthasar reports that dorsolateral tibial neurons have 5 to 10 finer dendritic trunks, of which 1 or 2 are thicker (principal dendrites); central tibial neurons usually have about 4 to 7 dendritic trunks of relatively larger caliber; peroneal neurons usually have 3 to 5 relatively even thicker trunks. He does not give values for these various trunk diameters, but measurements of his figures (in photographic enlargement) give diameters of about 19 μ for the larger dendritic trunks of peroneal neurons (presumably not chromatolytic in his Figs. 7a, b), and diameters from 12 to 20 μ for the principal dendrites of chromatolytic tibial neurons (his Figs. 3a and 7a, b). The smallest dendritic trunks of the chromatolytic tibial neurons appear to be around 4 to 7 μ in diameter. With such diameters, the three neuron types (cited above) all seem to imply values between 200 and 300 $\mu^{3/2}$ for the combined dendritic trunk parameter, in agreement with the results in Table 2.

Systematic Error. A serious possibility of systematic error is the possibility of swelling and/or shrinkage that may take place during various stages of death and fixation. There is evidence, for example, which indicates dendritic swelling in the cerebral cortex under conditions of anoxia (29); the possibility of such an effect in the spinal cord remains to be determined. On the other hand, histologists often estimate fixation shrinkage as much as 15 per cent (in linear dimensions) or more. There is the possibility of unknown osmotic shrinkage or swelling in Chu's preparations (4). With regard to peripheral branching, experienced anatomists appear to agree that the true branching must be more exten-

TABLE 2

MAMMALIAN MOTONEURONS

Mammal	Geometric quantities			Hypothetical estimates[h]			
	Dendrites $\Sigma d^{3/2}$ [a] (10^{-6} cm$^{3/2}$)	Soma S [b] (10^{-6} cm^2)	Ratio $\Sigma d^{3/2}/S$ (cm$^{-1/2}$)	(for $R_m = 4000\ \Omega$cm^2) ρ	R_N (megohms)	(for $R_m = 600\ \Omega$cm^2) ρ	R_N (megohms)
Human, adult (Chu)[c]							
Fig. 2	249	149	1.67	21	1.21	8.2	0.44
Fig. 3	205	129	1.59	20	1.47	7.8	0.53
Fig. 12	281	103	2.73	34	1.09	13.4	0.40
Fig. 13	226	109	2.07	26	1.35	10.1	0.50
Fig. 18	217	87	2.49	32	1.41	12.2	0.52
Fig. 21	244	98	2.49	32	1.26	12.2	0.46
Mean	237	112	2.17	27	1.30	10.6	0.48
Standard Deviation	27.1	22.7	0.47	5.9	0.14	0.23	0.05
Cat, adult							
(Haggar and Barr)[d]	204	94	2.17	28	1.49	11	0.55
(corrected for shrinkage)	261	130	2.01	25	1.17	10	0.43
(Fatt)[e]	226	107	2.11	27	1.35	10	0.50
Cat, "Standard Motoneurone"							
(Eccles, 1957)[f]	67	150	0.45	5.7	4.0	2.2	1.25
(Coombs, et al., 1959)[f]	78	150	0.52	6.6	3.5	2.6	1.13
Human, adult, chromatolytic (Chu)[c]							
Fig. 14	80	73	1.1	14	3.7	5.4	1.28
Fig. 15	104	126	0.83	10	2.8	4.1	0.93
Mean	92	100	0.92	12	3.2	4.5	1.09

TABLE 2 (*Continued*)

| | Geometric quantities | | | Hypothetical estimates[h] | | | |
	Dendrites $\Sigma d^{3/2a}$ (10^{-6} cm$^{3/2}$)	Soma S^b (10^{-6} cm^2)	Ratio $\Sigma d^{3/2}/S$ (cm$^{-1/2}$)	(for R_m = 4000 Ωcm^2) ρ	R_N (megohms)	(for R_m = 600 Ωcm^2) ρ	R_N (megohms)
Mammal							
Human, infant (Chu)[c]							
Fig. 1	100	63	1.59	20	3.0	7.8	1.08
Fig. 5	113	49	2.31	29	2.7	11.3	1.0
Fig. 6	135	76	1.78	22	2.2	8.7	0.81
Fig. 7	132	75	1.76	22	2.3	8.6	0.83
Fig. 20[g]	83	29	2.87	36	3.7	14.1	1.37
	(139)	(58)	(2.40)	(30)	(2.2)	(11.8)	(0.81)
Mean[g]	113	58	2.06	26	2.7	10.1	0.93
	(124)	(64)	(1.97)	(25)	(2.4)	(9.7)	(0.88)
Standard Deviation[g]	21.9	19.8	0.53				
	(16.6)	(11.3)	(0.36)				

[a] Combined dendritic trunk parameter, see Eq. [26] and [27]. The dendritic trunk diameters were measured at distances about 20 to 40 μ beyond their points of origin from the soma. This avoids most of the ambiguity due to sharp taper at dendritic origins. In many cases, the dendritic trunk is almost cylindrical from this point of measurement to the region where branching occurs; some swelling is often seen just before a branch point. These diameter values are subject to a measurement error of about 10 per cent; the possibility of systematic error is considered elsewhere.

[b] Estimate of soma surface area. The measurement consisted of estimating a major and a minor diameter (approximately perpendicular to each other). An attempt was made to exercise good judgment in adjusting the major diameter to include some allowance for proximal dendritic portions of particularly large diameter. The soma surface, S, was then estimated as π times the product of the major diameter and the minor diameter; this is an approximation to the surface area of an ellipsoid. Such estimates of soma surface area may well be subject to 25 per cent error or more, and it is not clear how they can be much improved upon without three-dimensional information. There is, of course, some arbitrariness in distinguishing between soma and proximal dendrites, because there is actually a transition from the large internal cross section of the soma, to the small internal cross section of a dendritic trunk.

TABLE 2 (*Continued*)

c Chu (4) presented photographs of human anterior horn cells isolated from fresh autopsy material. Although it is probable that the method of cell isolation resulted in breakage of peripheral dendritic branches, the dendritic trunks are probably all present. The origins of a few trunks may be hidden behind the soma, but most of them can be measured from the photographs. The number of dendritic trunks ranges from from 7 to 12; the apparent diameters range from about 2.5 to 10 μ for infants, and from about 4 to 15 μ for adults; there are a few 20-μ diameter trunks which bifurcate into smaller trunks after a short distance. Although these cells were not subject to fixation shrinkage, there remains a possibility of osmotic shrinkage or swelling; no attempt is made here to estimate this. Two sets of measurements were made several months apart; a comparison of these indicates reproducibility within about 10 per cent error.

d Haggar and Barr (18) presented in their Fig. 3, a photograph of a model of an adult cat motoneuron. This model represents a reconstruction from serial sections of 4-μ thickness. Thus, all of the dendritic trunks, regardless of their orientation relative to the plane of sectioning, have been included. Reasonably satisfactory measurements can be made from the photograph; however, a personal communication from Professor Barr provides the following approximate measurements from the actual model: the two large dendrites have diameters of about 16 and 19 μ; there are six small dendrites with an average diameter of about 4.5 μ; the mean diameter of the soma is about 50 μ. In estimating the soma surface area, I used a major diameter of 60 μ and a minor diameter of 50 μ. Professor Barr estimated the shrinkage produced by their histological methods as about 10 to 15 per cent, in terms of linear dimensions; the larger figure implies a correction factor of $(0.85)^{-3/2} = 1.28$ for the combined dendritic trunk parameter, and a factor of 1.38 for the soma surface area. Professor Barr also pointed out that the purpose of the model was illustrative rather than high precision. In view of the 200 × magnification used in the model, it seems reasonable to me to hope that the resulting measurements are subject to not more than about 10 per cent error.

e Fatt (11) presented in his Fig. 1, a camera lucida drawing of a large Golgi-stained neuron (presumably a motoneuron) in the ventral horn of an adult cat's spinal cord. Because the section was 0.25 mm thick, this should display all of the dendritic trunks, except those whose projections are hidden by the soma itself. Although Fatt makes no claim for high precision in the dendritic diameters of his camera lucida drawing, a photographic enlargement of his published figure was measured with the following results: the dendritic diameters in microns are about 14.2, 12.3, 11.3, plus two of 9.4 and two of 6.6; the soma major and minor diameters are about 95 and 40 μ. It is possible that these values should be increased to correct for shrinkage; it is also possible that 1 or 2 dendritic trunks are hidden by the soma. No correction has been made for these possibilities; consequently, the values given in the table are believed to be conservative (i.e., low rather than high).

f The "standard motoneurone" of Eccles (10) was based upon the illustrative example introduced by Cooms, Eccles, and Fatt (8). This consisted of a spherical soma, 70 μ in diameter, and six dendrites of 5 μ diameter and infinite length. A

TABLE 2 (*Continued*)

later version (7) added one more 5-μ diameter cylinder to take the axon into account. Both versions of this "standard motoneurone" are included for comparison with the measurements.

[g] Two sets of values are given for Chu's Fig. 20. The first set of values corresponds to the magnification (340) given in his figure legend. Because comparison of Fig. 20 with Figs. 5 and 21 suggests that this magnification might be incorrect, a second set of values (enclosed by parentheses) was calculated for magnification (240), which is the same as that for the adjacent Fig. 21.

[h] The dendritic to soma conductance ratio, ρ, is defined by Eq. [31], and the whole neuron resistance, R_N was calculated from Eq. [34]. It was assumed that the combined dendritic tree parameter, Eq. [26], could be approximated by the combined dendritic trunk parameter, expression [27]. This assumption is subject to modification as more complete information becomes available; it is based upon the theoretical considerations discussed in connection with Fig. 5 and Table 1, and upon a few branching measurements cited in this paper, below. It was also assumed that $C = 0.2 \ (\Omega cm)^{-1/2}$, which corresponds to R_i between 50 and 75 Ωcm; this provides no significant source of uncertainty. The 600 Ωcm^2 value for R_m corresponds to the latest estimate of Eccles and his collaborators (7), while the 4000 Ωcm^2 value was chosen to bring the calculated adult mean of Table 2 into approximate agreement with the mean R_N value obtained experimentally.

sive than that usually seen in histological preparations.[5] The difficulties include incompleteness of staining, loss into neighboring histological sections, and (in the case of Chu's preparations) loss by fragmentation.

It would be very unrealistic to assume that Table 2 is free of systematic errors. These values simply represent an attempt at a current best estimate, based on recent published evidence.

Comparison of Geometric Quantities

Several significant differences and similarities between the various neurons are suggested by inspection of Table 2. These have been tested for statistical significance by means of the "t" test (13), which is appropriate for such small samples on the usual assumption of unbiased sampling from an underlying normal distribution.

The two adult cat neurons are in good agreement with the sample of six adult human neurons. With respect to the values listed in Table 2, they may be treated as a combined sample from a single population. The t statistic, with 5 degrees of freedom, gives probabilities in the range 0.3 to 0.7 for such deviations.

Comparison of the six adult human cells with the five infant human cells reveals that the infant cells are significantly smaller. The average infant values for both $\Sigma d^{3/2}$ and S are about one half the average adult values. Values of the t statistic obtained for the difference between infant and adult means give a probability less than 0.001 for the $\Sigma d^{3/2}$ values, and a probability less than 0.01 for the S values, that these two samples would be obtained by chance from a single population. The good agreement between infant and adult mean values of the ratio, $\Sigma d^{3/2}/S$, indicates that $\Sigma d^{3/2}$ and S are comparable indices of neuron size. It also indicates a tendency to preserve this ratio and the related ratio, ρ, during growth.

Comparison of the two human chromatolytic cells with the six human adult cells reveals, contrary to the usual statements about degenerative swelling, that the abnormal dendrites are significantly smaller, and that the abnormal soma is also smaller, but not significantly so. In the case of the dendrites, the t statistic gives a probability less than 0.01 that such a deviation could have occurred by chance. This was an unexpected result in view of the usual references to degenerative swelling; Chu's

---

[5] It is a pleasure to acknowledge helpful discussions of this and related questions with Dr. Grant L. Rasmussen.

figure legends refer to a "swollen cell-body." In these two cases, at least, the swelling is an optical illusion due to dendritic shrinkage. These two cells may not correspond to the more acutely degenerate cells that have been studied electrophysiologically.

The "standard motoneurone" of Eccles (7, 10) is significantly different from both the adult and infant neurons in Table 2. It does not satisfy the usual statistical criteria for being a probable mean from these cell populations. Comparison of the $\Sigma d^{3/2}$ value (for either "standard motoneurone") with the group of eight adult neurons gives a value of the t statistic, which implies a probability less than 0.001 for chance occurrence of such a deviation. The "standard motoneurone" value for the ratio, $\Sigma d^{3/2}/S$, is about one-fourth the mean value found for both adult and infant neurons; the t statistic gives a probability of less than 0.01 for chance occurrence of such a deviation. The "standard motoneurone" may not be significantly different from the two chromatolytic cells.

DENDRITIC DIAMETER CHANGE WITH BRANCHING

It is important to know how the value of $\Sigma d^{3/2}$ changes as one considers successive branchings in a dendritic tree. The value of B_0 for any given dendritic tree depends most strongly upon the first few branchings (i.e., of the trunk and major branches); this can be seen by considering the branching calculations summarized in Table 1, accompanying Fig. 5.

Obviously, careful measurements ought to be made with the most suitable obtainable histological preparations. A few tentative results are given here based upon some of the published histological illustrations already referred to. The examples shown here include only the first one or two branchings. They indicate that the value of $\Sigma d^{3/2}$ increases somewhat with branching. When measurements are extended to more peripheral branching, it is important to guard against spuriously low values; these could result from loss of branches due to thin sections, incomplete staining, or fragmentation.

Haggar and Barr's photograph (18) provides a little information about branching. The 16-μ trunk gives off two branches, 4.5 and 5 μ, while becoming itself reduced to 13 μ in diameter; thus the trunk $d^{3/2}$ value of 64 $\mu^{3/2}$ is exceeded by a larger $\Sigma d^{3/2}$ value of 67.7 $\mu^{3/2}$. There is also a 6.5-μ trunk which bifurcates into a 5- and a 4-μ branch; here the trunk $d^{3/2}$ value of 16.6 $\mu^{3/2}$ is exceeded by a larger $\Sigma d^{3/2}$ value of 19.2 $\mu^{3/2}$.

Chu's Fig. 3 (4) has a trunk at 6 o'clock which is about 10 μ in diameter and gives rise to two branches about 7.5 and 6 μ; farther out, these have become three branches about 6, 5, and 4.5 μ. The $\Sigma d^{3/2}$ value goes from about 31.5 $\mu^{3/2}$ for the trunk, to about 35 $\mu^{3/2}$ for the two and also the three branches. This cell also has a 9-μ trunk at 10 o'clock which gives rise to two branches about 7.5 to 5 μ, and then three branches about 5, 5, and 3.5 μ. The $\Sigma d^{3/2}$ values go from about 27 $\mu^{3/2}$ to about 32 $\mu^{3/2}$, and then to about 29 $\mu^{3/2}$.

Clearly, better and more extensive measurements are desirable. These measurements do suggest, when considered together with Fig. 5 and Table 1, that motoneuron dendritic branching may exceed the amount necessary to make $B_0 = 1$ and may thus make the combined denditric tree parameter greater than the combined dendritic trunk parameter. If this should prove to be the rule, then R_N values calculated for any given R_m (Table 2) will become smaller; conversely, larger R_m values will be implied by any given experimental R_N value.

HISTOLOGICAL QUESTIONS

These preliminary results raise a number of questions requiring further study. Among these are the following: How extensive is the peripheral branching of mammalian motoneuron dendrites? Will further study confirm that the value of $\Sigma d^{3/2}$ increases when calculated for successive branchings of a dendritic tree? For how many branchings can this be reliably tested? Can the shrinkage and/or swelling of dendrites resulting from death and fixation be reliably estimated? Can satisfactory methods be devised for histological measurement of the same cell upon which physiological measurements have been made? Will further study confirm that acute chromatolytic somas only appear to be swollen because of shrunken dendrites? Are there important geometric differences between acute and chronic chromatolytic cells? Will further study confirm the proportionality found (on the average) between soma surface area and the combined dendritic trunk parameter, during growth from infant to adult? Do similar relations hold for other types of neurons?

Results with Comments

The purpose here is to compare the anatomical information of Table 2 with electrophysiological measurements of whole neuron resistance, R_N, obtained with cat motoneurons. This leads to an estimated range of R_m values within which the unknown R_m value of mammalian motoneuron membrane is most likely to lie.

PHYSIOLOGICAL-ANATOMICAL MATCHING

Electrophysiological R_N *Values.* Frank and Fuortes (14) reported a mean value of 1.65 megohms for fifty-two cat motoneurons; the eleven values listed in column 8 of their Table I have a mean of 1.5 megohms, and a statistical variance whose best estimate is 0.32 (megohms)^2, implying a standard deviation of 0.57 megohm. More recent results,[6] obtained with larger tipped micropipettes, give a lower mean value of about 1.2 megohms.

The earlier measurements of Coombs, Eccles, and Fatt (8) have been extended by the results recently reported for twenty-five cat motoneurons by Coombs, Curtis, and Eccles (7). These twenty-five values have a mean of 1.14 megohms, and a statistical variance whose best estimate is 0.22 (megohms)^2, implying a standard deviation of 0.47 megohm.

Both sets of measurements lie in the range from 0.5 to 2.5 megohms. The ratio between the two variances is not statistically significant (13). When the eleven tabulated values of Frank and Fuortes (14) are compared with the twenty-five values of Coombs, Curtis, and Eccles (7), the *t* test gives a probability slightly greater than 0.05 that this much difference between means would occur by chance (13), if sampling were from a single normal population; i.e., the difference is probably not significant. The combined sample of thirty-six motoneurons has a mean of 1.25 megohms, and a variance whose best estimate is 0.27 (megohms)^2, implying a standard deviation of 0.52 megohm.

Comparison with Table 2. For $R_m = 4000$ Ωcm^2, the mean of the calculated R_N values for adult motoneurons in Table 2 agrees quite well with the above-mentioned physiological measurements. However, the variance of the calculated R_N values has a best estimate of 0.019 (megohms)^2, for the six adult human cells. This is smaller than the physiological variance by a factor of about 14. This variance ratio has a probability less than 0.01 of occurring by chance (13), if sampling were from a single normal population; i.e., this ratio is probably significant.

Variance Discrepancy. The problem is to find a satisfactory explanation for the fact that the spread of physiological values corresponds to nearly four times the spread in anatomical size. The most important variability in anatomical size is that of the combined dendritic parameter,

[6] Personal communication from Drs. Frank and Fuortes.

as may be seen from the large values found for the dendritic to soma conductance ratio, ρ, in Table 2. It is therefore relevant to note the possible importance of variability between motoneurons with respect to the extensiveness of their branching. This could produce a variability in the combined dendritic tree parameter that would be greater than that of the combined dendritic trunk parameter. This possibility, as well as the possibility of unknown selection in this small anatomical sample, can be checked by further histological study.

Another possibility is that there could be variability in R_m superimposed upon size variability. Unless direct evidence is obtained for this, I prefer the hypothesis that these cat motoneurons are closely similar in their passive membrane resistivity.

It is possible that the larger physiological variance is partly due to variability in experimental recording conditions and in physiological trauma. Such variability is difficult to assess. For example, it is known that small neurons are more liable to serious injury upon penetration by a micropipette than are the larger neurons. This would be expected to bias the physiological sample toward the larger cells in a given population; the largest R_N values would tend to be lost and low R_N values would predominate. Evidence in support of this is provided by the observation[7] that average R_N values fell when the tip size of the micropipette was increased. This effect would lower both the mean and the variance of R_N. The effect of injury upon cells included in the physiological sample would also be in the direction of low R_N values; this would also tend to lower the mean value obtained for R_N, but it would probably increase the variance. Occasionally, clogging of a micropipette tip can produce a high resistance value, but this effect is probably secondary to those already mentioned.[7] The net result of all these factors upon the variance of R_N is not clear. It may be expected that the mean value obtained for R_N will be lower than the "correct" value, but the magnitude of this discrepancy is not known.

MEMBRANE RESISTIVITY

Because of the uncertainties considered above, the membrane resistivity of cat motoneurons is probably best estimated in terms of a range of

[7] Personal communication from Drs. Frank and Fuortes. It is a pleasure to acknowledge helpful discussions of this and related questions with Drs. Frank and Fuortes.

values. On the basis of the evidence considered here, this range extends approximately from 1000 to 8000 Ωcm^2.

The low end of this range corresponds to the possibility that the lowest R_N values, around 0.5 megohm, actually represent the true resistance values of large cells with $D^{3/2}$ values around 300 $\mu^{3/2}$. The high end of this range corresponds to the possibility that the largest R_N values, around 2.5 megohms, actually represent the true resistance values of small cells with $D^{3/2}$ values around 180 $\mu^{3/2}$; see Fig. 6.

However, if the mid-range of the physiological samples corresponds with the mid-range of the anatomical sample, a value around 4000 to 5000 Ωcm^2 would be indicated for R_m. Then the R_N value of 1.2 megohms (7) would correspond to a $D^{3/2}$ value of about 250 $\mu^{3/2}$. The 1.65-megohm value of Frank and Fuortes (14) was obtained with finer microelectrodes and may have been less weighted for the largest motoneurons; thus, while a 250-$\mu^{3/2}$ value for $D^{3/2}$ would imply $R_m = 7000$ Ωcm^2 for this R_N value, a reduction of $D^{3/2}$ to 200 $\mu^{3/2}$ would imply $R_m = 4700$ Ωcm^2.

Such values for R_m are larger than the values of 500 (8), 400 (10), and 600 (7) Ωcm^2 proposed by Eccles and his collaborators. Most of this difference can be attributed to a difference in estimation of dendritic dimensions; see "standard motoneurone" in Table 2. This difference is surprising because essentially the same anatomical sources (2, 4, 18) were cited by Eccles (10, pp. 2–6) as the basis for his "standard motoneurone." The statistical improbability of this "standard motoneurone" is assessed on page 515 of this paper. All of these estimates share whatever systematic error may be present.

Dendritic to Soma Conductance Ratio

A range of probable values for this conductance ratio can be obtained by combining the R_m values, considered above, with the values found for the purely geometric ratio in Table 2. The geometric size ratio, Eq. [32], has a mean value of about 2.1 cm$^{-1/2}$, with a standard deviation of about 0.4, for the combined population of eight adult plus 5 infant mammalian neurons in Table 2. There seems to be no significant correlation between neuron size and the value of this ratio. Therefore, the most probable values of the conductance ratio, ρ, can be expected to lie in a range, plus or minus one standard deviation, for any particular value of R_m. Using Eq. [31], with $C = 0.2$ $(\Omega$cm$)^{-1/2}$, the following ranges of probable ρ values are obtained: at one extreme, with $R_m = 1000$ Ωcm^2, this range extends approximately from 10 to 16; at the other extreme, with $R_m =$ 8000 Ωcm^2, this range extends approximately from 31 to 47; for the mid-range of 4000 to 5000 Ωcm^2, this probable range of ρ values extends approximately from 21 to 35.

All of these values are significantly larger than the value of 2.3 used by Eccles and his collaborators (7, 8, 10); see especially (7, p. 518). This discrepancy merits explicit mention, because of the interpretations which have been based upon the 2.3 value; it may be attributed to the difference between the "standard motoneurone" and the measurements summarized in Table 2; these differences have already been commented upon above. The factor of about 10 between this 2.3 value and the mid-range, 21 to 35, cited above, can be seen (in Table 2) to be composed of two factors: a factor of about 4 in the geometric ratio, $\Sigma d^{3/2}/S$, and a factor of about 2.5 in the value of $\sqrt{R_m}$.

Large values of ρ provide a measure of the dominance of dendritic properties over somatic properties in determining various whole neuron properties of motoneurons. Clearly, the conductance is predominantly dendritic. The above values further strengthen the case (24, 26) for dendritic dominance in the passive transient response of the motoneuron membrane to a current step applied at the soma. The case for dendritic dominance in the modulation of a facilitatory synaptic potential also depends upon large ρ values; this leads naturally to a possible functional distinction between dendritic and somatic synaptic excitation: the larger and slower dendritic contribution would be well suited for fine adjustment of central excitatory states, while the relatively small number of somatic synaptic knobs would be well suited for rapid triggering of reflex discharge. Such implications will be developed further in a subsequent paper.

Discussion
GENERALITY OF THE THEORY

The theory and the resulting method of analysis are clearly more general than the particular applications presented as Results. The applicability of the theory to motoneurons is not contingent upon the correctness of the particular anatomical and physiological estimates presented here; the possibility of systematic error has been pointed out; as better data become available, these can be fed into the general theoretical results. The same method of analysis is also applicable to other types of neurons. Of particular interest are the dendritic trees of Purkinje cells and of pyramidal cells, both of which have been subjected to recent quantitative study.

Diffusion Analogy. All of the theoretical results obtained in this paper are also applicable to the diffusion of material (without convection) from a steady source within the soma to a constant low extracellular concentration, or to diffusion from a constant high extracellular concentration to a steady sink within the soma. In this context, the intracellular source could represent either metabolic production of a substance within the soma, or active inward transport across the soma membrane; similarly, the intracellular sink could represent either metabolic consumption of a substance within the soma, or active outward transport across the soma membrane. Free diffusion along the dendritic core and across the soma and dendritic membrane would be assumed.

. For example, Eq. [31] could be used to calculate the dendritic to soma ratio for steady diffusional flux under the above-mentioned conditions; it is necessary only to replace the ratio, R_m/R_i, by the ratio, D/P, where D is the intracellular diffusion coefficient (cm^2/sec), and P is the membrane permeability (cm/sec). Thus, for $D = 10^{-5}$ cm^2/sec and $P = 10^{-7}$ cm/sec (34) the average neuron of Table 2 would give a value of about 31 for this diffusional flux ratio. Such diffusional considerations may be relevant to an understanding of factors governing neuronal development and metabolism.

Assessment of Simplifying Assumptions

Isopotentiality of the External Medium. The mathematical theory makes use of the assumption of extracellular isopotentiality. It is obvious that this assumption does not correspond strictly to the situation in nature, and it is desirable to assess the magnitude of discrepancies that might result from this. The gray matter does not provide an infinite conductivity; it is not even a homogeneous conducting medium. The heterogeneity of the interneuronal space is currently under active study (33). This heterogeneity may not produce very much distortion of the extracellular potential field, because the connectivity of the interstitial space must be much more extensive and of finer grain in three dimensions than it appears in a single plane. Thus, it may be hoped that little error results from considering the medium to be homogeneous with an apparent extracellular specific resistance, R_e, that is subject to physical measurement. The gray matter of cat cortex has been found to have an apparent R_e of about

222 Ωcm (16), or approximately four to five times the value of mammalian Ringer (28, p. 470).

For steady radial current flow from inside a spherical soma to a distant external electrode, the potential, V_e, just outside the membrane equals

$$V_e = i \int_b^\infty \frac{R_e}{4\pi r^2} dr = \frac{iR_e}{4\pi b}$$

where i is the total radial current and b represents the radius of the sphere. The potential drop, V, across the membrane resistance is simply

$$V = iR_m/(4\pi b^2).$$

Therefore, the ratio of V_e to V is equal to

$$V_e/V = bR_e/R_m.$$

For $b = 30 \times 10^{-4}$ cm, $R_e = 222$ Ωcm and $R_m = 4000$ Ωcm², it follows that $V_e/V = 1.5 \times 10^{-4}$; thus V_e differs negligibly from zero, for present purposes.

A similar calculation for a cylindrical membrane, with integration from $r = a$ to $a \times 10^{-3}$, gives the result

$$V_e/V = 6.9aR_e/R_m.$$

For $a = 5 \times 10^{-4}$ cm, $R_e = 222$ Ωcm and $R_m = 4000$ Ωcm², it follows that $V_e/V = 1.9 \times 10^{-4}$; here V_e also differs negligibly from zero.[8]

In the early theory of axonal electrotonus, the difficulty of treating the external potential field was recognized by Hermann (19), and was solved for certain boundary conditions, by Weber (30). This mathematical problem has also been studied by Weinberg (31); it involves infinite series of Bessel functions. These complications are usually avoided by limiting consideration either to the case of an axon placed in air or in oil, or to an external volume conductor whose conductivity may be regarded as effectively infinite.

---

[8] These quantitative considerations were also verified by means of a resistance-capacitance network analog constructed and tested by A. J. McAlister (21). The first analog assumed zero external resistance. Extension to the case of an external medium with finite resistance was accomplished by adding an external resistance network in which the radial increments in resistance were calculated to correspond to cylindrical symmetry in a volume; this type of external resistance network was suggested by K. S. Cole during discussions participated in by W. H. Freygang, Jr., K. Frank, A. J. McAlister, and W. Rall. The experimental tests also revealed a negligible longitudinal gradient of external potential.

Formal solutions of the external field surrounding a spherical neuron with or without cylindrical dendrites have recently been obtained, and will be presented separately.

Isopotentiality of Soma Membrane. Virtual isopotentiality of the soma interior, under resting conditions, has been assumed since the earliest intracellular electrode studies (3). However, the assumption of approximate isopotentiality during the flow of applied or active membrane current is more recent. A theoretical basis for it was provided first for a hypothetical spherical soma;[9] when the electrotonic potential distribution is expanded in terms of Legendre polynomials, it turns out that the higher order terms, which represent the nonuniformity of the electrotonic potential, are smaller than the uniform (zero order) component by a factor whose order of magnitude is $b(R_e + 2R_i)/R_m$, where b is the radius of the sphere. This factor is less than 10^{-3} for mammalian motoneurons. Intuitively, this means simply that the resistance to current flow across the soma membrane is much greater than the resistance to current flow between different points interior (or different points exterior) to the soma membrane. This assumption of soma membrane isopotentiality during current flow was implicit in the calculations of (8), and it has recently become explicit in the discussion of mammalian motoneurons (7, 10, 12, 15, 17, 21, 23–26).

When dendritic current is taken into account, soma isopotentiality does not hold as precisely as for the spherical nerve model. Consider, for example, the unfavorable case of an asymmetric neuron with an intracellular electrode at one end of an elongated soma (or even in a proximal dendrite) and with most of the major dendrites arising at the other end of the soma. If, for example, the soma has major and minor diameters of 90 and 40 μ, and if twenty times more steady current flows across the soma to the dendrites than flows across the soma membrane, then using $R_i = 50$ Ωcm and $R_m = 4000$ Ωcm², it can be calculated that the steady potential drop between the two ends of this soma would be about 2 per cent of the steady electrotonic potential of the soma membrane.

Uniform Membrane Resistivity. The value of R_m has been assumed to be the same for the entire soma-dendritic membrane. This is not necessary; the theoretical solutions could be carried out with a different R_m value for the soma and for each cylindrical branch component. In

---

[9] Preliminary results were presented in 1953 (22), 1955 (23), and 1957 (*Abstracts of National Biophysics Conference,* p. 58); full details have not been published.

particular, since G_N is dominated by the combined dendritic input conductance, the whole neuron value is not very sensitive to postulated changes in the R_m value of just the soma. For example, if we begin with $\rho = 25$, halving the somatic R_m value (12) would reduce R_N by only 4 per cent; reduction of the somatic R_m value by a factor of 10 would reduce R_N by 26 per cent.

The fact that synaptic knobs are distributed in high density over both soma and dendritic membrane surfaces,[10] and the fact that these knobs are packed very close to the membrane surface,[11] suggests that the soma dendritic membrane might have a true resistivity, for unit area, that is lower than the effective value which includes the heterogeneity of the external surface and external volume. Therefore, it should be emphasized that all of the theory and numerical estimates of the present paper are concerned with the effective value of R_m.

APPENDIX 1. DEFINITION OF SYMBOLS

V_e	= extracellular electric potential	G_∞	= input conductance of infinitely extended cylindrical trunk (Eq. [10])
V_i	= intracellular electric potential	R_i	= specific resistance of the internal medium (Ω cm)
V_m	= $V_i - V_e$ = membrane potential	R_m	= resistance across a unit area of membrane (Ω cm^2)
E	= resting membrane potential, and EMF	d	= diameter of cylinder (cm)
V	= $V_m - E$ = electrotonic potential	r_m	= $R_m/\pi d$ = membrane resistance for a unit length of cylinder (Ω cm)
x	= distance along a dendrite, measured from soma		
V_0	= electrotonic potential at $x = 0$	r_i	= $4R_i = \pi d^2$ = internal resistance per unit length of cylinder (Ω cm^{-1})
i_m	= membrane current density, expressed per unit length of cylinder		
I	= internal (axial) current	λ	= $[r_m/r_i]^{1/2}$ = characteristic length of cylinder (cm)
I_0	= internal current at $x = 0$; dendritic input current		
R_D	= V_0/I_0 = dendritic input resistance		= $[(R_m/R_i)(d/4)]^{1/2}$
		d_0	= diameter of trunk
G_D	= I_0/V_0 = dendritic input conductance	λ_0	= characteristic length of trunk

[10] See Rasmussen in Ref. (32).
[11] See, for example, Palay in Ref. (32).

APPENDIX 1 (*Continued*)

L_0	= length of trunk
B_0	= branching factor (see Eq. [12])
x_1	= value of x at which trunk gives rise to k branches
d_{1k}	= diameter of kth branch arising at $x = x_1$
λ_{1k}	= characteristic length of this kth branch
L_{1k}	= length of this kth branch
B_1	= branching constant at $x = x_1$ (see Eqs. [2] and [16] to [18])
I_1	= internal current at $x = x_1$
V_1	= electrotonic potential at $x = x_1$
x_{2k}	= value of x at end of kth branch arising at $x = x_1$

V_{2k}	= electrotonic potential at $x = x_{2k}$
x_j	= value of x at a general branch point
d_{jk}	= diameter of kth branch arising at $x = x_j$
λ_{jk}	= characteristic length of this kth branch (Eq. [21])
L_{jk}	= length of this kth branch
B_j	= branching constant at $x = x_j$ (see Eq. [19])
$B_{(j+1)k}$	= branching constant at end of kth branch arising at $x = x_j$
d_{j-1}	= diameter of cylinder from which branches arise at $x = x_j$

The following apply to whole neurons:

I_A	= total steady current applied from interior to exterior of neuron
R_N	= V_0/I_A = whole neuron resistance
G_N	= I_A/V_0 = whole neuron conductance
S	= soma surface area
G_S	= S/R_m = some membrane conductance
G_{Dj}	= dendritic input conductance of jth trunk
B_{0j}	= weighting factor of jth trunk at $x = 0$
d_{0j}	= diameter of trunk
$D^{3/2}$	= $\sum_j B_{0j}(d_{0j})^{3/2}$ = combined dendritic tree parameter; compare with combined dendritic trunk parameter, expression [27], and combined dendritic input conductance (Eq. [24])
C	= $(\pi/2)(R_i)^{-1/2}$ (see Eqs. [10] and [24] to [26])
ρ	= ratio of combined dendritic input conductance to soma membrane conductance (Eq. [31]).

References

1. ARAKI, T., and T. OTANI, Response of single motoneurons to direct stimulation in toad's spinal cord. *J. Neurophysiol.* **18**: 472-485, 1955.

2. BALTHASER, K., Morphologie der spinalen Tibialis- und Peronaeus-Kerne bei der Katze. *Arch. Psychiatr., Berl.* **188**: 345-378, 1952.

3. BROCK, L. G., J. S. COOMBS, and J. C. ECCLES, The recording of potentials from motoneurones with an intracellular electrode. *J. Physiol., Lond.* **117**: 431-460, 1952.

4. CHU, L. W., A cytological study of anterior horn cells isolated from human spinal cord. *J. Comp. Neur.* **100**: 381-414, 1954.

5. COLE, K. S., and A. L. HODGKIN, Membrane and protoplasm resistance in the squid giant axon. *J. Gen. Physiol.* **22**: 671-687, 1939.

6. COOMBS, J. S., D. R. CURTIS, and J. C. ECCLES, Time courses of motoneuronal responses. *Nature, Lond.* **178**: 1049-1050, 1956.

7. COOMBS, J. S., D. R. CURTIS, and J. C. ECCLES, The electrical constants of the motoneurone membrane. *J. Physiol., Lond.* **145**: 505-528, 1959.

8. COOMBS, J. S., J. C. ECCLES, and P. FATT, The electrical properties of the motoneurone membrane. *J. Physiol., Lond.* **130**: 291-325, 1955.

9. DAVIS, L., JR., and R. LORENTE DE NÓ, Contribution to the mathematical theory of the electrotonus. *Stud. Rockefeller Inst. M. Res.*, **131**: 442-496, 1947.

10. ECCLES, J. C., "The physiology of nerve cells," Baltimore, Johns Hopkins, 1957.

11. FATT, P., Electrical potentials occurring around a neurone during its antidromic activation. *J. Neurophysiol.* **20**: 27-60, 1957.

12. FATT, P., Sequence of events in synaptic activation of a motoneurone. *J. Neurophysiol.* **20**: 61-80, 1957.

13. FISHER, R. A., and F. YATES, "Statistical table for biological, agricultural and medical research," New York, Hafner, 1949.

14. FRANK, K., and M. G. F. FUORTES, Stimulation of spinal motoneurones with intracellular electrodes. *J. Physiol., Lond.* **134**: 451-470, 1956.

15. FREYGANG, W. H., JR., and K. FRANK, Extracellular potentials from single spinal motoneurons. *J. Gen. Physiol.* **42**: 749-760, 1959.

16. FREYGANG, W. H., JR., and W. M. LANDAU, Some relations between resistivity and electrical activity in the cerebral cortex of the cat. *J. Cellul. Physiol.* **45**: 377-392, 1955.

17. FUORTES, M. G. F., K. FRANK, and M. C. BECKER, Steps in the production of motoneuron spikes. *J. Gen. Physiol.* **40**: 735-752, 1957.

18. HAGGAR, R. A., and M. L. BARR, Quantitative data on the size of synaptic end-bulbs in the cat's spinal cord. *J. Comp. Neur.* **93**: 17-35, 1950.

19. HERMANN, L., Ueber eine Wirkung galvanischer Ströme auf Muskeln und Nerven. *Pflügers Arch.* **6**: 312-360, 1872 (ref. pp. 336-343).

20. HODGKIN, A. L., and W. A. H. RUSHTON, The electrical constants of a crustacean nerve fibre. *Proc. R. Soc., Ser. B., Biol. Sc., Lond.* **133**: 444-479, 1946.

21. MCALISTER, A. J., Analog study of a single neuron in a volume conductor. *Naval M. Res. Inst., Research Reports* **16**: 1011-1022, 1958.

22. RALL, W., Electrotonic theory for a spherical neurone. *Proc. Univ. Otago M. School* **31**: 14-15, 1953.

23. RALL, W., A statistical theory of monosynaptic input-output relations. *J. Cellul. Physiol.* **46**: 373-411, 1955 (ref. p. 403).

24. RALL, W., Membrane time constant of motoneurons. *Science* **126**: 454, 1957.

25. RALL, W., Mathematical solutions for passive electrotonic spread between a neuron soma and its dendrites. *Fed. Proc., Balt.* **17**: 127, 1958.

26. RALL, W., Membrane potential transients and membrane time constant of motoneurons. *Exp. Neur.* **2**: 1960 (in press).

27. RAMÓN Y CAJAL, S., "Histologie du système nerveux de l'homme et des vertébrés," vol. 1, Paris, Maloine, 1909.

28. TASAKI, I., E. H. POLLEY, and F. ORREGO, Action potentials from individual elements in cat geniculate and striate cortex. *J. Neurophysiol.* **17**: 454-474, 1954.
29. VAN HARREVELD, A., Changes in volume of cortical neuronal elements during asphyxiation. *Am. J. Physiol.* **191**: 233-242, 1957.
30. WEBER, H., Ueber die stätionaren Strömungen der Elektricität in Cylindern. *Borchardt's J. Math.* **76**: 1-20, 1873.
31. WEINBERG, A. M., Weber's theory of the kernleiter. *Bull. Math. Biophysics* **3**: 39-55, 1941.
32. WINDLE, W. F. (ed.), "New research techniques of neuroanatomy," Springfield, Illinois, Thomas, 1957.
33. WINDLE, W. F. (ed.), "Biology of neuroglia," Springfield, Illinois, Thomas, 1958.
34. ZWOLINSKI, B. J., H. EYRING, and C. E. REESE, Diffusion and membrane permeability. *J. Phys. Colloid. Chem.* **53**: 1426-1453, 1949.

Membrane Potential Transients and Membrane Time Constant of Motoneurons (1960), *Exptl. Neurol.* 2:503–532

Wilfrid Rall

This paper is concerned with the interpretation of passive membrane potential transients produced in a neuron when intracellular microelectrodes are used to apply current across the soma membrane. It is also concerned with the specific problem of estimating the nerve membrane time constant from experimental transients in neurons having extensive dendritic trees. When this theory is applied to the most recent results published for cat motoneurons, the resulting membrane time constant estimates are significantly larger than the values estimated by Eccles and collaborators. The time course of soma membrane potential is solved for a variety of applied currents: current step, brief pulse of current, sinusoidal current, voltage clamping current, and a current of arbitrary time course. The sinusoidal case provides a theoretical basis for a purely electrophysiological method of estimating the fundamental ratio between combined dendritic input conductance and soma membrane conductance. Also included is the time course of passive decay to be expected to follow various soma-dendritic distributions of membrane depolarization or hyperpolarization. The discussion includes an assessment of the observations, hypotheses, and interpretations that have recently complicated our understanding of synaptic potentials in cat motoneurons. It appears that electrotonic spread between the dendrites and soma can account for the observations which led Eccles and collaborators to postulate a prolonged residual phase of synaptic current in cat motoneurons.

Introduction

The experimental recording of motoneuron membrane potential transients resulting from the application of an electric current step across the soma membrane is one of the remarkable recent achievements made possible by intracellular microelectrodes (1, 6, 7, 19). A correct inter-

It is a pleasure to acknowledge the stimulation provided by discussion with many colleagues. Suggestions made by Dr. J. Z. Hearon led to some of the more generalized mathematical results. Preliminary results (25) were obtained while the author was in the Biophysics Division, Naval Medical Research Institute, Bethesda, Maryland.

pretation of these experimental results is important because it provides an estimate of the membrane time constant; this, in turn, has implications for the interpretation of synaptic potentials and for theoretical concepts of synaptic excitation and inhibition.

The fact that a large portion of the applied electric current must spread (electrotonically) from the neuron soma into its several dendritic trees was neglected in the first interpretations of such experimental transients. It is now becoming clear that this dendritic current is of primary importance in the estimation of motoneuron membrane properties (25, 28).

Synaptic Potential Decay and Membrane Time Constant. During the 10 years from 1946 to 1956, a rather simple and useful concept of the "synaptic potential" was developed by Eccles and his collaborators (2, 9, 12, 13). It was held that synaptic activation causes the motoneuron membrane to undergo a brief "active" phase of depolarization; when below the threshold for reflex discharge, this depolarization was assumed to undergo a passive decay having an exponential time constant of about 4 msec. The brief "active" phase was found to persist for not more than 0.5 msec (2, 13), an interval later revised to 1.2 msec (9); it was believed to result from a large nonselective increase in the ionic permeability of the motoneuron membrane (9). Because the subsequent synaptic potential decay was assumed to be passive,[2] and because the depolarization was implicitly assumed to be effectively uniform over the neuron surface,[3] this decay was expected to have an exponential time constant equal to the membrane time constant, $\tau = R_m C_m$, of the resting membrane. The average value of this τ was thus found to be about 4 msec, with a range from about 3 to 5 msec for cat motoneurons (13, pp. 116 and 142).

Rapid Transients Misinterpreted. In 1956, unexpectedly rapid membrane potential transients were recorded by Frank and Fuortes (19), and confirmed by Eccles and collaborators (6, 14). These transients were produced experimentally by the application of a current step across the soma membrane; their rapid time course was misinterpreted as evidence

---

[2] The word "passive" is used to imply that the membrane resistance, capacity, and electromotive forces all remain constant at their physiological resting values.

[3] This assumption of uniform distribution deserves explicit mention. A simple exponential decay is not to be expected when the dendritic depolarization is significantly different from that of the soma. The effect of nonuniform depolarization is represented mathematically in Eq. [23] and is illustrated graphically in Fig. 4.

for a membrane time constant that was significantly smaller than the time constant of synaptic potential decay; the values reported for τ were 1 to 1.4 msec (19) and 2.5 msec (6, 14).

If these values had correctly represented the true membrane time constant, they would have made the earlier simple concept of the synaptic potential untenable. Thus, Frank and Fuortes concluded that the long duration of the synaptic potential "is not a consequence of the time constant of the membrane itself, but rather of a similarly long-lasting change occurring elsewhere" (19, p. 468). Coombs, Curtis, and Eccles (6) developed a more detailed explanation; they calculated a hypothetical time course of synaptic current that was assumed to be necessary to account for the synaptic potential. Using their 2.5-msec time constant, they obtained a hypothetical time course that was characterized by a prolonged residual phase of current following the brief early phase of current; this hypothetical time course has been widely illustrated (6; 14, Figs. 11 and 23; 15, Fig. 2; 16, Fig. 5). Fatt (17), on the other hand, preferred to preserve the hypothesis that the "active" phase of depolarization is brief; he assumed that synaptic potential decay would be dominated by the dendritic membrane time constant which he assumed to be longer than that of the soma. Assuming that a large amount of the synaptic potential is generated in the dendrites, he suggested that electrotonic spread from dendrites to soma would cause the dendritic membrane time constant to dominate the decaying phase observed at the soma.

Dendritic Electrotonus Accounts for Rapid Transient. The apparent need for these various hypotheses was then shown to have resulted from a misinterpretation of the experimental results. It was pointed out in a preliminary communication (25), that when the transient characteristics of the motoneuron dendrites are taken into account, the recently obtained experimental transients agree quite well with theoretical predictions based upon the older membrane time constant value of around 4 msec. Briefly, this follows from the fact that the electrodes do not apply the current directly across the extensive dendritic surfaces; the current is applied across the soma membrane and must spread electrotonically into the dendrites. When these dendrites are approximated as cylinders of infinite length, it follows that the dendritic contribution to the motoneuron potential transient should be expected to resemble the uppermost curve in Fig. 1; this transient is already well established in the theory of axonal electrotonus (11, 21); it can be expressed $erf \sqrt{t/\tau}$. This transient is significantly faster than the simple exponential transient, $1 - e^{-t/\tau}$ (see lowermost curve in Fig. 1), that would be expected in the case of uniformly applied current.

The resultant whole neuron transient recorded across the soma membrane can be expected to represent a combination of these dendritic and somatic components. This transient function depends upon the relative weights given to the dendritic and somatic contributions. These weights depend upon the steady state ratio between the current flowing into all

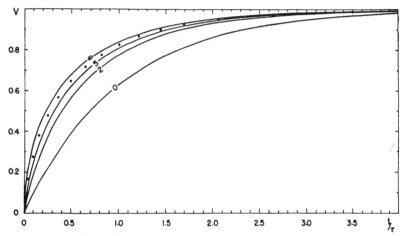

FIG. 1. Transients of passive soma membrane potential when a constant current step is applied across the soma membrane at zero time. The electrotonic potential, V, is expressed relative to its final steady value during constant applied current. Time is expressed relative to the membrane time constant. Curves are drawn for $\varrho = 0$, 2, 5, and ∞; the dots correspond to $\varrho = 10$. The uppermost curve, $\varrho = \infty$, represents the limiting case in which the dendrites are completely dominant. The lowermost curve, $\varrho = 0$, represents the limiting case of a soma without dendrites.

dendrites and the current flowing across the soma membrane (27, 28). The dependence of the resultant transient upon this ratio, ϱ, is illustrated in Fig. 1; it is expressed mathematically in Eq. [9] of the Appendix.

Although estimates of this dendritic-to-soma ratio vary (7, 25, 28), they all imply some degree of dendritic dominance, for motoneurons in cat and in man. The "standard motoneurone" of Eccles and his collaborators implies a ratio of 2.3 (7); however, the sample of motoneurons analyzed by Rall (28) suggests that values of this ratio are more likely to lie in the range from 21 to 35; known uncertainties permit an even wider range of values extending from about 10 to 47 (28, pp. 519-520).

The method of membrane time constant estimation used below has the advantage of being applicable over this entire range of dendritic dominance (i.e., for ratios from 2 to 50). Results obtained by this method support the conclusions of the preliminary note (25): the rapid experimental transients (6, 14, 19) do not conflict significantly with the old estimate of about 4 msec for the cat motoneuron membrane time constant; these transients do not force abandonment of the concept of passive synaptic potential decay.

Reinterpretations. The need to take the dendritic contribution into account has recently been accepted by Coombs, Curtis, and Eccles (7). Consequently, their membrane time constant estimate has been revised upwards (7), and the magnitude of their hypothetical residual synaptic current has been revised downwards (10). Nevertheless, these authors still find their membrane time constant estimates too small to be consistent with a passive synaptic potential decay (7, 10); also, they appear to regard their interpretations of several related experiments as evidence in support of their hypothetical residual synaptic current (10). Alternative interpretations of their experiments are considered below in the Discussion.

Assumptions and Method

It is assumed that a majority of readers will be more interested in a descriptive presentation of the theoretical results than in the details of the mathematical derivations. Consequently, the mathematical treatment has been condensed and placed in an Appendix. It should be emphasized that the method of this research actually depends upon the following logical sequence: Select simplifying assumptions which facilitate mathematical treatment without losing too much that is physiologically essential. Deduce the theoretical properties of this model in general, and also for special cases of current physiological interest. Demonstrate the implications of these theoretical results for the interpretation of recent experimental data.

The theoretical analysis is applied to an idealized model of a neuron possessing several branching dendritic trees. It is assumed that the membrane potential is effectively uniform over the soma surface, and that the extracellular gradients of electric potential can be neglected in the treatment of dendritic membrane electrotonous. These two assumptions, together with other assumptions used to idealize the geometric and passive electric membrane properties of neurons, have been given detailed presentation and assessment elsewhere (27, 28); previous Figs. 1, 2 and 5 (28) can be used to help visualize the spread of electric current in terms of the formal model.

Results

MEMBRANE TIME CONSTANT ESTIMATION

Analysis of Transient Obtained with Current Step Applied to Soma. The estimation procedure presented here is a rather simple and practical procedure that has the following advantages: it utilizes a linear plot of the experimental results; it thus permits full use of all reliable portions of the experimentally recorded transient; however, any obviously unreliable portion of the experimental transient need not be used; also, this method does not depend upon the prior assumption of any particular ratio between the dendritic and somatic contributions to the transients.

This method does require that the experimental records exhibit a noise level sufficiently low to permit reasonably reliable measurements of the slope, dV/dt, at various times after the onset of the current step. Given these measurements, the procedure is the following:

$$\text{plot log } \{\sqrt{t} \ (dV/dt)\}, \text{ versus } t.$$

Subject to qualifications (expressed below), these points should fit a straight line; when calculated with natural logarithms, the negative slope of this line gives the reciprocal of the membrane time constant, τ.

The theoretical basis for this procedure (and its qualifications) is provided by Eqs. [12, 13, 15] of the Appendix. For the limiting case of complete dendritic dominance, Eq. [13] shows that the above procedure applies without any qualifications. For lesser dendritic dominance (i.e., values of ϱ greater than 2 but less than infinity) the error resulting from use of the same plotting procedure can be calculated from Eq. [15]; this error can be shown to be small at times for which the quantity, $\varrho \sqrt{t/\tau}$, is not too small. Graphical illustration of this is provided by the (dashed) curves in the lower left part of Fig. 2, for $\varrho = 5$ and 2; a value of 7 msec was used for τ to simplify comparison with the plotted data in Fig. 2. It can be seen that there is little error at times greater than $\tau/2$, when $\varrho = 5$; the error is less for larger values of ϱ. Even for the low value, $\varrho = 2$, the curve between $t = \tau$ and 2τ is almost straight and has a slope which is about 5 per cent less steep than that for $\varrho = \infty$. Consequently, the same simple plotting procedure is useful when the value of ϱ is unknown but can reasonably be assumed to be greater than 2;

whenever ϱ is known, the correction can be calculated. For the limiting case of a soma without dendrites ($\varrho = 0$), Eq. [12] reduces to Eq. [14], and a linear relation exists between $\log(dV/dt)$ and t.

Illustrative Application to Cat Motoneurons. This linear plotting procedure was applied to some of the experimental transients published recently by Coombs, Curtis, and Eccles (7). The left half of Fig. 2 summarizes the applied current step analysis of one of their motoneurons (7, Figs 3 and 5); the right half of Fig. 2 summarizes both a current step and a current pulse analysis of a different motoneuron (7, Fig. 6). Photographic enlargements of the published figures were used; the slope, dV/dt, was measured at intervals of 1 msec. In the case of applied current steps, the natural logarithm of $\sqrt{t}(dV/dt)$ was plotted as ordinate against time as abscissa; these points are shown as open circles in Fig. 2.

The three sets of open circles (in the left half of Fig. 2) correspond to three different amplitudes of current, 6, 8, and 10 x 10^{-9} amperes, applied as steps to a single motoneuron (7, Fig. 5). The three corresponding sets of crosses represent the same data after correction for an estimated 500-msec time constant in the experimental recording system; see figure legend for details. The straight lines drawn through the circles and crosses were fitted by the method of least squares.[4] The three sets of crosses fit slopes corresponding to τ values of 7.1, 8.1, and 7.3 msec, respectively; the weighted mean of these values yields a best estimate of 7.5 msec for the membrane time constant of this motoneuron.[5]

From their analysis of the same transients, Coombs *et al.* estimated a τ value of 5.1 msec for this motoneuron (7, Table 3 with Figs. 3 and 5); their estimate is about 30 per cent below that obtained here. Even if this motoneuron were to have the small dendritic-to-soma ratio, $\varrho = 2$,

[4] Equal weighting was assumed for the ordinates (expressed as logarithms). This is equivalent to the not unreasonable assumption that the errors in slope measurement tend to be proportional to the magnitude of the slope (i.e., a constant coefficient of variation).

[5] This weighted mean has a standard error of about 0.2 msec. Such a mean is justified because the differences between the three component τ values are not statistically significant; the three standard errors are 0.28, 0.33, and 0.22, respectively; the largest difference between the three τ estimates yields a t value of 2.3, which is less than that required for significance at the 2 per cent level. The corresponding difference for the uncorrected slopes (open circles) gives a t value of 3.6, which exceeds that required for significance at the 1 per cent level, and nearly reaches the 0.1 per cent level.

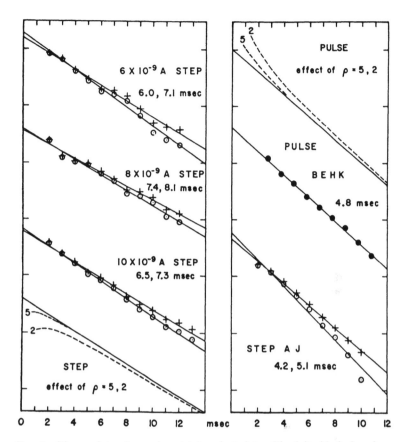

FIG. 2. Linear plots of experimental transient data. The left side is based upon transients obtained with applied current steps of three different amplitudes in a single neuron (7, Fig. 5); the right side is based upon experiments with a different motoneuron, that was subjected to both pulses and steps of applied current (7, Fig. 6). The open circles (both left and right) represent current step experiments; their ordinates represent the natural logarithm of the product $\sqrt{t}(dV/dt)$; their abscissae represent time from onset of the applied step. The crosses include a correction for the time constant of the recording system; see below in this figure legend. The straight lines represent least square fits;[4] the value of τ corresponding to each slope is stated in the figure. The filled circles represent current pulse experiments (7, Fig. 6, curves B, E, H, K); their ordinates represent the natural logarithm of the product, $\sqrt{t}(-dV/dt) / (1 + \tau/2t)$; correction for the recording system time constant is negligible in this case; the abscissae represent time from the mid-point of the pulse. The (dashed) curves at lower left illustrate the effect of $\varrho = 5$, and 2 to be expected with the step transient plotting procedure (see text); the (dashed) curves in the upper right illustrate the corresponding effect to be expected with the pulse

the corresponding 5 per cent slope correction (lower left of Fig. 2), would reduce the 7.5-msec estimate by less than 0.4 msec; however, the value of ϱ is likely to be greater than 10 (28), and the corresponding correction would be negligible.

In the right half of Fig. 2, the open circles and crosses summarize a similar analysis for a different motoneuron (7, Fig. 6, records A and J). Although the circles exhibit a systematic deviation from a straight line relation, this is not true of the crosses, which include a correction for an estimated 200-msec time constant in the experimental recording system; see figure legend for details. The least square fit through the crosses yields a membrane time constant estimate of 5.08 msec, with a standard error of about 0.13 msec.[6] This estimate is not significantly different from that obtained with a pulse analysis on the same motoneuron (filled circles of Fig. 2, explained below).

Transient Following Application of a Brief Current Pulse. When a brief pulse of current is applied across the soma membrane, the decay of the disturbance can be approximated quite well by that which would be theoretically expected to follow an instantaneous current pulse; the

---

[6] Combs, Curtis, and Eccles (7, Table 3) did not publish their estimate for this motoneuron. However, application of their estimation procedure to the step transients (7, Fig. 6, records A and J), seems to yield a value between 3.4 and 3.6 msec; this is about 30 per cent below the estimate obtained here.

---

transient plotting procedure (see text). The unit of the ordinate scale is one (i.e., the natural logarithm of e).

Correction for instrumental time constant: Coombs, Curtis, and Eccles state that a time constant of at least 200 msec was always present in their recording system (7, p. 507). The correction formula to use is $dV/dt = dU/dt + U/\tau_r$, where V represents the true transient voltage, U represents the distorted recording, and τ_r represents the time constant of the recording system. When U reaches its extremum, $dU/dt = 0$, and $\tau_r = U/(dV/dt)$. Neglecting other possible complications, such as electrode polarization and local response, it follows from this, and from Eq. [13], that τ_r can be estimated as $\sqrt{\pi \tau_m}\, t^* \, e^{t^*/\tau_m}$, where t^* represents the time at which $dU/dt = 0$, and τ_m is the membrane time constant. A 200-msec time constant was estimated for (7, Fig. 6), because records A to J appear to reach their extrema at times between 10 and 15 msec (corresponding to τ_r between 90 and 310 msec), and because the control records (C to L) exhibit a slope corresponding approximately to $\tau_r = 200$ msec. The value of τ_r appropriate to (7, Fig. 5) is considerably less certain because these are tracings that already include some correction; in view of this, and because the extrema of records J and K (7, Fig. 3) correspond to τ_r in the approximate range from 150 to 700 msec, it was decided that a correction for $\tau_r = 500$ msec would represent a reasonable compromise.

approximation is quite good except at very short times after the pulse. This is illustrated by the theoretical curves in Fig. 3, where the calculations were simplified by assuming complete dendritic dominance. The passive responses have been calculated for square current pulses of several durations (by means of Eq. [10]), and for an instantaneous pulse (by

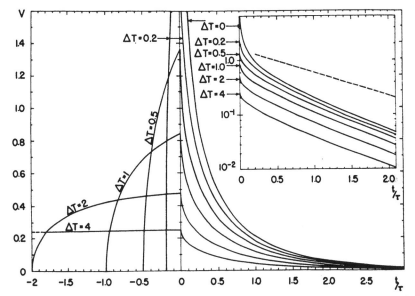

FIG. 3. Transients of passive soma membrane potential when a square pulse of current is applied across the soma membrane. Zero time corresponds to the instant when current is turned off. Pulse durations compared are $\Delta(t/\tau) = 4$, 2, 1, 0.5, 0.2, and instantaneous ($\Delta T = 0$). The amplitude of each current has been adjusted to make each pulse deliver the same amount of charge. The ordinate value, 1.0, represents the steady state value of V during a constant current having the same amplitude as that of the $\Delta T = 1.0$ pulse. Dendritic dominance has been assumed here. The inset presents the same curves with logarithmic scaling of the ordinates; the dashed line displays the corresponding slope for simple exponential decay, $e^{-t/\tau}$.

means of Eq. [17]). All amplitudes have been scaled to provide the same amount of charge displacement in every case. The logarithmically plotted inset (in Fig. 3) shows that the decay rates of neighboring curves differ rather little at times greater than $\tau/2$. Furthermore, the agreement between the instantaneous pulse curve and the shorter square pulse curves becomes excellent (for times greater than $\tau/2$) when the origin of the instantaneous pulse curve is shifted to the mid-point of each pulse duration; this is important for location of $t = 0$ when fitting experimental results.

Procedure for Brief Pulse Analysis. When a pulse is very brief and dendritic dominance can be assumed, a linear plotting procedure can be based upon Eq. [18] of the Appendix. The procedure is the following:

$$\text{plot log } [\sqrt{t}(-dV/dt)/(1 + \tau/2t)], \text{ versus } t.$$

When the correct value of τ is used in the factor, $(1 + \tau/2t)$, the plotted points can be expected to fit a straight line; the negative slope (calculated with natural logarithms) gives the reciprocal of τ. This procedure thus requires that a tentative value of τ be used in the factor, $(1 + \tau/2t)$, to obtain a preliminary plot of the data. With the resulting estimate for τ, the factor $(1 + \tau/2t)$ can be recalculated and the plotting procedure can be repeated. In practice, few repetitions of the procedure will be found sufficient.

Errors resulting from lesser dendritic dominance can be calculated from Eqs. [18] and [19]; graphical illustrations of such errors are provided by the (dashed) curves in the upper right part of Fig. 2, for $\varrho = 5$ and 2; a value of 5 msec was used for τ. There is little error at times greater than $\tau/2$, when $\varrho = 5$ or greater. For the low value, $\varrho = 2$, the curve between $t = \tau$ and $t = 2\tau$ is almost straight and has a slope which is about 5 per cent steeper than that for the $\varrho = \infty$. Errors associated with finite pulse duration were considered above, with Fig. 3.

Illustration of Brief Pulse Analysis. This procedure was applied to a set of experimental transients published by Coombs, Curtis, and Eccles (7, Fig. 6, records, B, E, H, K). At intervals of 1 msec, these slopes were measured in photographic enlargement, and averaged over the four curves. Then, using the procedure described above, the points shown as filled circles were plotted in Fig. 2; correction for the estimated 200-msec time constant in the experimental recording system is negligible in this case. The least square fit through these points yields a membrane time constant estimate of 4.84 msec, with a standard error of about 0.14 msec. This does not differ significantly from the estimate obtained with the step analysis on the same motoneuron (STEP AJ, crosses in Fig. 2). If these two estimates are given equal weight, a best estimate of about 5.0 msec is obtained for the membrane time constant of this motoneuron.[6]

Assessment of Motoneuron Membrane Time Constant Estimates. The experimental results of Coombs, Curtis, and Eccles (7) provide a valuable sample of eighteen carefully studied motoneurons. Although it would obviously be desirable to perform similar linear plots for all eighteen of their motoneurons, the two cases analysed here (Fig. 2) suggest that there is a significant difference between the method of membrane time constant estimation used by them, and the method presented here. In these two cases, their method yields estimates that are about 30 per cent below those obtained here. If these should prove to be representative of the entire sample, it would follow that the average membrane time constant estimate of this sample should be increased from 3.1 msec to about 4.4 msec. This would suggest that the present method of estimation yields membrane time constant values about 75 per cent greater than the earlier method of Coombs, Curtis, and Eccles (6, 14), which took no account of dendritic transient characteristics. This should not, however, be used as the basis for a computational short cut, such as, for example, an increase of the correction factor, 1.2, used by Coombs, Curtis, and Eccles (7, pp. 518-519) to a larger value of 1.75; some hazards of such short cuts are noted in the fine print below.

The apparent simplicity of the estimation procedure used by Coombs, Curtis, and Eccles (7) should be weighed against the following disadvantages. Their procedure depends upon their assumption of one particular degree of dendritic dominance, $\varrho = 2.3$, based upon their "standard motoneurone." The measurement of half decay times is complicated by uncertainties in the asymptotic baseline and by the fact that this transient does not possess a characteristic time for half decay. Because of the second difficulty, these authors (7, p. 519) recommend the measurement of two successive half decay times commencing at $t = 0.6\tau$; however, τ is not known in advance, and in their Fig. 5 their arrows reveal that their measurements commenced at about 2 msec, in spite of a τ value of 5.1 msec (their estimate) or 7.5 msec (estimate of this paper); such an error would be expected to result in a low estimate. Also, the device of averaging two successive "half times" is equivalent to halving a single "quarter time"; the accuracy of this "quarter time" depends upon the accuracy of two points together with the accuracy of the baseline used; all information contained in the experimental transient, but not fully contained in this "quarter time," is effectively disregarded by their procedure.

With regard to questions of statistical significance, the eighteen estimates of Coombs, Curtis, and Eccles (7, Table 3, column 5) have a mean of 3.14 msec, and a standard deviation of 1.01, implying a value of 0.24 for the standard error of the mean. Relative to these statistics, an application of the "t" test for the significance of a difference between this mean and a larger true mean gives the following result: if this mean is 25 per cent below the true mean, the difference corresponds to significance at the 0.001 level. Such significance levels are subject to the usual qualifications, and they should be considered together with the sources of error described above.

Application of Voltage Clamp. If it is assumed possible to apply a perfect voltage step across the entire soma membrane, then the time course of the current that must be supplied by the electronic clamping circuit would provide a valuable means of estimating the membrane time constant. Because the soma membrane capacity would have to be charged instantaneously, the transient time course of the applied current would be determined by the dendrites. Thus, the membrane time constant of the dendrites could be determined separately from the soma, and independently of ϱ.

The linear plotting procedure in this case would be the following:

$$\text{plot log } [t^{3/2}(-dI_A/dt)] \text{ versus } t,$$

where I_A represents the applied current. This procedure follows from Eq. [25] of the Appendix. It should be added that a mathematically more complicated result must be used if there is a significant amount of series resistance between the neuron membrane and the regions where the constant voltage difference is maintained.

PASSIVE DECAY OF SOMA-DENDRITIC POLARIZATION

The time course of passive decay from an initial soma-dendritic membrane depolarization (or hyperpolarization) depends upon the initial distribution of the disturbance over the soma-dendritic surface. Graphical illustration of this is provided by Fig. 4, which is based upon Eqs. [22] and [23]. The upper curve ($a = 0$) represents a simple exponential decay following a uniformly distributed initial depolarization. The two lower curves show the more rapid decay, to be expected at the soma, when the initial depolarization of the dendrites is reduced (as an exponential function of distance from the soma); see figure legend. The effect illustrated in Fig. 4 is relevant to synaptic potential decay if this is assumed to be a passive electrotonic process following a brief depolarization. For example, the relative rates of EPSP decay and IPSP decay reported by Curtis and Eccles (10), would fit the hypothesis that IPSP initiation is confined more closely to the soma than is EPSP initiation; see Discussion.

In contrast to these cases, a slower passive decay would be expected at the soma following an initial depolarization that is greater in the dendrites than in the soma.

SINUSOIDAL APPLIED CURRENT AND DENDRITIC DOMINANCE

Here is described the manner in which the application of sinusoidal current[7] across the soma membrane may provide a means of estimating

[7] It was suggested to me by Dr. L. Stark, that the soma-dendritic analysis be extended to include the sinusoidal case.

dendritic dominance quite independently of anatomical information. The fundamental parameter of dendritic dominance is the ratio, ϱ, of combined dendritic input conductance to soma membrane conductance (28); see also (7, 8, 25, 26). Previous estimates of this ratio have had to depend upon calculations which combine anatomical information obtained

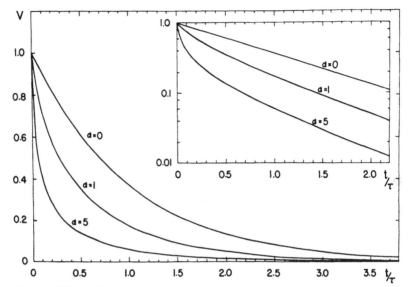

FIG. 4. Effect of initial distribution of soma-dendritic depolarization upon the time course of passive decay to be expected at the soma. The initial distribution is assumed to be $V(X,0) = e^{-ax/\lambda}$, for the three cases, $a = 0$, 1, and 5; the case, $a = 0$, represents a uniform distribution; when $a = 1$, 63 per cent of the dendritic depolarization is distributed proximally to $x = \lambda$; when $a = 5$, the total amount of dendritic depolarization is further reduced by a factor of 5, and 63 per cent of this is distributed proximally to $x = 0.2\lambda$. The logarithmically plotted inset permits an easier comparison of the three rates of decay. In contrast to this figure, when depolarization is least near the soma, Eqs. [22] and [23] imply that the rate of decay at the soma is slower than for the uniform case.

from one sample of neurons with electrophysiological information from another sample of neurons (28, pp. 508, 517-520).

Essentially, the experiment would consist of applying a sinusoidal current across the soma membrane, at several different frequencies, and recording the oscillatory electrotonic potential that is developed across the soma membrane. It would be anticipated, intuitively, that at low frequencies there must be significant current spread into the dendrites, while at high frequencies most of the current would flow across the soma membrane capacity. For very high frequencies, the current would be almost entirely capacitive; in other words, the phase angle between current and voltage would be very close to 90°. For very low frequencies, the current would be almost entirely resistive, implying a phase angle close to zero.

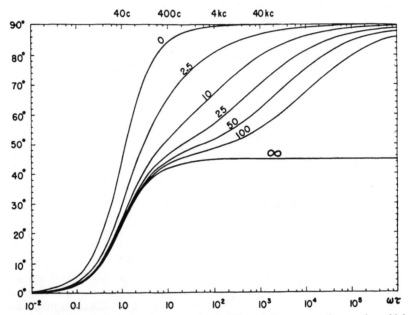

FIG. 5. Theoretical relation between phase shift and frequency when a sinusoidal current is applied across the soma membrane, for $\varrho = 0$, 2.5, 10, 25, 50, 100, and ∞. Zero phase angle implies a whole neuron impedance that is effectively a pure resistance; the 90° value corresponds to effectively pure capacitance. The $\omega\tau$ scale can be used for any τ value, the frequencies at the top of the figure apply when τ is 4 msec. This is based upon Eq. [29].

The transition from zero phase angle to 90° phase angle is displayed graphically in Fig. 5; phase angles are plotted against a logarithmic scale of frequency, for several dendritic to soma conductance ratio values, $\varrho = 0$, 2.5, 10, 25, 50, 100, and infinity. It can be seen that these curves offer a basis for distinguishing electrophysiologically between different values of ϱ.

These curves were calculated from Eq. [29] of the Appendix. A simple method of calculating ϱ from such experimental data is provided by the formula, Eq. [30], obtained by a rearrangement of the first equation. These equations were derived from the assumption of a passive membrane impedance composed of a pure resistance and pure capacitance in parallel; possible complications from additional reactive components have been considered and judged likely to require only a small correction to the midrange illustrated in Fig. 5; see Appendix. Complications resulting from physical instrumentation also may have to be taken into account.

Discussion

ELECTROPHYSIOLOGICAL ESTIMATION OF NEURON PARAMETERS

Estimation of ϱ and τ Independently of Anatomy. The theoretical formulations presented in this paper provide the basis for electrophysiological estimation of the membrane time constant, $\tau = R_m C_m$, and of the dendritic to soma conductance ratio, ϱ, both independently of anatomical data. In principle, simultaneous best estimates of both ϱ and τ could be obtained from good experimental data of the kind corresponding to Figs. 1 and 5. In practice, when there is good reason to believe that ϱ is greater than 2, it is simplest to make a first estimate of τ by the method of Fig. 2; then, using this value of τ, estimate ϱ by the method of Fig. 5. After ϱ has been estimated, the estimate of τ can be reexamined to see if successive approximations are required.

Validation of Sinusoidal Method. The sinusoidal method for estimating ϱ has not yet been tested, and the possibility of unanticipated difficulties must not be overlooked. However, the theoretical results of the preceding paper (28; cf. also 7), provide the means for an independent estimate of ϱ; this is based upon anatomical data in combination with a measurement of R_N. Comparisons would ideally be carried out under conditions where the electrode placement can be confirmed visually, and the soma dendritic dimensions of the same cell can be obtained under essentially the same conditions; obvious candidates are cells in tissue culture, possibly cells in tissue slices, and also cells such as the crustacean stretch receptors.

Estimation of R_m and C_m Depends on Anatomy. Although it now appears to be possible to estimate ϱ and τ independently of anatomical data, the same cannot be said for the membrane constants R_m and C_m, which apply to unit area. In order to estimate R_m from the whole neuron resistance, R_N, it is not sufficient to have the value of ϱ; it is also necessary to know either the soma surface area, or a combined dendritic size parameter (28).[8] The corresponding analysis of axons by Hodgkin and Rushton (21) demonstrated how four electrical constants can be determined from four electrical measurements. However, in that case it was also necessary to supplement the electrical measurements with an anatomical measurement (axon diameter) before the fundamental parameters, R_m, C_m and R_i could be estimated. In the soma-dendritic problem, the value of R_i is not regarded as a serious source of uncertainty and a reasonable value is assumed (28). Thus, the most essential motoneuron parameters may be given as R_m, C_m (or τ) and ϱ, plus a suitable measure of neuron size.

Hypothesis Advanced by Fatt

When the apparent discrepancy between synaptic potential decay and the erroneously low membrane time constant was first being discussed, Fatt (17, pp. 74 and 79) suggested that soma-dendritic electrotonic coupling might account for this discrepancy. This suggestion is in agreement with the present work. More particularly, Fatt's hypothesis was that the dendritic membrane has a larger R_m value than the soma. Assuming a uniform membrane capacity everywhere, this would result in a larger membrane time constant in the dendrites than in the soma. This hypothesis is not in conflict with the present results and interpretations. In view of the large dendritic to soma conductance ratio found, it can be said that the experimental results are determined mainly by the dendritic membrane and that a smaller value for the somatic τ and R_m would have little effect. Fatt gave two reasons for postulating smaller somatic values. Such somatic R_m values would correlate with a membrane threshold difference postulated to exist between soma and dendrites; this remains a possibility. Also, a smaller somatic τ value was intended to account for the rapid soma membrane potential transients observed with an applied current step; Fig. 1 shows that this assumption is not necessary when ϱ is large.

Hypotheses Advanced by Eccles and Collaborators

Because of their 2.5-msec time constant estimate, Coombs, Curtis, and Eccles were led to postulate a prolonged residual phase of synaptic cur-

---

[8] For neurons whose dendrites dominate the whole neuron conductance, it would be wiser to use a combined dendritic size parameter, especially if ϱ has been estimated by the sinusoidal method. This is because we do not yet know how much of the soma surface behaves as though it lies at $X = 0$ in the electrophysiological determination of ϱ. Once this question has been answered experimentally, it may be possible to simplify the procedure by using an appropriate estimate of the soma surface area.

rent (6, 14, 15, 16). It was subsequently postulated that this residual current is due to continued action of a negatively charged transmitter substance, and that the action of an applied hyperpolarizing current is to accelerate the removal of this transmitter substance from the synaptic cleft (14, pp. 63-64; 10, p. 543).

Although these authors have now accepted the necessity of considering dendritic electrotonous in the estimation of the motoneuron membrane time constant, they have explicitly objected to the suggested consequences (25), namely a membrane time constant of about 4 msec, and the removal of the need for a hypothetical prolongation of synaptic current time course. Their revised estimate of the average membrane time constant is 3.1 msec, with a range from 1.8 to 5.1 msec (7); this value allows them to interpret experiments which they find difficult to interpret with a 4-msec value (7, p. 526). However, there is now good reason to believe that even their revised membrane time constant estimates (7) are too low by a significant amount; see pp. 513 and 514.

The hypothetical time course of synaptic current, which originally showed a significant residual phase (6, 14, 15, 16), has now been revised by Curtis and Eccles (10) to a time course showing a much smaller residual phase than before. As explained in the fine print below, this calculated residuum does not establish the existence of actual residual synaptic currents; a very similar calculated residuum could be obtained in the complete absence of actual residual synaptic current.

Other evidence offered by Curtis and Eccles (10) in support of their hypothetical residual synaptic current is also considered in the fine print below. It appears that the various observations upon which Curtis and Eccles have based their arguments can be explained, at least approximately, by giving adequate consideration to electrotonic spread between dendrites and soma. Thus it would seem that the evidence presented by these authors (10) does not establish the existence of significant residual synaptic currents in these motoneurons.

Hypothetical Synaptic Current Time Course. The formula used by Curtis and Eccles (10) to calculate this current time course is equivalent to the well-known differential equation for current flow through a parallel resistance and capacity; this equation can be expressed $I = V/R + C(dV/dt)$. The validity of its application to the present problem depends fundamentally upon two requirements: The synaptic current must be uniformly distributed over the soma and dendrites; and the correct value for the membrane time constant must be used. Although Curtis and Eccles (10, p. 531) mention these requirements, it seems unlikely that either requirement has been adequately satisfied in their applications of this formula.

Even if the assumption of uniformly distributed synaptic current were valid, computation with a membrane time constant estimate, τ_e, that is significantly different from the true value, τ, would be expected to result in a computational artifact. Thus, in the complete absence of residual synaptic current, a uniform passive decay would imply that the formula, $V/\tau_e + dV/dt$, has a time course proportional to the expression, $(\tau - \tau_e)e^{-t/\tau}$. This equals zero only when τ_e equals τ. When τ_e is significantly smaller than τ, this artifact has a positive time course somewhat similar to that originally presented (6, 14, 15, 16) as evidence for residual synaptic currents.

With regard to the assumption of a uniform synaptic current distribution, these authors themselves (10, pp. 533-534, 541-542) suggest that the synaptic current is "largely generated by synapses in proximity to the soma." If this is true, their simple formula cannot be expected to yield synaptic current; it yields something best regarded as an analytical artifact. During a completely passive decay following brief synaptic current, the time courses of V and dV/dt to be expected at the soma must resemble Eqs. [23, 24]. As illustrated in Fig. 4, such passive decay is more rapid than for the uniformly distributed case. It can be shown that the formula, $V/\tau_e + dV/dt$, yields only negative values when τ_e equals τ; however, when τ_e is smaller than τ, this analytical artifact can have negative values during the first few milliseconds (after the brief large current) and then have positive values for the remainder of the decay. This artifact can account, at least approximately, for the "trough," the "reversal of current," and the "low residuum" obtained by Curtis and Eccles (10). Consequently, none of these features should be assumed to represent synaptic current; the "trough" and the "reversal" can be attributed to electrotonic spread from soma to dendrites, as was noted also by Curtis and Eccles (10, p. 541); the positive "residuum" can be attributed to calculation with a low estimate of the membrane time constant.

Comparison of EPSP and IPSP. Curtis and Eccles (10, p. 542) base one of their arguments upon the observation that IPSP decay is faster than EPSP decay. Such observations can be explained simply if one assumes that IPSP initiation is confined more closely to regions near the soma than is EPSP initiation. An illustration of such a difference is provided by Fig. 4; for example, the middle curve could represent an EPSP decay, and the lowest curve could represent an IPSP decay; the uppermost curve represents the simple exponential decay of a uniform disturbance. The logarithmically plotted inset shows that such IPSP decay would be faster than both of the other decays at all times; also, the decay following a brief pulse applied to the soma (see Fig. 3), is very similar to the lowest curve in Fig. 4. Curtis and Eccles (10, p. 542) reject an explanation of this kind on inadequate grounds. Although their τ_{IPSP} and τ_{EPSP}, as well as their τ_m, must be viewed with reservations (because they all appear to be based upon half decay times of curves that must not be assumed to be exponential), the following tentative interpretations would seem reasonable: the fact that their τ_{IPSP} is considerably smaller than the true τ_m, and that it is slightly larger than their estimate of τ_m, is what would be expected if the IPSP is initiated mainly near the soma; also, their larger τ_{EPSP} values may be fairly close to the true τ_m, suggesting that a significant amount of EPSP initiation probably takes place in the dendrites as well as the soma. It may be concluded that the more rapid rate of IPSP decay does not establish a need for prolonged residual synaptic current to explain EPSP decay.

Antidromic Interactions with Synaptic Potentials. Curtis and Eccles (10) base another argument for prolonged residual synaptic current upon their observation of a rebuilding of EPSP following its destruction by an antidromic impulse. Prior to 1956 the same type of experiment was used as evidence for the brevity of synaptic current (2, 9, 13); however, after the 2.5-msec membrane time constant was announced, Eccles (14, pp. 35-36) reinterpreted "small effects" that had been dismissed previously. These small residual depolarizations "are now regularly observed in all experiments in which the conditions are rendered specially favorable by the large size of the EPSP and the low noise level of the intracellular recording (10, pp. 535-536).

There is an alternative explanation for such observations. It is necessary only to assume that at least part of the dendritic surface does not have its synaptic potential destroyed by antidromic invasion; this surviving depolarization would then spread electrotonically to the soma. This suggestion has features in common with the ideas of Fatt (17, p. 74); it is mentioned and rejected by Curtis and Eccles (10, p. 542) on what appear to be inadequate grounds. Although Fatt did place emphasis upon dendritic synapses, this electrotonic explanation would be applicable even if dendritic synaptic activity were not predominant. In view of this alternative explanation, this complicated observation does not establish the existence of a prolonged residual synaptic current.

Effect of Hyperpolarizing Current upon EPSP Decay. The shortening of the time course of an EPSP, generated during the flow of hyperpolarizing current, was first reported and discussed by Coombs, Eccles, and Fatt (9). After the 2.5-msec time constant was announced, Eccles (14, pp. 62-64) postulated that the action of the hyperpolarizing current is to remove or loosen a negatively charged transmitter substance from the sub-synaptic membrane; this action would reduce the postulated residual synaptic currents. These hypotheses are restated by Curtis and Eccles (10, pp. 543-544), who also remark that "no explanation seems to be available for these results if, as suggested by Rall (1957), τ is as long as τ_{EPSP} and there is no residual transmitter action" (10, p. 542). Such an explanation is given below.

It is simplest, but not necessary, to consider an excitatory conductance increase (14, Figs. 22 and 56) to be distributed uniformly over the soma and dendritic membrane; then a purely passive decay would be a simple exponential with the time constant of the membrane. Even in this case, the synaptic current density would not be uniformly distributed when this conductance increase occurs during application of steady hyperpolarizing current. Because such hyperpolarizing current is applied across the soma membrane, the steady state hyperpolarization of the membrane must be greatest at the soma and must decrease electrotonically with distance along the dendrites. Under such conditions, both the density of synaptic current and the amount of depolarization caused by the brief excitatory conductance increase must be greatest at the soma. This nonuniformity will cause a more rapid EPSP decay of the kind illustrated in Fig. 4. Mathematical justification for the applicability of Eq. [23] and of Fig. 4 to the present problem is given in the Theoretical Appendix, following Eq. [23]. A similar argument applies also when the membrane conductance increase is itself not uniformly distributed; the apparent EPSP decay would be expected to be more rapid in the presence of hyperpolarizing current than in its absence. Similar arguments apply to the case of after-hyperpolarization following a spike (10, pp. 541-543); however this case is complicated by increased membrane conductance and by uncertainties about the amount of dendritic invasion by the spike.

The effects described above must contribute to the acceleration of EPSP decay observed during such hyperpolarization. Whether this effect can account completely for the observed phenomenon must be answered by future research. It is possible that additional complications will have to be taken into consideration. At present, the evidence does not appear to require postulation of significant residual synaptic current, or postulation of a negatively charged transmitter substance that is loosened or removed by the hyperpolarizing current (10, 14).

GENERALITY OF THE THEORY

The theoretical results in the Appendix are more general than most of the applications presented as results in the body of this paper. The theory can be applied to passive membrane responses in other neurons. Applied disturbances need not be limited to steps, pulses, and sinusoidal variation; they can also be applied currents or voltages of arbitrary time course. The transient response is obtained not only for the soma, but also for various distances along a dendritic tree. The theory can also be generalized to include the passive membrane response to various soma-dendritic distributions of synaptic current (27, pp. 520-523).

THEORETICAL APPENDIX

The necessary assumptions, definitions, and symbols have been listed and discussed elsewhere (27, 28). A derivation of the fundamental equations can be found in (27, pp. 484-488, 517-523) and in the classical papers on axonal electrotonus (11, 21). Here we begin with the partial differential equation

$$\partial^2 V/\partial X^2 = V + \partial V/\partial T \qquad [1]$$

where $X = x/\lambda$, $T = t/\tau$, and $V \equiv V_m - E$ is the electrotonic potential. The point, $X = 0$, represents the soma-dendritic junction; all dendritic trunks have a common origin there; the soma is treated as a lumped membrane impedance at $X = 0$.[9] The variable, X, represents "electro-

[9] The lumped soma membrane corresponds to the simplifying assumption of soma isopotentiality. During steady state soma-dendritic electrotonus, the error in this assumption may be as large as 2 per cent (8, p. 523). A larger error can occur during the early part of a transient; however, such transient nonuniformity over the soma surface tends to decay with a microsecond time constant (23, 24); see also *Abstracts of National Biophysics Conference*, 1957; full details have not yet been published. The transient error was also found to be small in tests made with a resistance-capacitance network analog, by McAlister (22).

tonic distance" along a dendritic cylinder. When changes in λ are taken into account at points of dendritic branching, Eq. [1] is applicable to an entire dendritic tree, provided that all branch points satisfy the criteria for $B_j = 1$; see (28, pp. 499-501).

When current is applied across the membrane at $X = 0$, the amount of this current must equal the sum of the somatic current and the combined dendritic current. This continuity condition implies

$$I_A = (1/R_s)(V + \partial V/\partial T) + (\varrho/R_s)(-\partial V/\partial X), \text{ at } X = 0,$$

where I_A is the applied current, R_s is the soma membrane resistance, and ϱ represents the ratio between the combined dendritic input conductance and the soma membrane conductance.[10] Rearrangement results in the soma-dendritic boundary condition

$$\partial V/\partial X = (1/\varrho)[V + \partial V/\partial T - I_A R_s], \text{ at } X = 0. \qquad [2]$$

The other boundary condition is that V remains bounded as X approaches infinity.

This boundary value problem can be solved by methods making use of the Laplace Transformation (3, 4). Using the notation of Churchill (4), Eqs. [1] and [2] became transformed to

$$d^2v/dX^2 = (s + 1)\, v - V(X,0) \qquad [3]$$

and

$$dv/dX = (1/\varrho)[(s + 1)v - V(X,0) - i_A R_s], \text{ at } X = 0, \qquad [4]$$

where v and i_A represent Laplace transforms of $V(X,T)$ and $I_A(T)$, and $V(X, 0)$ represents the initial condition of $V(X,T)$.

When the initial condition is zero, this boundary value problem is satisfied by

$$v(X,s) = \frac{C_o(\varrho + 1)\ f(s)e^{-X\sqrt{s+1}}}{s + 1 + \varrho\sqrt{s+1}}, \qquad [5]$$

---

[10] The combination of all dendritic transient current into a single expression is strictly valid only when all of the dendrites (whether extended cylinders or branching trees) have the same separate transient response characteristic at $X = 0$. This does not require the several dendrites to be of the same diameter. It does require them to be electrotonically equivalent to cylinders of the same electrotonic ($X = x/\lambda$) length. For the solutions given in this Appendix, this electrotonic length is assumed to be effectively infinite. If, instead, finite electrotonic length is explicitly assumed, the boundary value problem is changed and a different class of solutions must be used. Some solutions of this class have been illustrated (26); details will be presented elsewhere.

where $f(s)$ is the Laplace transform of the time course, $F(T)$, of the applied current, and C_o is a constant defined by

$$C_o F(T) \; = \; I_A R_N \; = \; I_A R_s/(\varrho + 1). \qquad [6]$$

This definition has the merit that C_o equals the steady electrotonic potential at $X = 0$ during a constant applied current; this is because the steady resistance, R_N, of the whole neuron is smaller than that of the soma, by the factor, $(\varrho + 1)$; see (28).

The general solution above, Eq. [5], is still in terms of Laplace transforms; after inverse Laplace transformation, we can express this general result in the following form

$$V(X,T) \; = \; C_o F(T) \; * \; K(X,T) \qquad [7]$$

where the right hand side represents a concise notation for the convolution operation (4, pp. 35-41), and

$$K(X,T) \; = \; (\varrho + 1) e^{\rho X + (\rho^2 - 1)} \; erfc\left[\frac{X}{2\sqrt{T}} + \varrho \sqrt{T}\right]; \qquad [8]$$

see Churchill's Transform No. 87 and his Operation No. 11 (4); the complementary error function, abbreviated $erfc$, is defined, expanded, and tabulated by Carslaw and Jaeger (3, Appendix II).

There are two simple physical interpretations that can be given for the function, $K(X,T)$. It expresses the transient (passive electrotonic) response when $F(T)$ is a very brief pulse, i.e., "unit impulse" (4, 20) applied at $T = 0$. Also, when $F(T)$ is a unit step applied at $T = 0$, $K(X,T)$ defines the time derivative, dV/dT, of the response, as a function of X and T.

Equations [7] and [8] express a general result of considerable power. On the one hand, it can be reduced to numerous simpler special cases; on the other hand, it can serve as the basis for numerical calculation of $V(X,T)$ from any given $F(T)$, and conversely.

The simplest special cases can be obtained by various combinations of setting $X = 0$, $\varrho = 0$ or $\varrho = \infty$, and making $F(T)$ a unit step function or a unit impulse function. When $F(T)$ is a unit step applied at $T = 0$, $f(s) = 1/s$; also, with certain qualifications (4, 20), when $F(T)$ approximates a unit impulse (instantaneous monophasic pulse) applied at $T = 0$, we can treat $f(s)$ as equal to unity.

Soma Response to Applied Current Step. We set $X = 0$ and $f(s) = 1/s$ to obtain

$$V(0,T) \; = \; \frac{C_o}{\varrho - 1}\left[\varrho \; erf \sqrt{T} - 1 + e^{(\rho^2 - 1)T} \; erfc(\varrho \; \sqrt{T})\right] \qquad [9]$$

This is illustrated in Fig. 1 for several values of ϱ. When $\varrho = \infty$, this simplifies to

$$V(0,T) \ = \ C_0 \ erf \ \sqrt{T} \ ; \qquad\qquad [10]$$

this limiting case can be interpreted as "dendrites without soma" (25), or in other words, complete dendritic dominance; this equation agrees with results previously obtained for axons (11, 21), for a constant current step applied at $X = 0$. The other limiting case, $\varrho = 0$, can be interpreted as a "soma without dendrites" (25); in this case

$$V(0,T) \ = \ C_0(1 - e^{-T}); \qquad\qquad [11]$$

this is the well-known result for the application of a constant current step to a lumped resistance in parallel with a lumped capacity, where $T = t/\tau$ and $\tau = RC$.

Soma dV/dt for Applied Current Step. As a basis for linear plotting of data, we make use of the corresponding time derivatives. From Eq. [9] we obtain

$$dV/dt \ = \ C_0 \left[\frac{\varrho + 1}{\tau} \right] e^{(\varrho^2 - 1)t/\tau} \ erfc \ (\varrho \sqrt{t/\tau}). \qquad [12]$$

When $\varrho = \infty$, this simplifies to

$$dV/dt \ = \ \frac{C_0 e^{-t/\tau}}{\sqrt{\pi \tau t}}, \qquad\qquad [13]$$

and when $\varrho = 0$,

$$dV/dt \ = \ (C_0/\tau)e^{-t/\tau}. \qquad\qquad [14]$$

The deviation of Eq. [12] from Eq. [13] can be assessed. Rearrangement of Eq. [12] gives

$$\sqrt{\pi t} \ (dV/dt)e^{+t/\tau} \ \propto \ \varrho \ \sqrt{\pi t/\tau} \ e^{\varrho^2 t/\tau} \ erfc \ (\varrho \sqrt{t/\tau}). \qquad [15]$$

It can be shown (3, Appendix II) that the expression on the right differs from unity by less than 0.02 when $\varrho \sqrt{t/\tau}$ is greater than 5, and by about 0.1 when $\varrho \sqrt{t/\tau} = 2$; see illustration in Fig. 2, lower left.

Brief Current Pulse Applied to Soma. Assume $F(T)$ to be sufficiently brief that $f(s) = 1$. Then $V(X,T)$ is proportional to $K(X,T)$ of Eq. [8]. When $\varrho = \infty$, this simplifies to

$$V(X,T) \ = \ \frac{C_0}{\sqrt{\pi T}} e^{-\frac{X^2}{4T} - T}, \qquad\qquad [16]$$

which agrees with an earlier result for cylinders provided by Hodgkin (18, p. 363). When also $X = 0$,

$$V(0,T) = \frac{C_0 e^{-T}}{\sqrt{\pi T}} \qquad [17]$$

and

$$dV/dt = \frac{-C_0 e^{-t/\tau}}{\sqrt{\pi \tau t}} \left(1 + \frac{\tau}{2t}\right). \qquad [18]$$

Eq. [17] has been used for the $\Delta T = 0$ curve in Fig. 3, and Eq. [18] has been used as the basis for linear plotting of experimental pulse data in Fig. 2. When ϱ is not effectively infinite, the time derivative at $X = 0$ is more general than Eq. [18]; then

$$dV/dT = C_0(\varrho + 1)e^{-T}\left[(\varrho^2 - 1)e^{\varrho^2 T}erfc\ (\varrho\sqrt{T}) - \frac{\varrho}{\sqrt{\pi T}}\right]. \quad [19]$$

When $\varrho\ \sqrt{t/\tau}$ is not too small, we can use the asymptotic expansion (3, Appendix II) to obtain

$$dV/dT = \frac{-C_0(\varrho + 1)e^{-T}}{\varrho\ \sqrt{\pi T}}\left[1 + \frac{(\varrho^2 - 1)}{2\varrho^2\ T} - \frac{3(\varrho^2 - 1)}{4\varrho^4\ T^2}\cdots\right]$$

The limit of this expression, as $\varrho \to \infty$, is Eq. [18]. Such deviations are illustrated in Fig. 2, upper right.

Soma-Dendritic Response to Current Step. For a current step applied at the soma, $f(s) = 1/s$ in Eq. [5]. If we do not set $X = 0$, the inverse Laplace transformation is more complicated than those considered previously. The problem can be solved by noting that

$$\frac{\varrho^2 - 1}{\sqrt{s}\ (s - 1)(\sqrt{s} + \varrho)} = \frac{\varrho}{\sqrt{s}\ (s - 1)} + \frac{1}{\sqrt{s}\ (\sqrt{s} + \varrho)} - \frac{1}{s - 1}$$

and then using Carslaw and Jaeger's transforms, Nos. 13, 19, and 30 (3). The final result can be expressed

$$V(X,T) = \frac{C_0}{2}\left[e^{-X}\ erfc\ \left(\frac{X}{2\sqrt{T}} - \sqrt{T}\right) - \left(\frac{\varrho + 1}{\varrho - 1}\right)e^X\ erfc\right.$$
$$\left.\left(\frac{X}{2\sqrt{T}} + \sqrt{T}\right)\right] + \left(\frac{C_0}{\varrho - 1}\right)e^{\varrho X + (\varrho^2 - 1)T}\ erfc\ \left(\frac{X}{2\sqrt{T}} + \varrho\sqrt{T}\right)$$
$$[20]$$

For the limiting special case, $\varrho = \infty$, Eq. [20] simplifies to the result previously obtained for axons (21, Eq. 4.1) and (11, p. 452, Eq. 36b).

Nonzero Initial Condition. When $V(X,0)$ is not zero in Eqs. [3, 4], the solution, Eq. [5], must be modified. In particular, if

$$V(X,0) = Ae^{-aX}$$

we obtain

$$v(X,s) = (\varrho + 1)C_o\left[\frac{f(s)e^{-X\sqrt{s+1}}}{s+1+\varrho\sqrt{s+1}}\right] + \left[\frac{A}{s+1-a^2}\right]\left[e^{-aX} - \frac{a(\varrho+a)e^{-X\sqrt{s+1}}}{s+1+\varrho\sqrt{s+1}}\right].$$

The inverse Laplace transformation can be obtained by noting that

$$\frac{\varrho^2 - a^2}{\sqrt{s}\,(s-a^2)(\sqrt{s}+\varrho)} = \frac{\varrho}{\sqrt{s}\,(s-a^2)} + \frac{1}{\sqrt{s}\,(\sqrt{s}+\varrho)} - \frac{1}{s-a^2}$$

and then using Carslaw and Jaeger's transforms, Nos. 13, 19, and 30 (3). The final result can be expressed

$$V(X,T) = C_oF(T) * K(X,T)$$

$$+ (A/2)e^{-aX+(a^2-1)T}\left[1 + erf\left(\frac{X}{2\sqrt{T}} - a\sqrt{T}\right)\right]$$

$$+ (A/2)\left(\frac{\varrho+a}{\varrho-a}\right)e^{aX+(a^2-1)T}\,erfc\left(\frac{X}{2\sqrt{T}} + a\sqrt{T}\right)$$

$$- \left(\frac{Aa}{\varrho-a}\right)e^{\varrho X+(\varrho^2-1)T}\,erfc\left(\frac{X}{2\sqrt{T}} + \varrho\sqrt{T}\right) \qquad [21]$$

where $K(X,T)$ is given by Eq. [8].

The same method can be used to generate results for more complicated initial conditions provided these can be expressed as a linear combination of exponential terms like the one considered above.

Passive Decay from Brief Depolarization. Consider passive decay from a soma-dendritic depolarization (or hyperpolarization). If this depolarization can be represented as the initial condition

$$V(X,0) = Ae^{-aX} + B \qquad [22]$$

and there is no current being applied at $X = 0$, then Eq. [21] implies a passive decay with a time course at $X = 0$ that can be expressed

$$V(0,T) = \frac{A}{\varrho-a}\left[\varrho e^{(a^2-1)T}\,erfc\,(a\sqrt{T}) - ae^{(\varrho^2-1)T}\,erfc\,(\varrho\sqrt{T})\right] + Be^{-T}. \qquad [23]$$

This time course is illustrated graphically in Fig. 4, for three values of a, with $B = 0$; of course, the exponential rate of decay that would be associated with B is the same as that associated with A when $a = 0$.

Equation [23] also expresses the time course following a very brief synaptic current pulse whose soma-dendritic density is proportional to Eq. [22]. Although this can be appreciated intuitively, it is demonstrated mathematically by the agreement between Eq. [23] and a similar result obtained by another approach (27, pp. 520-523). If such a soma-dendritic distribution of depolarizing current were instantaneously applied (at $T = 0$) during a maintained steady application of hyperpolarizing current at $X = 0$, this would be equivalent to setting $F(T) = 1$, in Eq. [21], and adding $C_o e^{-X}$ to the initial condition of Eq. [22]. It follows from Eqs. [21, 7, 8, 9], that the time course, $V(0,T) — V(0,\infty)$, of return to steady state hyperpolarization, is identical with the right side of Eq. [23]. This result is relevant to the interpretation of certain experiments (10); see Discussion, where it is important to note that the distribution of synaptically induced depolarization is different in the presence and absence of applied hyperpolarization.

The time derivative of Eq. [23] is needed in another part of the Discussion; it can be expressed

$$dV/dt = \frac{A}{\tau(\varrho - a)} \left[\varrho(a^2 - 1)e^{(a^2-1)T} \, erfc \, (a\sqrt{T}) - \right.$$

$$\left. a(\varrho^2 - 1)e^{(\varrho^2-1)T} \, erfc \, (\varrho\sqrt{T}) \right] — (B/\tau)e^{-T} \qquad [24]$$

Voltage Step Applied to Soma. We assume that a voltage step, V_A, is applied across the membrane at $X = 0$ and $T = 0$. This implies the Laplace transformed boundary condition

$$v(0,s) = (V_A — E)/s,$$

where E is the resting potential, and $V(X,0)$ is assumed zero before the step. It follows, therefore, from Eq. [5], that

$$f(s) \propto 1 + \frac{1}{s} + \frac{\varrho\sqrt{s+1}}{s}.$$

The first two terms correspond to the instantaneous current and the steady current that must be supplied to the soma; the last term corresponds to the current being supplied to the dendrites. This implies that after the initial instant,

$$I_A \propto erf\sqrt{T} + \frac{e^{-T}}{\sqrt{\pi T}} + \text{constant};$$

see Churchill's Transform No. 38 and Operation No. 11 (4).

Thus, the time derivative of applied current after the initial instant has a time course given by

$$dI_A/dt \ \propto \ - \ (e^{-t/\tau})/(t^{3/2}) \tag{25}$$

Sinusoidal Current Applied Across Soma Membrane. Here we make use of the relation between Laplace transform admittance functions and the complex admittance of a-c steady state analysis (20, p. 176; 29, pp. 24-31). Assuming a passive membrane consisting of pure resistance in parallel with pure capacitance, the complex a-c admittance, Y_m, per unit area of membrane, is related to the membrane conductance, G_m, per unit area as follows

$$Y_m/G_m = 1 + j\omega\tau \tag{26}$$

where $\tau = R_m C_m$ is the membrane time constant, $j = \sqrt{-1}$, and $\omega/2\pi$ is the frequency in cycles per second. If we set $X = 0$ in Eq. [5], the resulting expression implies an admittance function proportional to the expression $s + 1 + \varrho \sqrt{s + 1}$. This implies a complex a-c admittance

$$Y_N = [G_N/(\varrho + 1)][Y_m/G_m + \varrho \sqrt{Y_m/G_m}] \tag{27}$$

for the whole neuron during steady state a-c current application across the membrane at $X = 0$.

By using the identity

$$\sqrt{1 + j\omega\tau} = \sqrt{r}\, e^{j\theta/2} = \sqrt{(r + 1)/2} + j\sqrt{(r - 1)/2}$$

it follows from Eqs. [26] and [27], that

$$Y_N = [G_N/(\varrho + 1)][1 + \varrho \sqrt{(r + 1)/2} + j(\omega\tau + \varrho \sqrt{(r - 1)/2})] \tag{28}$$

where

$$r = \sqrt{1 + \omega^2\tau^2}.$$

This complex admittance implies a phase angle

$$\psi = \arctan\left[\frac{\omega\tau + \varrho \sqrt{(r - 1)/2}}{1 + \varrho \sqrt{(r + 1)/2}}\right] \tag{29}$$

for the whole neuron. This is the relation illustrated in Fig. 5, for several values of ϱ. An explicit expression for ϱ in terms of $\omega\tau$ and $\tan \psi$ can be obtained by a rearrangement of Eq. [29]; this gives

$$\varrho = \sqrt{2(r - 1)}\left[\frac{\omega\tau - \tan \psi}{\omega\tau \tan \psi - (r - 1)}\right]. \tag{30}$$

The sensitivity of the dependence of ϱ upon values of $\omega\tau$ and ψ can be characterized as follows: when $\omega\tau$ and $\varrho \sqrt{\omega\tau}$ are both large compared with unity, and ψ has moderate values (from about 60° to about 75°), an error of 20 per cent in the value of $\omega\tau$ would cause 10 per cent error in the value calculated for ϱ; also, an error of 1 degree in the value of the phase angle, ψ, would cause 10 per cent error in the value calculated for ϱ.

Two possible complications should be mentioned. Application to experimental results may require that phase shift resulting from the physical instrumentation be included in the theoretical formulation. Also, Drs. K. S. Cole and R. FitzHugh have called my attention to the possibility that the soma-dendritic membrane impedance may contain additional reactive components like those of squid membrane. In the case of squid giant axons, three such reactances have been characterized. Of these, the one corresponding to the "sodium-on" process of the Hodgkin and Huxley model, is the most important for the present problem. This reactance can be treated as either a capacitance with series resistance, or a negative inductance with negative series resistance; at 6.3° C, it has a time constant of about 0.24 msec, associated with a resistance of about 2.3×10^3 Ωcm^2 (Cole and FitzHugh, personal communication; also see 5). When Eqs. [26] to [30] are modified to include this reactance, calculations with squid membrane parameters indicate a difference of about 1 degree in the phase angle for a frequency of 1 kilocycle per second and $\varrho = 10$; higher frequencies result in smaller differences. Furthermore, it is possible that the motoneuron membrane exhibits less of this reactance than does squid membrane; experimental evidence from cat motoneurons provides some support for this possibility (personal communication with K. Frank).

References

1. Araki, T., and T. Otani, Response of single motoneurons to direct stimulation in toad's spinal cord. *J. Neurophysiol.* **18**: 472-485, 1955.

2. Brock, L. G., J. S. Coombs, and J. C. Eccles, The nature of the monosynaptic excitatory and inhibitory processes in the spinal cord. *Proc. Roy. Soc. London B* **140**: 170-176, 1952.

3. Carslaw, H. S., and J. C. Jaeger, "Conduction of heat in solids," London, Oxford, 1959.

4. Churchill, R. V., "Operational mathematics," New York, McGraw-Hill, 1958.

5. Cole, K. S., "Electro-ionics of nerve action." Naval. Med. Res. Inst., Lecture and Review Series, No. 54-6, 1954.

6. Coombs, J. S., D. R. Curtis, and J. C. Eccles, Time courses of motoneuronal responses. *Nature* **178**: 1049-1050, 1956.

7. Coombs, J. S., D. R. Curtis, and J. C. Eccles, The electrical constants of the motoneurone membrane. *J. Physiol. London* **145**: 505-528, 1959.

8. COOMBS, J. S., J. C. ECCLES, and P. FATT, The electrical properties of the moto-neurone membrane. *J. Physiol. London* **130**: 291-325, 1955.

9. COOMBS, J. S., J. C. ECCLES, and P. FATT, Excitatory synaptic action in moto-neurones. *J. Physiol. London* **130**: 374-395, 1955.

10. CURTIS, D. R., and J. C. ECCLES, Time courses of excitatory and inhibitory synaptic actions. *J. Physiol. London* **145**: 529-546, 1959.

11. DAVIS, L., JR., and R. LORENTE DE NÓ, Contribution to the mathematical theory of the electrotonus. *Studies Rockefeller Inst. Med. Research* **131**: 442-496, 1947.

12. ECCLES, J. C., Synaptic potentials of motoneurones. *J. Neurophysiol.* **9**: 87-120, 1946.

13. ECCLES, J. C., "The neurophysiological basis of mind," London, Oxford Univ. Press, 1953.

14. ECCLES, J. C., "The physiology of nerve cells," Baltimore, Johns Hopkins Press, 1957.

15. ECCLES, J. C., Excitatory and inhibitory synaptic action. *Harvey Lectures* **51**: 1-24, 1957.

16. ECCLES, J. C., Neuron Physiology. *Handbook Physiol., Sec. 1*, **1**: 59-74, 1959.

17. FATT, P., Sequence of events in synaptic activation of a motoneurone. *J. Neurophysiol.* **20**: 61-80, 1957.

18. FATT, P., and B. KATZ, An analysis of the end-plate potential recorded with an intra-cellular electrode. *J. Physiol. London* **115**: 320-370, 1951.

19. FRANK, K., and M. G. F. FUORTES, Stimulation of spinal motoneurones with intracellular electrodes. *J. Physiol. London* **134**: 451-470, 1956.

20. GARDNER, M. F., and J. L. BARNES, "Transients in linear systems," New York, Wiley, 1942.

21. HODGKIN, A. L., and W. A. H. RUSHTON, The electrical constants of a crustacean nerve fibre. *Proc. Roy. Soc. London B* **133**: 444-479, 1946.

22. MCALLISTER, A. J., Analog study of a single neuron in a volume conductor. *Naval Med. Research Inst.*, Research Report NM 01 05 00.01.01, 1958.

23. RALL, W., Electrotonic theory for a spherical neurone. *Proc. Univ. Otago Med. School.* **31**: 14-15, 1953.

24. RALL, W., A statistical theory of monosynaptic input-output relations. *J. Cellular Comp. Physiol.* **46**: 373-411, 1955 (ref. p. 403).

25. RALL, W., Membrane time constant of motoneurons. *Science* **126**: 454, 1957.

26. RALL, W., Mathematical solutions for passive electrotonic spread between a neuron soma and its dendrites. *Federation Proc.* **17**: 127, 1958.

27. RALL, W., Dendritic current distribution and whole neuron properties. *Naval Med. Research Inst.*, Research Report NM 01 05 00.01.02, 1959.

28. RALL, W., Branching dendritic trees and motoneuron membrane resistivity. *Exp. Neurol.* **1**: 491-527, 1959.

29. TUTTLE, D. F., JR., "Network synthesis," Vol. I, New York, Wiley, 1958.

3 INTERPRETING EXTRACELLULAR FIELD POTENTIALS FROM NEURONS WITH DENDRITIC TREES

3.1 Introduction by Donald R. Humphrey

Rall, W. (1962). Electrophysiology of a dendritic neuron model. *Biophys. J.* 2:145–167.

"Electrophysiology of a Dendritic Neuron Model" (Rall 1962) was at the time a remarkable paper, but it is even more so in retrospect. It was presented first at a Symposium on Mathematical Models and Biophysical Mechanisms, held at the International Biophysics Congress in Stockholm in 1961, and published subsequently in the proceedings of the symposium in the *Biophysical Journal*. With simple but elegant illustrations, Rall outlines in this paper a mathematical model of the neuron that, in this and subsequent forms, has allowed neuroscientists to address fundamental questions about the properties of nerve cells that were previously intractable. To appreciate the significance of this and related work by Rall of about the same time (Rall 1959, 1960, 1961), it is helpful to know the scientific milieu in which it emerged. Only 15 years had elapsed since the classic experiments by Hodgkin and Rushton (1946) on electrotonus in crustacean nerve fibers. Only ten years had elapsed since the prize-winning experiments by Hodgkin and Huxley (1952a,b) on the ionic bases of the action potential, and those by Fatt and Katz (1951) on the end-plate potential. In all these classic experiments, the core conductor (cable) model was used as a theoretical tool to estimate membrane parameters or to relate ionic currents and membrane potentials. But there was no hint in any of these papers as to how the model might be extended to studies of the electrophysiology of neurons, where branching dendrites and complex geometries appeared, for all but the simplest of applications, to be well beyond the scope of available theory.

Yet there was clearly a need for an appropriate model of the neuron. Anatomical data had established that dendrites were the major recipients of synaptic input in the central nervous system, where dendritic surface areas are 10 to 100 times those of the soma (Ramón y Cajal 1909; Fox and Barnard 1957; Sholl 1955; Young 1958). And though only a few years had elapsed since the first intracellular recordings from spinal motoneurons (e.g., Brock et al. 1953; Frank and Fuortes 1955; Eccles 1957), a large body of evidence had accumulated about the electrophysiological properties of these cells. Yet there was no clear vision as to how these data might be used to answer many fundamental questions about cellular function. For example, are dendritic membranes passive or excitable (e.g., Fatt 1957; Freygang and Frank 1959; Nelson and Frank 1964)? If dendritic membranes are passive, are the synapses on distal parts effective in modulating neuronal excitability; that is, what is the effective electrotonic length constant of a cell's dendritic tree (Eccles 1964; Rall 1967)? How are excitatory and inhibitory synapses distributed over the soma-dendritic surface of spinal motoneurons, and how do their effects sum at cellular trigger zones (Smith et al. 1967)? Finally, how could one interpret the extracellular potentials that are generated by neurons to approach these and other important questions (Fatt 1957; Rall 1962; Nelson and Frank 1964; Humphrey 1976)?

In this and related papers, Rall set forth the elements of a dendritic neuron model that allowed quantitative approaches to these and many other fundamental questions. Though it was necessary to make simplifying assumptions about dendritic branching in this initial formulation, the major geometrical features of the neuron were captured. Moreover, this model led to the development of more sophisticated, compartmental models, which can be extended to cases of unequal dendritic branching (e.g., Rall 1964). During the next decade, the basic model outlined in this paper was used to address the fundamental questions about spinal motoneurons previously enumerated (Nelson and Frank 1964; Burke 1967; Smith et al. 1967; Rall 1967); to determine the biophysical factors that contribute to a dominance of synaptic over action-potential currents in the generation of electroencephalographic potentials (Humphrey 1968); to relate intracellular and extracellular potentials in stellate-shaped and in cortical pyramidal cells (Nelson and Frank 1964; Humphrey 1968, 1976); to estimate the excitability of the dendrites of cerebellar Purkinje cells (Llinas et al. 1968a,b); and, perhaps most significantly, to provide the first direct evidence for functional dendrodendritic synapses in the mammalian nervous system (Rall and Shepherd 1968).

The work summarized in this and in other papers by Rall over the next decade is thus a landmark in computational neuroscience; indeed, the full potential of his theoretical insights have yet to be reached. It is a distinct privilege, therefore, to introduce this classic paper to the reader, and to be among the many researchers who know Wil Rall as a friend and as a neuroscientist of the highest stature.

References

Brock, L. G., Coombs, J. S., and Eccles, J. C. (1953). The recording of potentials from motoneurons with an intracellular electrode. *J. Physiol.* (Lond.), 122:429–461.

Burke, R. E. (1967). Composite nature of the monosynaptic excitatory postsynaptic potential. *J. Neurophysiol.*, 30:1114–1137.

Eccles, J. C. (1957). *The Physiology of Nerve Cells*. Baltimore: Johns Hopkins Univ. Press.

Eccles, J. C. (1964). *The Physiology of Synapses*. New York: Academic Press.

Fatt, P. (1957). Electric potentials occurring around a neurone during its antidromic activation. *J. Neurophysiol*, 20:27–60.

Fatt, P., and Katz, B. (1951). An analysis of the end-plate potential recorded with an intra-cellular electrode. *J. Physiol.* (Lond.), 115:320–370.

Fox, C. A., and Barnard, J. W. (1957). A quantitative study of the Purkinje cell dendritic branchlets and their relationship to afferent fibers. *J. Anat. Lond.*, 91:299–313.

Frank, K., and Fuortes, M. G. F. (1955). Potentials recorded from the spinal cord with microelectrodes. *J. Physiol.* (Lond.), 130:625–654.

Freygang, W. H., Jr., and Frank, K. (1959). Extracellular potentials from single spinal moto-neurons. *J. Gen. Physiol.*, 42:749–760.

Hodgkin, A. L., and Huxley, A. F. (1952a). Currents carried by sodium and potassium through the membrane of the giant axon of Loligo. *J. Physiol.* (Lond.), 117:449–472.

Hodgkin, A. L., and Huxley, A. F. (1952b). A quantitative description of membrane current and its application to conduction and excitation in nerve. *J. Physiol.* (Lond.), 117:500–544.

Hodgkin, A. L., and Rushton, W. A. H. (1946). The electrical constants of a crustacean nerve fiber. *Proc. Roy Soc. B. Lond.*, 133:444–479.

Humphrey, D. R. (1968). Re-analysis of the antidromic cortical response. II. On the contribu-tion of cell discharge and PSPs to the evoked potentials. *Electroenceph. Clin. Neurophysiol.*, 25:421–442.

Humphrey, D. R. (1976). Neural networks and systems modeling. In *Biological Foundations of Biomedical Engineering*, ed. by J. Kline. Boston: Little, Brown and Company.

Llinás, R., Nicholson, C., Freeman, J., and Hillman, D. E. (1968a). Dendritic spikes and their inhibition in alligator Purkinje cells. *Science*, 160:1132–1135.

Llinás, R., Nicholson, C., and Precht, W. (1968b). Preferred centripetal conduction of den-dritic spikes in alligator Purkinje cells. *Science*, 163:184–187.

Nelson, P. G., and Frank, K. (1964). Extracellular potential fields of single spinal moto-neurons. *J. Neurophysiol.*, 27:913–927.

Rall, W. (1959). Branching dendritic trees and motoneuron resistivity. *Exp. Neurol.*, 1:491–527.

Rall, W. (1960). Membrane potential transients and membrane time constant of motoneu-rons. *Exp. Neurol.*, 2:503–532.

Rall, W. (1961). Theory of physiological properties of dendrites. *Ann. N.Y. Acad. Sci.*, 96:1071–1092.

Rall, W. (1962). Electrophysiology of a dendritic neuron model. *Biophys. J.*, 2:145–167.

Rall, W. (1964). Theoretical significance of dendritic trees for neuronal input-output rela-tions. In *Neural Theory and Modeling*, ed. R. Reiss. Stanford, CA: Stanford Univ. Press.

Rall, W. (1967). Distinguishing theoretical synaptic potentials computed for different soma-dendritic distributions of synaptic input. *J Neurophysiol.*, 30:1138–1168.

Rall, W., and Shepherd, G. M. (1968). Theoretical reconstruction of field potentials and dendrodendritic synaptic interactions in olfactory bulb. *J. Neurophysiol.*, 31:884–915.

Ramón y Cajal, S. (1909). *Histologie du Système Nerveux de l'Homme et des Vertébrés*. Vol. 1. Paris: Maloine.

Sholl, D. A. (1955). The surface area of cortical neurons. *J. Anat. Lond.*, 89:571–572.

Smith, T. G., Wuerker, R. B., and Frank, K. (1967). Membrane impedance changes during synaptic transmission in cat spinal motoneurons. *J. Neurophysiol.*, 30:1072–1096.

Young, J. Z. (1958). Anatomical considerations. *EEG Clin. Neurophysiol., Suppl.* 10:9–11.

Editorial Comment with an Excerpt from Rall (1992)

Rall, W. (1992). Path to biophysical insights about dendrites and synaptic function. In *The Neurosciences: Paths of Discovery II*, ed. F. Samson and G. Adelman. Boston: Birkhauser.

Because of space limitations we have chosen not to reprint this paper by Rall (1962b). The paper's first half reviewed the modeling perspective gained in several earlier papers (Rall 1957, 1959, 1960, 1962a). The second half presented new results on computed extracellular potential fields and transients. Some of these were published only in that paper, while others were included in Rall 1977, which also is not reprinted in this collection. In order to describe explicitly these computed extracellular potentials here, we include two illustrations from the Rall 1962b, together with some explanatory commentary.

At the time of these extracellular field computations (early 1960s), neurophysiologists were taught that a positive extracellular voltage, recorded relative to a distant (indifferent) electrode, signifies that the recording electrode is located near nerve membrane acting as a current source (i.e., outward membrane current), and that a negative extracellular voltage signifies that it is located near nerve membrane acting as a current sink (i.e., inward membrane current). Although this does hold true for an axon, the fact that this simple rule does not hold for a neuron with several dendrites was clearly demonstrated by these computed results. This was important to the interpretation of recorded extracellular potentials from cat spinal cord, in response to antidromic activation of a single motoneuron (Fatt 1957; Nelson and Frank 1964).

Rall's insights about these spinal cord extracellular potentials are well explained by the following excerpts taken from an essay (Rall 1992).

My dendritic modeling efforts also followed a parallel path that was concerned with extracellular potentials. In 1960, with the help of Ezra Shahn and Jeanne Altmann, I computed extracellular potential fields of simplified dendritic neurons, for the instant of peak action potential in the soma membrane, assuming one or more long dendritic cylinders with passive membrane properties (details can be found on pages 156–163 of Rall 1962b). This required considerable physical labor, because it involved piece-meal computations using large batches of punched cards with an IBM-650 computer. We hand-plotted equi potential contours for the case of a single passive dendrite and a case of seven passive dendrites [shown here as figure 1]. We found the extracellular potential field to be negative (relative to a distant reference electrode) everywhere near the soma and proximal dendrites, and found only weakly positive sleeves surrounding distal dendritic membrane. The physical intuitive explanation of this is that the soma surface provides the sink for all of the extracellular current, which converges radially into the soma; if the sources were all at infinite distance, the equi-potential contours would be spherical

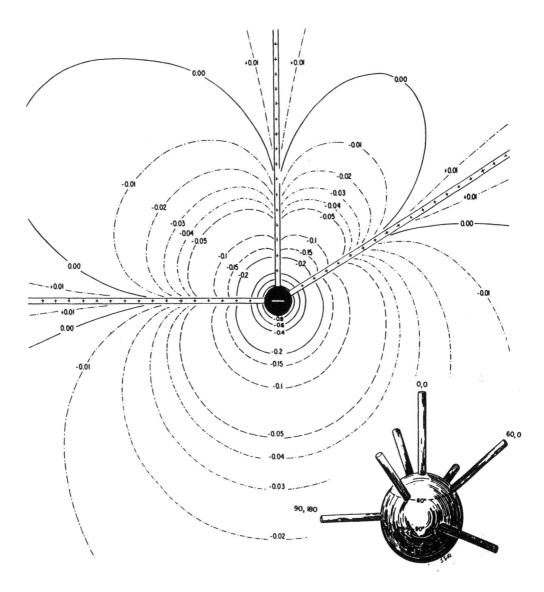

Figure 1
Computed isopotential contours for a spherical soma with seven cylindrical dendrites, of which only three can be seen in the plane shown at upper left. As indicated by the inset at lower right, three dendrites were equally spaced at 60 degrees from the polar axis, and three more dendrites were equally spaced at the equator. The three-dimensional equipotential surfaces are shown cut by a plane that includes the polar axis, one 60-degree dendrite, and one 90-degree dendrite. The soma was the sink for extracellular current current; the dendritic cylinders were distributed sources of extracellular current matching the passive electrotonic spread along the dendrites at the time of the peak of the somatic antidromic action potential. Here, the dendritic length constant was set equal to 40 times the somatic radius. The numbers labeling the contours correspond to the quantity $V_e/(I_N R_e/4\pi b)$, where I_N is the total current flowing from dendrites to soma, R_e represents the extracellular volume resistivity, and b represents the soma radius. For the particular case of the peak somatic action potential in a cat motoneuron, this numerical quantity expresses the value of V approximately in millivolts. This is because of the following order of magnitude considerations: I_N is of the order 10^{-7} A, because the peak intracellular action potential is of the order 10^{-1} V, and the whole neuron instantaneous conductance is of the order 10^{-6} siemens; also, $R_e/4\pi b$ is of the order 10^4 ohms, because the soma radius, b, lies between 25 and 50 μm, and the effective value of R_e probably lies between 250 and 500 ohm cm; see Rall 1962b for more detail. This appeared first as figures 8 and 9 of Rall 1962b; the combined figure appeared as figure 14 of Rall 1977.

surfaces, all of them negative (relative to a distant reference electrode), with the greatest negativity at the soma surface; the negative magnitude would fall off inversely with radial distance (a Coulomb potential). However, the current sources are actually distributed (at a low surface density) over the widely distributed dendritic surface; alone, this low density source current would produce a small positive potential relative to a distant sink. But, because proximal dendritic locations are actually near the soma, the small positive source component is outweighed by the much larger negative potential associated with the radial current into the soma sink. Thus, the extracellular potential is negative at a proximal dendritic source location (an explicit numerical example can be found on pages 158–160 of Rall 1962b). This new physical intuitive insight was important because it had been conventional dogma to say that an extracellular positivity is always associated with a current source (as is indeed true for an axon). The new insight holds for dendritic neurons, and especially for multipolar dendritic neurons. It follows, of course, that when the soma membrane is a source of extracellular current to all of the dendrites, the extracellular potential (relative to a distant reference electrode) is then positive everywhere except for sleeves of weak negativity associated with distal dendrites.

Also around this time, I discussed with Karl Frank and Philip Nelson the problems of interpreting extracellular potential transients generated by antidromic activation of a single motoneuron in cat spinal cord (Nelson, Frank, and Rall 1960; Rall 1962b; Nelson and Frank 1964; see also Fatt 1957). They performed careful experiments in which they recorded the evoked potential transients at many different locations; for locations near the soma, their larger transient (the AB spike) was diphasic, consisting of a brief large negative spike followed by a smaller and slower positive phase, as illustrated by the theoretical curve at lower left in figure 2. Paul Fatt and others had interpreted such diphasic transients as evidence for action potential propagation in the dendrites. However, my computations demonstrated that this transient could be successfully simulated with a model that assumed the dendritic membrane to be entire passive (figure 2) (additional details are provided by pages 160–163 of Rall 1962b). This computation did not prove the dendrites to be passive, but it did help to tip the scales in a careful discussion of the issues (see Nelson and Frank 1964).

This new result was included in presentations at the first International Biophysics Congress, held at Stockholm in 1961. It depends on the fact that an action potential involves two active phases: rapid membrane depolarization by active inward Na^+ ion current, and then rapid membrane repolarization by active outward K^+ ion current. When the dendritic membrane is assumed to be passive, the impulse cannot propagate actively in the dendrites. However, the rapid active membrane repolarization at the soma does produce a reversal in the direction of current flow between the soma and dendrites. In the computed diphasic $(-, +)$ extracellular voltage transient (lower left in figure 2) the large negative peak corresponds to extracellular current flowing radially inward from the passive dendritic membrane to the actively depolarizing soma membrane; then, the subsequent, smaller positive phase corresponds to reversed extracellular current flow, from the rapidly repolarizing soma membrane radially outward to the passively depolarized dendritic membrane. This insight was essential to the interpretation of antidromically evoked extracellular potential transients in cat spinal cord (Nelson and Frank 1964), and also later, in the olfactory bulb of rabbit (Rall and Shepherd 1968).

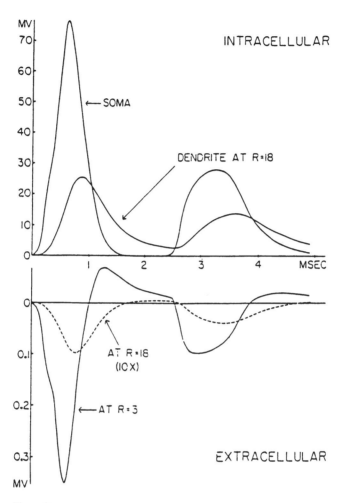

Figure 2
Computed theoretical relation between intracellularly recorded and extracellularly recorded antidromic action potentials, as a function of time.

Uppermost curves: Intracellular potential vs. time. The large-amplitude intracellular curve was given; it corresponds to experimental intracellular recordings made by Nelson and Frank (1964); the full-sized "AB spike" was believed to represent antidromic invasion of both axon hilloc and soma membrane, while the subsequent, smaller "A spike" was believed to represent a spike at the axon hilloc that fails to invade a refractory soma membrane. The lower-amplitude intracellular curve represents the theoretical effect of passive electrotonic spread into a dendritic cylinder of infinite length, computed for a dendritic location at a radial distance $R = 18$, that is, 18 times the soma radius (this corresponds to a dimensionless electrotonic distance of 0.425 from the soma, or about 600 μm in the examples considered).

Lowermost curves: Extracellular potential vs. time. The extracellular curves were computed on the assumption of radial symmetry. The curve for a radial distance $R = 3$ has a shape that is very similar to that at $R = 1$, except the amplitude is about 5 times less. The dashed curve, for a radial distance $R = 18$, has had its amplitude multiplied by 10 to aid the comparison of shape; see Rall 1962b for more detail.

This figure appeared first as figure 11 of Rall 1962b, and also as figure 13 of Rall 1977.

References

Fatt, P. (1957). Electric potentials occurring around a neurone during its antidromic activation. *J. Neurophysiol.*, 20:27–60.

Nelson, P. G., and Frank, K. (1964). Extracellular potential fields of single spinal motoneurons. *J. Neurophysiol.*, 27:913–927.

Nelson, P. G., Frank, K., and Rall, W. (1960). Single spinal motoneuron extracellular potential fields. *Fed. Proc.*, 19:303.

Rall, W. (1957). Membrane time constant of motoneurons. *Science*, 126:454.

Rall, W. (1959). Branching dendritic trees and motorneuron resistivity. *Exp. Neurol.*, 1:491–527.

Rall, W. (1960). Membrane potential transients and membrane time constant of motoneurons. *Exp. Neurol.*, 2:503–532.

Rall, W. (1962a). Theory of physiological properties of dendrites. *Ann. N.Y. Acad. Sci.*, 96:1071–1092.

Rall, W. (1962b). Electrophysiology of a dendritic neuron model. *Biophys. J.*, 2:145–167.

Rall, W. (1977). Core conductor theory and cable properties of neurons. In *Handbook of Physiology, Cellular Biology of Neurons*, ed. E. R. Kandel, J. M. Brookhardt, and V. M. Mountcastle. Bethesda, MD: American Physiological Society.

Rall, W. (1992). Path to biophysical insights about dendrites and synaptic function. In *The Neurosciences: Paths of Discovery, II.*, ed. F. Samson and G. Adelman. Boston: Birkhauser.

Rall, W., and Shepherd, G. M. (1968). Theoretical reconstruction of field potentials and dendrodendritic synaptic interactions in olfactory bulb. *J. Neurophysiol*, 31:884–915.

4 COMPARTMENTAL METHOD FOR MODELING NEURONS, AND THE ANALYSIS OF DENDRITIC INTEGRATION

4.1 Introduction by Idan Segev

Rall, W. (1964). Theoretical significance of dendritic trees for neuronal input-output relations. In *Neural Theory and Modeling*, ed. R. F. Reiss. Palo Alto: Stanford University Press.

This paper (Rall 1964) is one of the most significant landmarks in the modern era of computational neurosciences. Here, Rall first introduced the compartmental modeling approach, which is now widely used for simulating electrical and chemical signaling both at the level of dendritic (and axonal) trees and at the level of networks of neurons. The paper is of special significance for me personally because the compartmental modeling technique has become the primary method in my theoretical studies.

In his previous work, Rall introduced the cable theory for dendritic neurons and solved analytically cases of idealized, passive trees. However, the electrical consequences of complex spatiotemporal patterns of synaptic input impinging on dendritic trees could not be explored analytically, so numerical techniques were necessary. Rall introduced the compartmental modeling method, which, in principle, allows computation of voltage and current spread in nonidealized, and hence biologically realistic, trees, with any specified voltage- and time-dependent membrane nonlinearities. Rall used digital computers to implement this approach, carefully choosing examples that focus on the nonlinear interactions between synaptic inputs in passive dendritic trees and on their effect on the resultant somatic potential. The principles that emerged from these simulations have shaped many of our current ideas about the computational capabilities of neurons. The implications of the method for experimental neurobiologists were also immense. By making possible comparison of experimental findings with model predictions, the method allowed Rall and his colleagues (Rall et al. 1967) to estimate important biophysical parameters for the modeled α motoneurons (see also Barrett and Crill 1974; Fleshman et al. 1989; Jack et al. 1975; Stratford et al. 1989; and a recent review by Rall et al. [1992]).

After presenting compartmental models formally, Rall solved the system of equations numerically and explored the nonlinearity produced by patterns of synaptic inputs distributed in a passive dendritic tree. Because synaptic inputs were modeled as transient conductance changes, the shunting effect inherent to the mechanism of synaptic inputs was explicitly considered in the models. Rall showed that for excitatory inputs, summation of excitatory postsynaptic potentials (EPSPs) may deviate markedly from linearity when the synapses are electrically adjacent, but that the effects of brief synapses that are located at electrically remote distal dendritic branches sum almost linearly. Hence, when the tree receives spatially distributed excitatory synaptic activity, it tends to operate as a linear summing device, whereas when these inputs are spatially clustered, the tree operates in its nonlinear regime.

Another point Rall highlights in his simulations is the importance of the spatial (and temporal) organization of inhibitory and excitatory inputs for dendritic computation. He showed that, as a general rule, an excitatory input is most efficiently reduced by an inhibitory input when the latter is placed between the excitatory synapse and the target (output) site (e.g., the soma and axon hillock). The optimal location depends on several factors, such as the electrotonic structure of the tree, the time course and magnitude of the synaptic conductance involved, and the activation time of inhibition and excitation. The idea that strategic placement of inhibitory and excitatory inputs and temporal relation between these inputs can implement a wide repertoire of input-output operations was later explored more fully by Jack et al. (1975), Koch et al. (1983), and Segev and Parnas (1983). Although not explicitly discussed, perhaps Rall's most significant contribution in this paper was the demonstration that the single neuron can be computationally a very powerful unit. In a simple and elegant example he demonstrated that, by virtue of its distributed (nonisopotential) electrotonic structure, the neuron becomes sensitive to the temporal sequence of inputs and, as explored later by Erulkar et al. (1968) and by Torre and Poggio (1978), the neuron could act as a device that computes the direction of motion. This nontrivial computation was implemented by a neuron model consisting of a straight chain of 10 compartments, with compartments 2–9 each receiving a transient excitatory input. The depolarization at the model soma (compartment 1) was computed for two different temporal sequences of synaptic activation. One sequence starts at the distal compartment (9) and proceeds successively to activate more proximal synapses. The second sequence follows the reverse order in time (i.e., compartments $2 \rightarrow 9$). Rall showed that the distal-to-proximal sequence would produce a larger somatic depolarization compared to the depolarization resulting from the reverse sequence. The output of this neuron is, therefore, sensitive to the spatiotemporal direction of synaptic activation. It essentially becomes a directionally sensitive unit.

Finally, Rall showed that because of the electrotonic structure of neurons, excitatory potentials originating at the dendrites are expected to have multiple time courses when measured at the soma. Distal dendritic inputs result in broad (and more delayed) EPSPs as compared to the earlier, faster-rising, and narrower EPSPs due to proximal inputs. The functional significance of these differences was briefly discussed. In one mode of neuronal operation, the smooth, relatively "sluggish" EPSPs from distal inputs might set the background (subthreshold) depolarization at the soma, while the proximal inputs, when precisely timed, would trigger the axonal spikes. In this way the neuron may operate as an integrator for distal inputs and as a coincidence detector for the proximal inputs. Rall also discussed another possible mode of behavior, in which background synaptic activity is sufficient to cause a rhythmic discharge at the axon. In this case, inhibition near the soma could block axon firing over specific periods, thereby "shaping" the temporal pattern of the neuron's output.

In retrospect, in addition to specific contributions previously discussed, this paper marked three more general pioneering advances for neuronal modeling. First, Rall shows the potential power of digital computers in exploring and explaining physiological problems; in the mid-1960s digital computers were only rarely used in biology. Second, Rall brought his background from the inanimate world of physicists and engineers to bear on problems of physiological systems. Third, Rall showed great vision by suggesting computational approaches to modeling aspects of neurons that could not *yet* be measured, such as the detailed dimensions of dendrites. Unlike many physicists who are satisfied with simple cases that allow "pretty" analytical solutions, Rall sought to understand the rich, but complicated, possibilities that nonlinear systems typically introduce, and he developed sophisticated *numerical* methods to achieve this goal.

During this "decade of the brain," computers have become an essential tool in neurobiology, and detailed compartmental models of diverse types of neurons are constantly under construction. Sophisticated software tools for implementing compartmental techniques (e.g., NEURON, GENESIS, NODUS, AXONTREE, MNEMOSIS) have been developed (see reviews by Segev et al. [1989] and De Schutter [1992]). This theoretical approach has been proven to be extremely useful for probing the computational role of dendrites and of dendritic spines (see reviews by Mel [1994] and Segev [1995]) and exploring their possible significance for plastic processes in dendrites (review by Koch and Zador [1993]).

Sometimes neuronal models become too complicated, and we do well to heed the message implicit in Rall's approach to modeling. He started with the simplified, idealized case and used it as a reference. Then he added complexities to the model, one at a time. Following theoretical explorations of the models, he formulated the main principles that govern their behavior and then used these to build reduced models that retain the essential properties of the complex models. Rall's work teaches that this path, from the simple to the complex to the reduced, can be a real route to understanding.

I conclude this introduction with a personal comment about Wil Rall. When I came to the NIH as a postdoctoral fellow in 1982, I was rather overwhelmed by my move to the United States. Feeling that I had little to offer the renowned Rall, I feared that he would be disappointed by my ignorance. Even though, from our previous written correspondence (which he always wrote by hand), I could sense his warmth and kindness, I was still extremely tense. When I finally met him I was amazed, and still am, at how modest and generous Wil is. He respects his colleagues whatever their status, and he considers their ideas, however naive. He listens! It was a most important lesson for me, and a crucial step toward independence, to see how Wil, with all his powerful physical insights and his mathematical tools, is self-confident enough to reexamine his thinking and reevaluate his conclusions again and again in light of our discussions. This is the ultimate expression of intellectual honesty. Few are fortunate to have such a mentor and a friend as Wil Rall.

References

Barrett, J. N., and Crill, W. E. (1974). Specific membrane properties of cat motoneurones. *J. Physiol. (Lond.)* **239**:301–324.

De Schutter, E. (1992). A consumer guide to neuronal modeling software. *TINS* **15**:462–464.

Erulkar, S. D., Butler, R. A., and Gerstein, G. L. (1968). Excitation and inhibition in Cochlear nucleus. II. Frequency-modulated tones. *J. Neurophysiol.* **31**:537–548.

Fleshman, J. W., Segev, I., and Burke, R. E. (1989). Electrotonic architecture of type-identified α-motoneurons in the cat spinal cord. *J. Neurophysiol.* **60**:60–85.

Jack, J. J. B., Noble, D., and Tsien, R. W. (1975) *Electric Current Flow in Excitable Cells.* Oxford: Oxford University Press.

Koch, C., Poggio, T., and Torre, V. (1983). Nonlinear interaction in dendritic tree: Localization, timing and role in information processing. *PNAS* **80**:2799–2902.

Koch, C., and Zador, A. (1993). The function of dendritic spines: Devices subserving biochemical rather than electrical compartmentalization. *J. Neurosci.* **13(2)**:413–422.

Mel, B. W. (1994). Information processing in dendritic trees. *Neural Computation.* In press.

Rall, W. (1964). Theoretical significance of dendritic trees for neuronal input-output relations. In *Neural Theory and Modeling*, ed. R. F. Reiss. Palo Alto: Stanford University Press.

Rall, W. (1967). Distinguishing theoretical synaptic potentials computed for different soma-dendritic distribution of synaptic input. *J. Neurophysiol.* **30**:1138–1168.

Rall, W., Burke, R. E., Holmes, W. R., Jack, J. J. B., Redman, S. J., and Segev, I. (1992). Matching dendritic neuron models to experimental data. *Physiological Reviews* **72**:S159–S186.

Rall, W., Burke, R. E., Smith, T. G., Nelson, P. G., and Frank, K. (1967). Dendritic location of synapses and possible mechanisms for the monosynaptic EPSP in motoneurons. *J. Neurophysiol.* **30**:1169–1193.

Stratford, K., Mason, A., Larkman, A., Major, G., and Jack, J. J. B. (1989). The modeling of pyramidal neurones in the visual cortex. In *The Computing Neuron*, ed. R. Durbin, C. Miall, and G. Mitchison. Reading, MA: Addison Wesley.

Segev, I. (1995). Dendritic processing. In *The Handbook of Brain Theory and Neural Networks*, ed. M. A. Arbib. Cambridge, MA: MIT Press. In press.

Segev, I., Fleshman, J. W., and Burke, R. E. (1989). Compartmental models of complex neurons. In *Methods in Neuronal Modeling: From Synapses to Networks*, ed. C. Koch and I. Segev. Cambridge, MA: MIT Press.

Segev, I, and Parnas, I. (1983). Synaptic integration mechanisms: A theoretical and experimental investigation of temporal postsynaptic interaction between excitatory and inhibitory inputs. *Biophys. J.* **41**:41–50.

Torre, V., and Poggio, T. (1978). A synaptic mechanism possibly underlying directional selectivity to motion. *Proc. R. Soc. Lond.* **B. 202**:409–416.

4.2 Theoretical Significance of Dendritic Trees for Neuronal Input-Output Relations (1964), in *Neural Theory and Modeling*, ed. R. F. Reiss, Palo Alto: Stanford University Press

Wilfrid Rall

Neural modelers have usually assumed that the synaptic input to a neuron can be treated as input delivered to a single point or a single summing capacitor. There has also been a tendency to assume that a combination of synaptic excitation and inhibition can be treated as a simple arithmetic sum of positive and negative input components. Both of these assumptions are oversimplifications. It is the purpose of this paper to draw attention to theoretical models which avoid these oversimplifications, and to present the results of computations designed to test the significance of what may be called spatiotemporal patterns of synaptic input.

It is a well-established anatomical fact that essentially all of the neurons in the gray matter of the vertebrate central nervous system have extensively branched dendritic receptive surfaces. Two examples of this (A and B) are illustrated in Fig. 1. The Purkinje cell of mammalian cerebellum (Fig. 1A) has a dendritic surface area that can be as much as one hundred times that of its cell body (estimate based upon the careful measurements of Fox and Barnard, 1957). Mammalian motoneurons (Fig. 1B) and pyramidal cells have dendritic surface areas that have been estimated to be ten to twenty times that of their cell bodies (Sholl, 1955; Aitken, 1955; Young, 1958; Schadé and Baxter, 1960, p. 175). Although the Purkinje cell is a special case, neural modelers should beware of schematic neurons (e.g., C, D, E, F) whose dendrites are either short and unbranched or completely missing. An excellent illustration and discussion of various dendritic branching patterns can be found in a recent paper by Ramon-Moliner (1962).

The entire dendritic surface of mammalian motoneurons is covered by a high density of synaptic connections (Wyckoff and Young, 1956; Rasmussen, 1957).[*] Thus there is little reason to doubt that the extensive dendritic surface of such neurons must be regarded as a receptive surface to which synaptic input is delivered from many afferent sources. In spite of differences between various

---

[*] These densities were estimated as 15 to 20 synaptic end-feet per 100 square micra of dendritic surface area. Motoneurons vary in size; the total dendritic surface of any one such neuron is of the order of 10^4 to 10^5 square micra. Such values imply that an individual motoneuron can be expected to receive from 1500 to 20,000 synaptic endings.

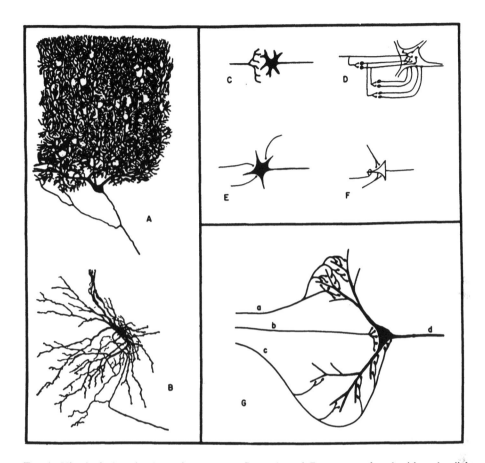

FIG. 1. Histological and schematic neurons. Parts A and B are reproduced with only slight modification from the classic histological work of Ramón y Cajal (1909); A represents a single Purkinje cell of adult-human cerebellum; B represents a single motoneuron of fetal-cat spinal cord. Parts C, D, E, F and G are schematic neurons with schematically indicated synaptic connections; they all represent neurons whose dendritic branching could be expected to resemble B. Part C represents a portion (redrawn) of a well-known diagram by Ramón y Cajal (1909) of a circumscribed reflex; D resembles a schematic drawing by Lorente de Nó (1938b); E resembles the schematic motoneurons of Lloyd (1941); F resembles the even more schematic symbols of McCulloch and Pitts (1943). Part G is also schematic; it is intended to show neither the full dendritic receptive surface of the neuron nor a full complement of synaptic connections to this surface; its purpose is to distinguish between three different patterns of synaptic connections, as discussed in the text.

types of central neurons with respect to both synaptic histology and unre-solved synaptic mechanisms, it seems reasonable to assume that all of their extensive dendritic surfaces serve a receptive function; see also Bishop (1956, 1958), Grundfest (1957), and Bullock (1959). Furthermore, many questions of synaptic mechanism can be bypassed if one is willing to assume that the effects upon the receptive surface can be treated as excitatory and inhibitory mem-brane-conductance changes; this approach is elaborated in a later section.

The schematic dendritic neuron of Fig. 1G helps to illustrate some of the questions we wish to consider. Three sets of synaptic endings are indicated; these are not intended to represent all synaptic connections with this neuron; neither should (a), (b), and (c) be taken literally as single afferent fibers. Here, (a) is meant to represent a group of afferent fibers whose synaptic connections are made predominantly over the peripheral dendritic surface; (b) represents a different group of afferent fibers whose synaptic connections are made predominantly over the surface of the neuron soma and dendritic trunks. A third group of afferent fibers (c) makes synaptic connections first with the dendritic periphery, but also, at successively later times, with successively less peripheral portions of the dendritic system, and finally with the soma. Separate synaptic activity in (a), (b), or (c) provides a simplified example of difference in *spatial* pattern of synaptic input; (c) also implies a particular spatio-temporal pattern. Various sequences of activity in various combinations of (a), (b), and (c) can provide a variety of spatio-temporal patterns of synaptic input.

In order to gain insight into the possible functional significance of various spatio-temporal patterns, we pose the following theoretical problem: develop and explore mathematical models which permit the calculation and comparison of the effects to be expected at a neuron soma for such varied patterns of synaptic activity.

A mathematical model to aid the exploration of the physiological implications of dendritic branching has been developed over the past several years (Rall 1957, 1959, 1960, 1962a, b). The 1959 paper presents and discusses the essential simplifying assumptions and makes a detailed effort to determine, for important model parameters, the ranges of values which would be consistent with available anatomical and electrophysiological evidence. This study provided evidence for a significant dominance of dendritic properties over somatic properties in determining various whole-neuron properties of mammalian motoneurons. It was pointed out (Rall, 1959, p. 520) that "this leads naturally to a possible functional distinction between dendritic and somatic synaptic excitation: the larger and slower dendritic contribution would be well suited for fine adjustment of central excitatory states, while the relatively small number of somatic synaptic knobs would be well suited for rapid triggering of reflex discharge."

A limited aspect of this problem, the passive decay of nonuniform membrane depolarization, was dealt with first (Rall, 1960, pp. 515–16 and 527–29). This was useful for a discussion of problems in the interpretation of experimentally observed synaptic-potential decay. This limited problem has the mathematical advantage that the nonuniformity occurs in the initial condition of the boundary-value problem; the linear partial differential equation remains homogeneous, and its constant coefficients are not affected by the nonuniformity. However, this mathematical simplification is lost when one wants to treat the onset of nonuniform synaptic activity or to treat various durations of sustained nonuniform synaptic activity. As will be shown below, such problems involve a perturbation of the system; not only does the differential equation become nonhomogeneous, but the value of an important coefficient is perturbed from its passive-membrane value. For each region of soma-dendritic receptive surface which receives significantly different synaptic activity, the magnitude of the perturbed coefficient and of the nonhomogeneous term of the partial differential equation will be different. The problem becomes a multi-region boundary-value problem. The particular case of two regions has been presented, together with its formal solution and with numerical examples (Rall, 1962a). One example of those results is included below (in Fig. 5); however, the details of the two-region boundary-value problem will not be reproduced here.

Spatiotemporal synaptic patterns involving multiple regions can be more conveniently handled by using a compartmental model of a dendritic system. The term "compartmental model" is borrowed from the fields of chemical kinetics and radioactive-tracer kinetics. The essential simplifying assumption is that spatial nonuniformity *within* regions (compartments) is completely neglected; nonuniformity is represented only by differences *between* regions (compartments). For nerve models, this means that one explicitly replaces a distributed-parameter transmission line with a lumped-parameter transmission line, a procedure that is commonly used for both diagrammatic and analog representations of transmission lines. Mathematically, the multi-region (partial-differential-equation) boundary-value problem is replaced by a system of ordinary differential equations which are linear and of first order. The formal mathematics and also computational methods for dealing with such systems are well developed. My acquaintance with this body of knowledge has benefited greatly from discussions with John Z. Hearon and Mones Berman. Particularly relevant papers, which also include references to the literature, are Hearon (1963) and Berman, Shahn, and Weiss (1962a, b).

Membrane Model

Equivalent Circuit. For the present discussion, a small uniform patch of dendritic membrane is represented by the equivalent circuit shown in Fig. 2. This is only a slight generalization of the models proposed by Fatt and Katz (1953) and Coombs, Eccles, and Fatt (1955). The background for such models

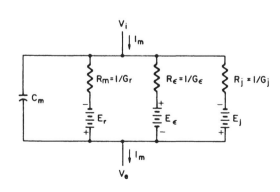

Fig. 2. Equivalent circuit for electric model of nerve membrane, where I_m is the membrane current density (i.e., current per unit area of membrane) flowing from the cell interior, at potential V_i, to the cell exterior, at potential V_e; C_m is the membrane capacitance per unit area; and G_r, G_ϵ, and G_j are separate parallel conductances per unit area, with their associated emf's designated as E_r, E_ϵ, and E_j. The subscripts r, ϵ, and j designate the conductance pathways associated with the resting membrane, with synaptic excitation, and with synaptic inhibition, respectively. Membrane potential is defined as $V_m = V_i - V_e$. The value of I_m is defined by Eq. 1 below; positive values of I_m indicate outward current.

is provided by the important papers of Hodgkin and Katz (1949), Fatt and Katz (1951), and Hodgkin and Huxley (1952); references to earlier literature can be found in these papers.

An essential feature of this model is that each of the three parallel conducting pathways contains its own series emf, which is assumed to remain constant. The resting conductance G_r is also assumed to remain constant; thus all voltage changes are treated as consequences of changes in the values of G_ϵ, G_j, and I_m. The resting state of the membrane is obtained when these three variables are all zero; then the membrane potential, defined as $V_m = V_i - V_e$, is equal simply to the resting emf E_r. When G_ϵ alone is increased from zero, this causes the value of V_m to move closer to that of E_ϵ; similarly, an increase of G_j alone causes a displacement of V_m toward E_j.

It is consistent with experimental evidence to regard E_r and E_j as around 70 to 80 mv negative (interior relative to exterior) and to regard E_ϵ as close to zero. Thus an increase in G_ϵ, assuming that V_m is initially close to E_r, makes V_m less negative; this is a positive displacement of V_m and is commonly described as depolarizing, because the absolute value of V_m is decreased. An increase in G_j, assuming that V_m is initially close to E_r and E_j, can either hyperpolarize, depolarize, or have no effect on, V_m; the direction of the change depends upon the sign of the difference, $E_j - V_m$.

Synaptic Input. Mechanisms of synaptic transmission will not be specified or discussed here. To focus attention upon spatiotemporal patterns of synaptic input, it is assumed that local changes in G_ϵ and G_j can be used as measures of local synaptic activity. Thus for a given portion of dendritic receptive surface area, ΔA, and for a given period of time, ΔT, we will think of the excitatory membrane conductance per unit area, G_ϵ, as roughly proportional to the number of synaptic excitatory events that occur over ΔA, during ΔT. Similarly, G_j shall be regarded as roughly proportional to the number of synaptic inhibitory events that occur over ΔA during ΔT. We will mention, but not elaborate on, the possible complications (1) that the elementary synaptic events might not be of equal magnitude, and (2) that a different type of inhibition could reduce G_ϵ rather than increase G_j. Here we will assume that synaptic input to a dendritic neuron can be specified as a set of G_ϵ and G_j values, each assumed to remain constant over specified ΔA for specified ΔT.

Voltage Dependence of Conductances. As presented below, the mathematical model depends upon the assumption that G_ϵ and G_j are independent of the membrane potential. This assumption confers the advantages of a differential equation having constant coefficients. The solution of the two-region boundary-value problem (Rall, 1962a) depends upon this assumption. It should be noted, however, that when one shifts emphasis from formal solutions to numerical computations with a compartmental model, it becomes practical to consider the possibility of testing the effects of mild voltage dependence. The assumption of complete voltage independence corresponds to the "electrical inexcitability" of Grundfest (1957). The assumption of a mild voltage dependence might provide a way of approximating the property of "decremental conduction" in the dendrites favored by Lorente de Nó and Condouris (1959, p. 612). Both of these cases can be distinguished from the full-blown time and voltage dependence assumed in the Hodgkin and Huxley (1952) model of the axonal nerve impulse. The approach of the present research is to explore questions of spatio-temporal pattern first with the simpler assumption (voltage-independent conductances). Later, it would be well to explore the differences obtained for various degrees of voltage dependence.

Mathematical Formulation of Membrane Model. The net current across a uniform patch of membrane is simply the algebraic sum of four component currents, one capacitive and three conductive; the density of this current (i.e., current per unit area of membrane) can be expressed as

$$(1) \qquad I_m = C_m \dot{V}_m + G_r(V_m - E_r) + G_\epsilon(V_m - E_\epsilon) + G_j(V_m - E_j),$$

where $\dot{V}_m$ represents the time derivative of membrane potential; the other symbols are all defined in Fig. 2 and its legend. To focus attention upon V_m as the dependent variable, this differential equation can be rearranged as follows:

$$(2) \quad \tau \dot{V}_m = -(1 + \mathscr{E} + \mathscr{J})(V_m - E_r) + I_m R_m + \mathscr{E}(E_\epsilon - E_r) + \mathscr{J}(E_j - E_r),$$

where the new variables $\mathscr{E}$ and $\mathscr{J}$, representing synaptic excitation and inhibition, are defined:

$$(2.1) \qquad\qquad \mathscr{E} = G_\epsilon/G_r = R_m/R_\epsilon,$$

$$(2.2) \qquad\qquad \mathscr{J} = G_j/G_r = R_m/R_j,$$

and where τ represents the membrane time constant:

$$(2.3) \qquad\qquad \tau = C_m/G_r = R_m C_m.$$

The introduction of $\mathscr{E}$ and $\mathscr{J}$ as new variables has several advantages; these quantities are dimensionless numbers which correspond to intuitively meaningful conductance ratios; they also provide a simple notation that is well suited for later compartmental assignment of subscripts.

Here we are concerned with the solution of the differential equation (2) for step changes in the values of $\mathscr{E}$, $\mathscr{J}$, and I_m. At first, I_m will be regarded as constant current applied across the patch of membrane by means of electrodes; later, I_m will include the net current supplied to one region of soma-dendritic membrane by neighboring regions or compartments. For periods of time during which $\mathscr{E}$, $\mathscr{J}$, and I_m remain constant (after a step change at time $t = 0$), the differential equation and its solution can be conveniently expressed in the reduced form

$$(3) \qquad\qquad \dot{v} = -\mu(v - v_s),$$

whose solution is

(4)
$$v = v_s - (v_s - v_0)e^{-\mu t},$$

where μ, v_s, and v_0 are constants and v is a transformed variable; v_0 is the value of v at $t = 0$; and v_s is the steady-state value approached by v for large t. The following definitions complete this formulation:

(5)
$$\mu = \frac{1 + \mathscr{E} + \mathscr{J}}{\tau} = \frac{G_r + G_\epsilon + G_j}{C_m},$$

(6)
$$v = \frac{V_m - E_r}{E_\epsilon - E_r},$$

(7)
$$v_s = \frac{\mathscr{E} + \beta\mathscr{J} + \chi}{1 + \mathscr{E} + \mathscr{J}},$$

with

(8)
$$\beta = \frac{E_j - E_r}{E_\epsilon - E_r},$$

and

(9)
$$\chi = \frac{I_m R_m}{E_\epsilon - E_r}.$$

This notation differs from, but remains consistent with, that of an earlier presentation (Rall, 1962a). As before, the dependent variable expresses the departure of the membrane potential from its resting value. By defining v as in Eq. (6), we normalize this variable so that $v = 1$ for $V_m = E_\epsilon$, and $v = 0$ for $V_m = E_r$; also, $v = \beta$ for $V_m = E_j$, and $\beta = -0.1$ for the particular example $E_\epsilon = 0$, $E_r = -70$ mv, and $E_j = -77$ mv.

Six examples of Eq. (4) are illustrated in Fig. 3. In all cases, the initial value, $v_0 = 0.1$, represents a preceding steady state. Curves A and D both correspond to a step increase of 0.5 in the value of $\mathscr{E}$ only, whereas curves C and F both correspond to a step increase of 0.5 in the value of $\mathscr{J}$ only (with $\beta = 0$), and curves B and E both correspond to a step increase of 0.5 in the values of both $\mathscr{E}$ and $\mathscr{J}$. In the original calculation (Rall, 1962a, Fig. 3) the initial values were $\mathscr{E} = \frac{1}{9}$, $\mathscr{J} = 0$, and $\chi = 0$ for curves A, B, and C, on the left; they were $\mathscr{E} = \frac{1}{3}$, $\mathscr{J} = 2$ (with $\beta = 0$), and $\chi = 0$ for curves D, E, and F, on the right; however, these same curves correspond equally well to other sets of initial values and to other step changes in the values of $\mathscr{E}$, $\mathscr{J}$, and χ.[*]

_____

[*] The values of three parameters are needed to determine a particular curve from Eq. (4). All six curves in Fig. 3 have in common the value $v_0 = 0.1$; thus they differ from each other only in the values of two independent parameters. It is convenient to regard the dimensionless rate constant $\mu\tau$ (see Eq. 5 and Eq. 12.1) as one independent parameter, and the initial slope $\tau(\dot{v})_0$ (see Eq. 11) as the other. Then the values of v_s and Δv_s are not independent; they are determined by Eq. (12). A difference in the value of a single independent parameter accounts for the difference between the two curves in each of the following pairs (A, D), (B, E), (C, F), (A, C), and (D, F). One of many possible sets of conditions corresponding to curve A is given by $\mathscr{E}_0 = 0.61$, $\mathscr{J}_0 = 0$, $\chi_0 = -0.45$, with the step $\Delta\chi = 0.45$, and $\mathscr{E}$ and $\mathscr{J}$ unchanged; another set is given by $\mathscr{E}_0 = 0.61$, $\mathscr{J}_0 = 2.25$ (with $\beta = -0.1$), $\chi_0 = 0$, with the step $\Delta\mathscr{J} = -2.25$, and $\mathscr{E}$ and χ unchanged.

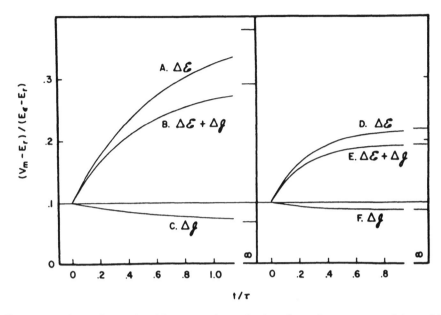

FIG. 3. Transients of v produced by a step change in the values of one or more of the variables $\mathscr{E}$, $\mathscr{J}$, and χ; see Eq. (4) and Eqs. (10)–(12). Values corresponding to each curve are listed below, where "slope" refers to the initial slope defined by Eq. (11):

Curve	$\Delta\mathscr{E}$	$\Delta\mathscr{J}$	Slope	Δv_s	$\mu\tau$
A	0.5	—	0.45	0.28	1.61
B	0.5	0.5	0.40	0.19	2.11
C	—	0.5	−0.05	−0.031	1.61
D	0.5	—	0.45	0.118	3.83
E	0.5	0.5	0.40	0.092	4.33
F	—	0.5	−0.05	−0.013	3.83

Linearity, Nonlinearity, and Related Properties. Several noteworthy properties of this membrane model are illustrated by Fig. 3; several of these are made both more explicit and more general by Eqs. (10)–(12) below. Algebraic manipulation of Eqs. (3), (5), and (7) yields for the change in slope (at $t = 0$) to be expected for any combination of step changes in the values of $\mathscr{E}$, $\mathscr{J}$, and χ at $t = 0$, the expression

$$(10) \qquad \tau(\Delta\dot{v})_0 = (1 - v_0)\Delta\mathscr{E} - (v_0 - \beta)\Delta\mathscr{J} + \Delta\chi,$$

where v_0 is the value of v at $t = 0$. If we assume a preceding steady state, it follows that a zero slope existed just before $t = 0$; also, $v = v_{0s}$ at $t = 0$; then Eq. (10) simplifies to

$$(11) \qquad \tau(\dot{v})_0 = (1 - v_{0s})\Delta\mathscr{E} - (v_{0s} - \beta)\Delta\mathscr{J} + \Delta\chi,$$

which expresses the initial slopes of Fig. 3. Also, it follows from Eq. (3) that the steady-state increment can be expressed as

$$(12) \qquad \Delta v_s = v_s - v_{0s} = \tau(\dot{v})_0/\mu\tau,$$

where $\tau(\dot{v})_0$ is given by Eq. (11) and $\mu\tau$ corresponds to constant values following the step at $t = 0$; that is,

$$(12.1) \qquad \mu\tau = 1 + \mathscr{E}_0 + \mathscr{J}_0 + \Delta\mathscr{E} + \Delta\mathscr{J}.$$

Linearity can be seen to hold in two restricted senses:

(i) The change of initial slope is shown by Eq. (10) to be a linear combination of the input increments, $\Delta\mathscr{E}$, $\Delta\mathscr{J}$, and $\Delta\chi$; however, the coefficients of this linear combination are different for every value of v_0. Thus in Fig. 3 curves B and E both have an initial slope equal to the sum of the separate slopes of curves A and C, or of curves D and F.

(ii) Linearity in the sense of summation of successive steps applies only to $\Delta\chi$; the contribution of $\Delta\chi$ in Eqs. (10) and (11) is independent of the value of v_0; also, the value of $\mu\tau$ in Eq. (12) is left unchanged by $\Delta\chi$. Successive increments in the value of $\mathscr{E}$ and $\mathscr{J}$ do not have this property, except for the special case of simultaneous $\Delta\mathscr{E}$ and $\Delta\mathscr{J}$ with the constraint that $\Delta\mathscr{J} = -\Delta\mathscr{E}$. The fundamental requirement for linear summation of successive steps is that the value of the rate constant μ remain unchanged.

Nonlinearity is present in the following two senses.

(iii) The steady-state increment (Eq. 12) cannot be expressed as a linear combination of $\Delta\mathscr{E}$, $\Delta\mathscr{J}$, and $\Delta\chi$ because $\Delta\mathscr{E}$ and $\Delta\mathscr{J}$ also appear in the value of the denominator, $\mu\tau$. This accounts for the differences between the left and right sides of Fig. 3, in spite of the matching initial slopes.

(iv) Successive increments in the value of $\mathscr{E}$ or of $\mathscr{J}$ do not sum linearly in their effects. Successive increases in the value of $\mathscr{E}$ are decreasingly effective because the successive values of v_0 in Eq. (10) increase and because the value of $\mu\tau$ in Eq. (12) increases; it follows also that successive decreases of $\mathscr{E}$ from an initially large value are increasingly effective. Successive increases in the value of $\mathscr{J}$ are decreasingly effective because the successive values of v_0 in Eq. (10) approach the value of β (i.e., V_m shifts toward E_j) and because the value of $\mu\tau$ in Eq. (12) increases; it follows also that successive decreases of $\mathscr{J}$ from an initially large value are increasingly effective.

At the risk of unnecessary repetition, it is noted that these nonlinearities exist without any added complication such as voltage dependence of conductances. They result from the fact that $\Delta\mathscr{E}$ and $\Delta\mathscr{J}$ are inputs of a different kind from $\Delta\chi$. A change in χ represents a change of input current to an unperturbed system. A change in $\mathscr{E}$ or $\mathscr{J}$ is a change in a conductance which is an element of the system; the system itself is perturbed; the value of a constant coefficient in the linear differential equation is changed; hence the simple superposition rules do not hold.

Dendritic Trees

Although a compartmental model of dendritic trees proves to be more flexible for treating variety both in spatiotemporal patterns of activity and in dendritic branching pattern, it seems desirable to consider first the distributed model of dendritic branching. The latter has the advantage of more immediate appeal to intuition and thus provides a bridge from familiar concepts of anatomy and physiology to the more abstract compartmental model.

Distributed Model. A theoretical model of dendritic branching depends upon a number of simplifying assumptions. A dendritic tree is assumed to consist of cylindrical trunk and branch elements; extracellular gradients of potential are assumed to be negligible; the membrane is assumed at first to be passive and uniform throughout the dendritic tree. Also, the distribution of membrane potential along each cylindrical branch element must satisfy the same partial differential equation that is well established for passive axonal membranes (Hodgkin and Rushton, 1946; Davis and Lorente de Nó, 1947). For each cylindrical element, this equation is of the form

$$\frac{\partial V}{\partial T} = \frac{\partial^2 V}{\partial X^2} - V,$$

where $V = V_{\mathrm{m}} - E_{\mathrm{r}}$ represents the deviation of the membrane potential from its resting value, $T = t/\tau$ expresses the time in terms of the passive-membrane time constant, and $X = x/\lambda$ expresses axial distance in terms of the characteristic length λ, which is proportional to the square root of the cylinder diameter. We require solutions for cylinders of finite length which satisfy boundary conditions determined by the physical requirement of continuity of axial current and of membrane potential at all points of junction between branches. A systematic method for satisfying these boundary conditions under steady-state conditions for any arbitrary branching pattern has been devised (Rall, 1959).

Class of Trees Equivalent to Cylinder. The exploration of transient solutions was facilitated greatly by a consideration of the class of dendritic trees which can be shown to be mathematically equivalent to a cylinder. Figure 4 shows one example of this class. Because this particular example displays symmetric branching, each daughter branch at every bifurcation has a diameter that is 63% of its parent diameter. It should be pointed out, however, that less-symmetric trees also belong to the class under discussion. The essential requirement is that the daughter diameters at each bifurcation satisfy the following constraint: the sum of their separate diameters raised to the $\frac{3}{2}$ power is equal to the parent diameter raised to the $\frac{3}{2}$ power. The mathematical argument (Rall, 1962a) will not be reproduced here; intuitively, this constraint resembles the familiar notion of impedance-matching.

It is a particularly simple and convenient property of this class of dendritic trees that equal increments of length in the equivalent cylinder correspond to equal increments of dendritic surface area. This is indicated in Fig. 4 by the dashed lines which divide the dendritic tree into five regions of equal dendritic surface area. This property provides a convenient scale, extending from a neuron's soma to its dendritic periphery, that can be used to define and compare various soma-vs.-dendrite distributions of synaptic activity.

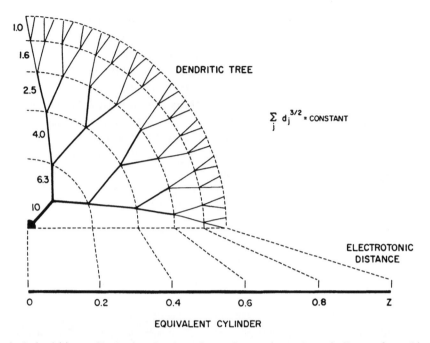

FIG. 4. A dendritic tree illustrative of a class of trees that can be mathematically transformed into an equivalent cylinder. The diagram corresponds to a specific numerical example (Rall, 1962a, Table I) of a symmetric tree with a radial extent of about 800 μ, and with cylindrical diameters decreasing from a trunk of 10 μ to peripheral branches of 1 μ. The dashed lines connect points having the same Z-value (electrotonic distance) in both tree and cylinder. Z is defined by

$$Z_2 - Z_1 = \int_{x_1}^{x_2} \frac{dx}{\lambda},$$

where x represents distance along successive cylindrical axes. λ, the characteristic length which changes with branch diameter, is defined as

$$\lambda = \sqrt{(R_m/R_i)(d/4)},$$

where R_i is the specific resistivity of the intracellular medium, d is the diameter of the cylinder, and the extracellular resistivity is assumed to be negligible.

Relation to Anatomy. The relation of such dendritic trees to anatomical evidence deserves brief comment, with respect both to the constraint upon branch diameter and to the electrotonic length of the equivalent cylinder. Inspection of the various dendritic branching patterns presented and discussed by Ramon-Moliner (1962) suggests that dendritic trees of the "tufted" type are less likely to satisfy the ($\frac{3}{2}$-power) constraint upon branch diameter than trees of the "radiate" type; however, this question has not yet been investigated in detail. Motoneurons of the spinal cord are of the radiate type; the constraint upon the $\frac{3}{2}$ power of branch diameters appears to be satisfied, to at least a rough first approximation, by some of the histological examples that have been studied (Rall, 1959; also unpublished analysis of measurements provided me by Aitken and Bridger, 1961). The same material has also been analyzed to obtain estimates of electrotonic length; when the value of Z (as defined in Fig. 4 above) is computed for all dendritic terminals, an appropriately weighted average of the values obtained for such a neuron typically lies in the range between $Z = 1$ and $Z = 2$. The order of magnitude of such estimates is important in determining that the dendritic periphery is much less functionally remote from the neuron soma than many neurophysiologists have assumed for over twenty years, from Lorente de Nó (1938a) through Eccles (1960, pp. 199–201).

Limitations of Equivalent-Cylinder Model. Although the equivalent-cylinder model has served a very useful purpose in studying dendritic trees, it has three significant limitations which can be overcome by going to a compartmental model. One limitation is the assumption of what might be called "electrotonic symmetry." Although the actual branch diameters and lengths need not be as symmetrical as the diagram in Fig. 4, all terminal branches must be assumed to end with the same Z-value (i.e., the same electrotonic distance from the soma). Furthermore, spatiotemporal disturbances in the equivalent cylinder can represent only those dendritic tree disturbances which can be assumed to be the same in all parts of the tree corresponding to any given Z-value. This assumption is readily fulfilled when a disturbance is initiated at the soma and spreads into a passive dendritic tree (e.g., Rall, 1960), or when synaptic activity is assumed to be distributed uniformly over all dendritic branches corresponding to a given range of Z-values (e.g., Rall, 1962a, and also Figs. 5, 6, and 7 below). However, this symmetry requirement is not satisfied by patterns of synaptic activity which feature significant differences between two or more branches that occupy the same range of Z-values.

An obvious limitation is the constraint upon the $\frac{3}{2}$ power of branch diameter. Some exceptions to this limitation can be represented by the more general class of dendritic trees that are equivalent to an exponential taper (see treatment of taper in Rall, 1962a); in some cases it may be useful to join two segments of different taper. However, as soon as more than two regions are required to express either complexity of taper or complexity of synaptic pattern, the rigorous solution of the boundary-value problem becomes even more complicated than in the two-region case. For practical purposes, this can be regarded as a third limitation: when more than two regions of cylinder or taper are required, it is simpler to go to a compartmental model.

Compartmental Model. A lumped-parameter transmission line is commonly used to introduce and develop the theory for the distributed-parameter case; successive subdivision of the lumps leads, in the limit, to the distributed case. Here, however, we retain the lumped-parameter approximation; each lump of membrane becomes a compartment; the rate constants governing exchange between compartments are proportional to the series conductance between them. A single compartment may correspond to a single dendritic branch, a group of branches, or just a segment of a trunk or branch element, according to the needs of a given problem. For problems compatible with the equivalent-cylinder constraints, the compartmental model is simply a straight chain of compartments of equal size; this case permits a comparison of predictions made with both kinds of models. Branching chains of compartments of unequal size can be used to approximate an unlimited variety of dendritic branching systems and of synaptic activity patterns.

The mathematical formulation of such a compartmental model consists of a system of ordinary differential equations which are linear and of first order. The ith compartment satisfies the equation

$$(13) \qquad \dot{v}_i = \sum_j \mu_{ij} v_j + f_i,$$

where

$$(14) \qquad f_i = (\mathscr{E}_i + \beta \mathscr{J}_i + \chi_i)/\tau,$$

and each of the coefficients μ_{ij}, represents a rate constant. When subscript j differs from subscript i, the value of the coefficient is always nonnegative, and the order of the subscripts has the meaning: from the jth compartment into the ith compartment. When subscript j equals subscript i, the coefficient μ_{ii} always has a negative value which represents the total rate of loss from the ith compartment. The values of these μ_{ii} and μ_{ij} are given by the expressions,

$$(15) \qquad \mu_{ii} = -(1 + \mathscr{E}_i + \mathscr{J}_i)/\tau - \sum_{j \neq i} \mu_{ij},$$

and

$$(16) \qquad \mu_{ij} = g_{ij}/c_i = g_{ji}/c_i \quad \text{for} \quad i \neq j,$$

where c_i represents the capacitance of the ith compartment, and $g_{ij} = g_{ji}$ represents the conductance between adjacent compartments. Where i and j do not represent directly connected compartments, g_{ij} is zero. It can be seen that the net current flow from the jth compartment to the ith compartment is given by the difference

$$c_i \mu_{ij} v_j - c_j \mu_{ji} v_i = g_{ij}(v_j - v_i).$$

For the special case of a straight chain of compartments each of which corresponds to an equal increment ΔZ of an equivalent cylinder, it can be shown that the result

$$(17) \qquad \mu_{ij} = \mu_{ji} = \tau^{-1}(\Delta Z)^{-2}$$

corresponds to treating all the c_i as equal to the capacitance of a ΔZ-length of equivalent cylindrical membrane and all the nonzero g_{ij} as equal to the core conductance of a ΔZ-length of equivalent cylinder. Furthermore, this result leads, in the limit, as ΔZ is made successively smaller, to the correct partial differential equation for the equivalent cylinder.

The symbols $\mathscr{E}$, $\mathscr{J}$, β, and τ have the same significance as earlier [see Eqs. (2)–(9)]; however, χ is here restricted to current that might be supplied to a compartment by means of electrodes. Subscripting of $\mathscr{E}$ and $\mathscr{J}$ is essential for synaptic patterns; β and τ could also be given subscripts, but they will be assumed, for present purposes, to be the same for all compartments.

Some Properties of Linear Compartmental Systems. For any given set of values of $\mathscr{E}_i$, $\mathscr{J}_i$, and χ_i, the linear system defined by Eqs. (13)–(16) is of the type discussed by Hearon (1963). The square matrix M, composed of the coefficients μ_{ij}, has two important properties discussed by Hearon. It has a strictly dominant diagonal composed of μ_{ii} that are all negative, and it has nonnegative off-diagonal elements whose values are so constrained by the connectivity of the system that the matrix is either symmetric to begin with (special case of Eq. 17), or symmetrizable because $c_i\mu_{ij} = c_j\mu_{ji}$. These properties of the matrix are sufficient to guarantee a number of important properties of the solutions of such a linear system. The roots of the matrix are all real and negative; this ensures that the solutions are bounded and nonoscillatory, and that the homogeneous problem (all $f_i = 0$) has no nonzero steady-state solution. For the nonhomogeneous problem, the steady-state solution is a vector which can be defined as $v(\infty) = -M^{-1}f$, where M^{-1} represents the inverse of M, and f is a constant vector composed of the f_i in Eqs. (13) and (14). As long as M and f remain unchanged, the transient behavior of the system, in passing from any given initial state toward its steady state, can be expressed as a linear combination of (decaying) exponentials, exp $(-m_i t)$, where $-m_i$ represents distinct roots of the matrix M. See Hearon (1963) for a discussion of multiple roots, separation of roots by the μ_{ii}, initial conditions permitting overshoot, and other related questions.

Whenever there is a step change in the value of $\mathscr{E}_i$ or $\mathscr{J}_i$, this has two effects upon Eq. (13). First, it perturbs the system by changing the diagonal element, μ_{ii}; this changes the matrix M and the values of its roots. Second, it changes the value of f_i; this, together with the change in M, causes a change in the steady state toward which the system now tends. In contrast, a change in only the value of χ_i would change f_i without changing the matrix M; in this case, the system itself is not perturbed.

The superposition properties of linear systems apply only to changes in f_i which are not associated with any change in the matrix M. When M remains unchanged, the system can be called a linear time-invariant system, or a constant-parameter linear system; see, for example, Mason and Zimmerman (1960, pp. 318–21). The point here is that we do not have such a system when changes occur in $\mathscr{E}_i$ or $\mathscr{J}_i$, except for the very special case where μ_{ii} remains constant because of equal and opposite changes in $\mathscr{E}_i$ and $\mathscr{J}_i$.

Method of Solution. For any given initial condition, with a constant f vector and a constant matrix M, it is possible to completely define the required transient solution. Numerical computation requires inversion of M and solution of its roots; standard procedures are available for this. However, for spatio-temporal patterns of synaptic activity which involve repeated stepwise perturbations of the system, a new transient solution with a new initial condition, a new constant f vector, and a new constant matrix M is required for each perturbation. An alternative numerical procedure replaces the set of differential equations with a corresponding set of difference equations. Beginning with the initial set of v_i, the change δv_i in each compartment is obtained from the difference equation for a short time increment, δt. As the computation progresses through successive δt's, the perturbations (changes in μ_{ii} and f_i) can be introduced at the times required by the synaptic-activity pattern being assumed. The results presented below were obtained by a numerical procedure of this kind. Use was made of a general computer program that has been developed by Berman, Shahn, and Weiss (1962a, b)* for a large variety of problems related to compartmental systems, as well as other systems; this program employs a fourth-order Runge-Kutta procedure for improving the accuracy of numerical solutions obtained for any specified time increment.

Results of Computations

Central vs. Peripheral Half of Tree. Consider a dendritic tree that is equivalent to a cylinder whose length equals one characteristic length, as in Fig. 4. We wish to compare the effect at the soma ($Z = 0$) of synaptic excitation (G_e) delivered only to the central half of the receptive surface (i.e., $Z = 0$ to $Z = 0.5$) with the effect of the same amount of synaptic excitation delivered only to the peripheral half (i.e., $Z = 0.5$ to 1.0). Curve A in Fig. 5 shows the effect of a step increase (from $\mathcal{E} = 0$ to $\mathcal{E} = 2$ at $t = 0$) confined to the central half, whereas curve C shows the effect of an equivalent step increase confined to the peripheral half; curve B corresponds to a uniform step ($\mathcal{E} = 1$) over the entire receptive surface. These curves were originally computed as solutions of a two-region boundary-value problem in a distributed-parameter system (Rall, 1962a). More recently, they were recomputed for a chain of ten equal

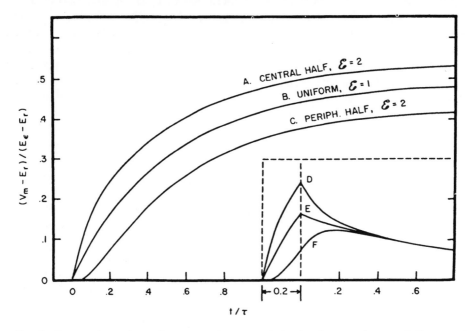

FIG. 5. Computed transients of soma membrane depolarization for step changes of G_e; central vs. peripheral half of dendritic tree; see text. Curves A and D are for $\mathcal{E} = 2$ over central half of receptive surface. Curves B and E are for $\mathcal{E} = 1$ over entire surface. Curves C and F are for $\mathcal{E} = 2$ over peripheral half of surface. Curves A, B and C are for an on-step; curves D, E, and F are for a square pulse (on-step followed by off-step).

* I wish to express my appreciation to Dr. Berman and Mrs. Weiss for their advice and help in the task of achieving compatibility between their program and the idiosyncrasies of my problems. The computations were done on the IBM 7090 at the National Bureau of Standards.

compartments, using Eqs. (13)–(15) and (17). Agreement was within 2%, indicating that errors due to compartmental lumping were not serious.

The early portions of curves D, E, and F are the same as those of curves A, B and C, because they are produced by the same on-step; after a time interval, 0.2τ, each on-step is followed by an off-step. Thus curves D, E, and F can be regarded as theoretical (excitatory) synaptic potentials (epsp) for the artificial assumption of a square $\mathscr{E}$ pulse. It can be seen that curve F rises more slowly to a later peak with an amplitude half that of curve D. Because the threshold for motoneuron reflex discharge has been found (experimentally) to correspond to soma-membrane depolarizations in the range between these peak amplitudes, it is clear that the differences between curves D, E, and F could be responsible for success or failure in the initiation of a propagated impulse.

In addition to the differences that have been noted for the effects of central vs. peripheral $\mathscr{E}$ steps and pulses, it is important to note that the asymptotic value of curve C is only about 20% less than that of curve A. This means that a sustained barrage of peripheral dendritic synaptic activity can have a very significant effect on the level of soma-membrane depolarization.*

Comparison of Four $\mathscr{E}$-Pulse Locations. To demonstrate the importance of specifying the spatiotemporal patterns of synaptic input, a specific numerical example will be presented in two stages. The first stage compares four different cases in which the same magnitude of excitatory conductance pulse is delivered to four different portions of the dendritic receptive surface of a neuron. A comparison of the transient soma-membrane depolarizations calculated for these four cases provides a more detailed demonstration of the effect of central vs. peripheral dendritic location than was demonstrated above for two regions. The second stage makes use of these same four input locations to compare two different spatiotemporal sequences of $\mathscr{E}$ pulses.

Computations were carried out for a straight chain of ten equal compartments ($\Delta Z = 0.2$ per compartment). Compartment No. 1 is regarded as the soma, and compartments 2, 3, $\cdots$, 10 are regarded as equal increments of dendritic surface area, arranged in sequence from dendritic trunks to dendritic periphery; see the diagram in the upper-right corner of Fig. 6.

All four of these curves display transient depolarization of the soma membrane. The magnitude and time of occurrence of the $\mathscr{E}$ pulse is the same in each case; perturbations A, B, C, and D differ only with respect to $\mathscr{E}$-pulse location, as indicated in the figure. Curve A displays the largest and earliest peak depolarization; it results from an $\mathscr{E}$ pulse in compartments 2 and 3, a dendritic location which would correspond to the trunks and portions of primary branches. Cases B, C, and D result from progressively more peripheral $\mathscr{E}$-pulse locations; these are intended to correspond to progressively more

---

* The curves in Fig. 5 correspond to an over-all electrotonic length equal to one characteristic length (i.e., the Z-values extend from 0 to 1.0). For the same geometry, a reduction in the estimated value of R_m/R_i by a factor of four would reduce the estimated values of λ by a factor of two; all Z-values would be doubled. Recalculation of these curves on this assumption would increase the steady-state asymptote of curve A from a value of 0.54 to a value of 0.65 and would decrease the asymptote of curve C from 0.43 to 0.33; also, the peak of D would increase from 0.24 to about 0.28, and the peak of F would decrease from about 0.12 to about 0.07; the decaying portions of D and F would come together (within 10%) only at about $t = \tau$

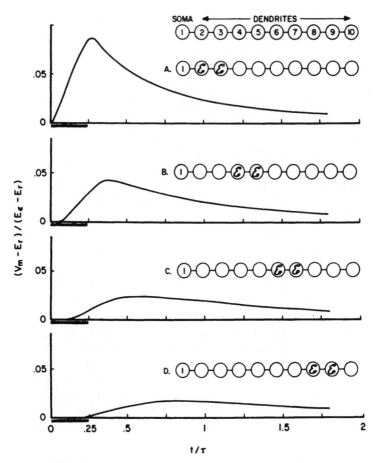

FIG. 6. Effect of $\mathscr{E}$-pulse location upon transient soma-membrane depolarization. The soma-dendritic receptive surface is divided into ten equal compartments ($\Delta Z = 0.2$) as shown, upper right. The four $\mathscr{E}$-pulse locations are shown in the diagrams beside the letters A, B, C, and D; in each case, $\mathscr{E} = 1$ in two compartments for the time interval indicated by the heavy black bars. These curves were drawn through computed values for time steps of 0.05τ. To convert to real time, a τ-value between 4 and 5 msec is appropriate for mammalian motoneurons.

peripheral distributions of restricted synaptic activity delivered to the dendritic receptive surface of a neuron. As a consequence of these locations, curves B, C, and D display progressively lower and later peaks;* these curves also display a progressive delay in their initial rise.

Each of these curves represents a theoretical synaptic potential (epsp) for the artificial assumption of a square $\mathscr{E}$ pulse. It does not seem likely that the differences between such synaptic potentials would be unimportant for neuronal input-output relations.

---

* The peak height of curve A is 0.085 at about $t = 0.25\tau$. For curve B, this is 0.042 at about $t = 0.4\tau$. Curve C has a wide peak of 0.023 centered at about 0.6τ. Curve D has a wide peak of about 0.017 centered at about $t = 0.8\tau$. At times after $t = 1.5\tau$, the decay of all four curves is approximately the same (within 10%); this is because the depolarization spreads and tends to become uniform over the soma dendritic surface as it decays.

Two Spatiotemporal Patterns.   Consider next a sequence of four successive $\mathscr{E}$ pulses where each individual $\mathscr{E}$ pulse has the same magnitude and duration as in Fig. 6. What kind of difference should be expected at the soma for the following two sequences of $\mathscr{E}$-pulse locations: sequence $A \to B \to C \to D$ (trunks first, dendritic periphery last) and $D \to C \to B \to A$ (dendritic periphery first, trunks last), where these letters refer to the four input locations (not the voltage transients) of Fig. 6? The computed transient soma-membrane depolarizations for these two cases are shown in Fig. 7. Curve $D \to C \to B \to A$ has a peak value of 0.152 which occurs close to $t = \tau$. Curve $A \to B \to C \to D$ has two peaks of 0.085, one near $t = 0.25\tau$ and a second near $t = 0.55\tau$. The decay of the curves is approximately the same (within 10%) after $t = 2\tau$.

It should be emphasized that these curves were not obtained by displacing and adding curves A, B, C, and D of Fig. 6; they represent the results of separate computations for the designated sequences of $\mathscr{E}$ pulses. It is clear that the effect at the soma of these two sequences is quite different. The $\mathscr{E}$-pulse sequence $A \to B \to C \to D$ achieves no significant increase of peak soma response over that achieved by $\mathscr{E}$ pulse A alone. In contrast, the $\mathscr{E}$-pulse sequence $D \to C \to B \to A$ achieves significant summation by almost doubling the peak soma response. Both sequences produce results that differ significantly

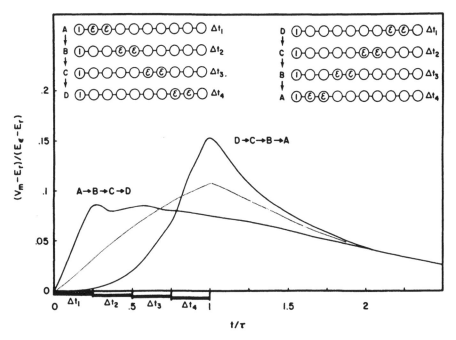

FIG. 7. Effect of two spatiotemporal sequences upon transient soma-membrane depolarization. Two $\mathscr{E}$-pulse sequences, $A \to B \to C \to D$ and $D \to C \to B \to A$, are indicated by the diagrams at upper left and upper right; the component $\mathscr{E}$-pulse locations are the same as in Fig. 6. The time sequence is indicated by means of the four successive time intervals, Δt_1, Δt_2, Δt_3, and Δt_4, each equal to $0.25\,\tau$. The magnitude, $\mathscr{E} = 1$, in two compartments is the same as in Fig. 6. The dotted curve shows the computed effect of $\mathscr{E} = 0.25$ in eight compartments (2 through 9) for the period $t = 0$ to $t = \tau$.

from the dotted curve, obtained when the spatiotemporal pattern is removed by averaging $\mathscr{E}$ over the eight compartments and four time intervals. Three conclusions seem warranted.

(i) A temporal sequence of $\mathscr{E}$ pulses does not result in a unique output unless the dendritic locations of these $\mathscr{E}$ pulses are specified.

(ii) For maximal peak of the soma-membrane depolarization, the peripheral dendritic $\mathscr{E}$ pulses should be delivered earlier than the proximal dendritic $\mathscr{E}$ pulses.

(iii) For rapid achievement and maintainance of a steady soma-depolarization level, a proximal dendritic $\mathscr{E}$ pulse followed by a prolonged sequence of peripheral dendritic $\mathscr{E}$ pulses would be very effective.

Effect of Inhibitory-Conductance Location. Consider the presence of a sustained inhibitory conductance during the occurrence of an $\mathscr{E}$ pulse. What difference in transient soma-membrane depolarization should one expect when the inhibitory perturbation is located peripherally or proximally in relation to $\mathscr{E}$-pulse location? The results of a relevant computation are presented in Fig. 8. For A the $\mathscr{J}$ location (compartments 9 and 10) is peripheral to the $\mathscr{E}$ pulse. For B the $\mathscr{J}$ location (compartments 5 and 6) is the same as the $\mathscr{E}$-pulse location. For C the $\mathscr{J}$ location (compartments 1 and 2) includes the soma and is proximal to the $\mathscr{E}$ pulse. The peak of curve B is 93% of the control peak, while

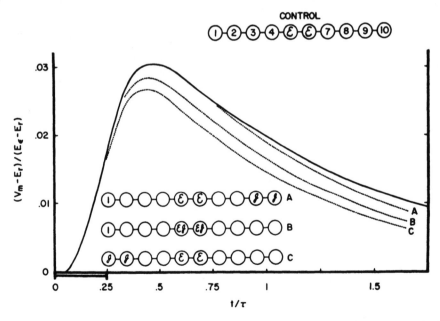

FIG. 8. Effect of inhibitory-conductance location upon transient soma-membrane depolarization. The continuous curve represents the uninhibited "control" transient in compartment 1 (i.e., the soma) for an $\mathscr{E}$ pulse in compartments 5 and 6, as shown in the diagram at upper right; $\mathscr{E} = 1$ for $\Delta t = 0.25\,\tau$, as in the two preceding figures. The dotted curves show the inhibitory effect of having $\mathscr{J} = 1$ in two compartments throughout the time shown; it was assumed for these particular computations that $E_j = E_r$. The $\mathscr{J}$ locations corresponding to curves A, B, and C are indicated by the three diagrams in the lower part of the figure.

that of curve C is about 88% of control. In another calculation with $\mathscr{I} = 10$, the peak corresponding to B dropped to 57% of control, while the peak corresponding to C dropped to 40% of control; even with $\mathscr{I} = 10$, the peak corresponding to A was 99% of control. Also, for $\mathscr{I} = 1$ in compartments 7 and 8, the computed peak was 99% of control. These results suggest a rather simple generalization. When the $\mathscr{I}$ location is peripheral to the $\mathscr{E}$-pulse location, the peak of the transient soma-membrane depolarization is not significantly reduced from the uninhibited control level; however, the declining phase of the soma transient is more rapid. When the $\mathscr{I}$ location is identical with, or proximal to, the $\mathscr{E}$-pulse location, the transient soma peak is reduced from its control level; this reduction is greatest when the $\mathscr{I}$ location includes the soma.

Some qualifications should be added immediately. These results were computed for a straight chain; other computations with branching systems have revealed situations in which a $\mathscr{I}$ location identical with a peripheral $\mathscr{E}$ location can produce more effective inhibition than an equal amount of sustained $\mathscr{I}$ at the soma. Such situations, and also the effect of E_j different from E_r, require further investigation. Furthermore, when $\mathscr{E}$ and $\mathscr{I}$ perturbations are both sustained, the steady-state results differ from those noted above for the peak of a brief transient; the effects due to peripheral $\mathscr{I}$ locations are less discriminated against. On the other hand, when $\mathscr{E}$ and $\mathscr{I}$ perturbations are both brief, their timing becomes very important and peripheral locations become less effective. Proximal $\mathscr{I}$ pulses are most effective when they are timed to center upon the peak depolarization at the $\mathscr{I}$ location; this means that for optimal effect a $\mathscr{I}$ pulse located as in C of Fig. 8 should be timed later than a $\mathscr{I}$ pulse located as in B of Fig. 8. Thus it should be clear that a strategically placed (spatiotemporally) $\mathscr{I}$ pulse can have a potent inhibitory effect.

Spatial Summation of Events in Peripheral Divisions of Tree. Here we present only one set of results obtained for a branching compartmental system. Computations were carried out for the nine-compartment system shown in Fig. 9; compartment 8 was taken to be the neuron soma, while compartments 1, 2, 3, and 4 represent four divisions of the dendritic periphery; transient membrane depolarization in compartment 8 was computed for various combinations of events in the four peripheral compartments. Curve A was computed for an instantaneous depolarization, $v = 0.5$, in any one of the four peripheral compartments; curve B was computed for a simultaneous pair of such events; curve C was computed for four simultaneous events of this kind. Except for inaccuracies in drawing these curves, the ordinates of B are twice those of A at all times; also, the ordinates of C are four times those of A at all times. Because the system is not perturbed, curves A, B, and C can be obtained equally well for other distributions of equal amounts of instantaneous depolarization in the peripheral compartments; for example, curve B would also result from $v = 1$ at $t = 0$ in any one peripheral compartment, or from some combination, such as $v = 0.1, 0.2, 0.3,$ and 0.4, in the four peripheral compartments. In contrast, curves D–H on the right all involve different perturbations of the system, but all are computed for $\Delta t = 0.25\tau$. Curve D was computed for an $\mathscr{E}$ pulse

($\mathscr{E} = 2$) in any one of the four peripheral compartments. Curve E was computed for a simultaneous pair of such $\mathscr{E}$ pulses in compartments 1 and 2; the peak amplitude of E is not twice, but 1.94 times, that of D; symmetry requires the same result if compartments 3 and 4 are substituted for 1 and 2; however, for compartments 1 and 4 (or 2 and 3, or 1 and 3, or 2 and 4) a slightly different curve (not shown) is obtained with a peak amplitude that is 1.99 times that of D. If, on the other hand, the pair of $\mathscr{E}$ pulses is combined in a single peripheral compartment (i.e., $\mathscr{E} = 4$) the summation is poorer, as shown by the dotted curve, G, whose peak is 1.83 times that of D. Curve F was computed for simultaneous $\mathscr{E}$ pulses (each $\mathscr{E} = 2$) in all four peripheral compartments; the peak amplitude of F is 3.84 times that of D; in contrast, when these four $\mathscr{E}$ pulses are combined in a single peripheral compartment (i.e. $\mathscr{E} = 8$), the summation is still poorer, as shown by the dotted curve H, whose peak is only 3.12 times that of D. In these calculations all compartments were assumed to be of the same size, corresponding to $\Delta Z = 0.2$, and all μ_{ij} were taken to be equal.

Once one has accepted the fact that linearity of summation of effects should not be expected for perturbations of the system, it is interesting to reflect on the significance of the results shown at the right in Fig. 9. These results show that, although the departure from linearity can become quite large when perturbations are superimposed upon the same compartment, the departure from linearity can be surprisingly small when brief perturbations occur in separate portions of·the dendritic periphery. The intuitive key to this phenomenon is the notion that separate location reduces the interference that each perturbation introduces into the effect from the other. Just as an $\mathscr{E}$ pulse in one peripheral compartment sums better (because it interferes less) with an $\mathscr{E}$ pulse in a different peripheral compartment than in the same compartment, so, also, a $\mathscr{J}$ pulse in one peripheral compartment is less effective in inhibiting the transient

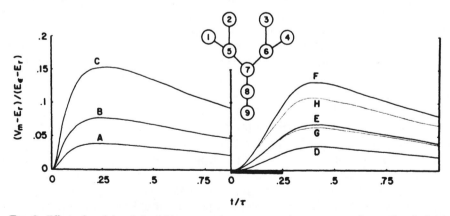

FIG. 9. Effect of peripheral dendritic summation upon transient soma-membrane depolarization. The left side of this figure illustrates linear summation for events which can be regarded either as initial conditions or as nearly instantaneous (at $t = 0$) depolarizations produced by very brief and very large applied currents. The right side of this figure illustrates various degrees of non-linearity in the summation of simultaneous $\mathscr{E}$ pulses having a duration $\Delta t = 0.25\tau$, as shown by the black bar.

due to an $\mathscr{E}$ pulse in a different peripheral compartment than in inhibiting the transient due to an $\mathscr{E}$ pulse in the same compartment.

Discussion

Although more computations will be required for exploring answers to a variety of further questions, the specific results presented and discussed above (Figs. 5–9) support the notion that spatial pattern and spatiotemporal pattern of synaptic activity must be taken into account by any comprehensive theory of neuronal input-output relations.

Dendritic Synaptic Functions. Dendritic branching provides a very large surface area which can receive synapses from many different afferent sources. Although individual brief events in the dendritic periphery suffer significant attenuation in the spread of their effects to the soma, the very large number of dendritic synapses (of the order 10^3 to 10^4) permits a ceaseless spatiotemporal spattering of synaptic events, the integration of which can provide a finely graded background level of depolarization (a biasing of neuronal excitatory state). The sluggish transient characteristic (compare curve D of Fig. 6 with curve A) provides for a smoothing of the temporal input pattern delivered to the dendritic periphery. An approximation to linear summation of $\mathscr{E}$-pulse effects is provided by separated peripheral dendritic locations (see Fig. 9); however, linear summation does not occur with common locations, whether central or peripheral. The effect of $\mathscr{I}$ location has been discussed above with Fig. 8.

Trigger Zone, Convergence Zone, and Soma. It is important to distinguish the soma from the concepts of the trigger zone and of the convergence zone, although they are often (at least implicitly) identified with each other, for convenience. In the case of motoneurons, the soma does represent the zone of dendritic convergence, and it is in this sense that the word *soma* has been used in this paper. The present theoretical results can be applied to other situations, such as receptor branches or the dendritic arborization from an apical dendrite, where the functionally important zone of convergence may be far from the soma. The situation is conceptually simplest when the trigger zone (for initiation of an impulse) is either at or near the convergence zone. This is generally assumed to be the case for motoneurons, except perhaps in those cases where the axon arises from a dendrite at some considerable distance from the soma. The possibility of two trigger zones, one for each of two different dendritic convergence zones, has been suggested for pyramidal cells (see Eccles, 1957, p. 226); particularly interesting to me is the suggestion that one of these (the more peripheral one) might serve a "booster" rather than an impulse-triggerng function (Spencer and Kandel, 1961). The importance of graded integration of synaptic activity in the dendrites, as contrasted with impulse generation and propagation in axons, has been increasingly emphasized in recent years (Bishop, 1956, 1958; Bullock, 1959; Grundfest, 1957).

Central vs. Peripheral Dendritic Function. For a neuron with a single trigger zone that can be identified with the soma and the zone of dendritic convergence, the theoretical results can be seen to suggest a general functional distinction between dendritic and somatic synaptic activity. In contrast with the relatively sluggish and finely graded depolarization that would spread to the trigger zone from the dendritic periphery, brief synchronous activity of a few synapses at or near the soma could produce precisely timed and relatively sharp depolarizations. These would be well suited to precisely timed triggering of axonal impulses; their amplitudes might well be too small to reach threshold without the help of earlier dendritic synaptic activity. Thus the dendritic activity could determine success or failure in the onward transmission of temporal synaptic patterns delivered at the soma. A different mode of behavior would result when sustained dendritic synaptic activity was sufficient to cause a rhythmic discharge of impulses (similar to the action of a generator potential in a sensory neuron); in such a case, synaptic inhibition at the soma could block the discharge of impulses over specific periods, or it could reduce the frequency of rhythmic discharge. An experimental example of this last effect is provided by the observations of Kuffler and Eyzaguirre (1955) on stretch receptor cells of crayfish. The differences in epsp time course presented in Figs. 5 and 6 are roughly similar to the differences reported by Fadiga and Brookhart (1960) for spinal motoneurons of the frog.

Implications for Theories of Nerve Networks. The incorporation of these results into a theory of nerve networks seems to lead to something more complicated than is usually assumed. In the case of the "neuronic equations" of Caianiello (1961, and this volume), the delayed-coupling coefficients (for h different from k, and r greater than zero) could be used to approximate the differences displayed here in Fig. 6; however, the assumed linear combination of inputs neglects the nonlinearities discussed above with Eqs. (10)–(12). A complete incorporation of the compartmental model would lead to four sets of equations: two sets would define all of μ_{ii} and f_i as linear combinations of input from all sources; another set would consist of systems of differential or difference equations, one for each compartmental neuron; and the fourth set would test the difference between depolarization and threshold at the trigger zone of each neuron.

Conduction Safety Factor with Branching. A question was asked regarding the electrotonic equivalence between a cylinder and a class of dendritic trees (see Fig. 4); the questioner felt, especially from the point of view of impulse propagation, that successive branching must, with the accompanying reductions of diameter, lead to a block of conduction; would this not conflict with the concept of electrotonic equivalence? The answer is that small branch diameter should not be expected to cause conduction block, when the $\frac{3}{2}$-power-of-diameter constraint (see Fig. 4, and Rall, 1962a) is satisfied at every branch point; the partial differential equation is the same for cylinder and tree, provided that distance is expressed as electrotonic distance, Z. For conditions of constant impulse-propagation velocity in a cylinder (Hodgkin and Huxley, 1952), one should expect the corresponding velocity in individual branches to decrease as the square root of branch diameter; (see Rall, 1962a, p. 1082). Furthermore, if branch diameters are smaller than required by the $\frac{3}{2}$-power constraint, the safety factor for impulse propagation into the small branches will increase, not decrease. A decrease of safety factor and an increased likelihood of conduction block would be expected when branch diameters exceeded the values required by the $\frac{3}{2}$-power constraint. For such cells (e.g., the Purkinje cell of Fig. 1A, and at least some of the "tufted" cells of Ramon-Moliner, 1962), this geometric polarity might account for a failure of impulses to invade dendritic trees, even if the membrane were electrically excitable; such cells also provide for powerful convergence from their dendritic periphery whether the spread is passive or by means of impulses. Such safety-factor considerations may be important at branched receptor terminals and at branched axonal terminals.

References

AITKEN, J. T., 1955. Observations on the larger anterior horn cells in the lumbar region of the cat's spinal cord, *J. Anat. (London)*, **89**, 571.

AITKEN, J. T., and J. E. BRIDGER, 1961. Neuron size and neuron population density in the lumbosacral region of the cat's spinal cord, *J. Anat. (London)*, **95**, 38–53.

BERMAN, M., E. SHAHN, and M. F. WEISS, 1962a. The routine fitting of kinetic data to models: a mathematical formalism for digital computers, *Biophys. J.*, **2**, 275–87.

BERMAN, M., M. F. WEISS, and E. SHAHN, 1962b. Some formal approaches to the analysis of kinetic data in terms of a linear compartmental system, *Biophys. J.*, **2**, 289–316.

BISHOP, G. H., 1956. Natural history of the nerve impulse, *Physiol. Rev.*, **36**, 376–99.

BISHOP, G. H., 1958. The dendrite: receptive pole of the neurone, *EEG Clin. Neuorophysiol.*, Suppl. No. 10, 12–21.

BULLOCK, T. H., 1959. Neuron doctrine and electrophysiology, *Science*, **129**, 997–1002.

CAIANIELLO, E. R., 1961. Outline of a theory of thought processes and thinking machines, *J. Theoret. Biol.*, **1**, 204–35.

COOMBS, J. S., J. C. ECCLES, and P. FATT, 1955. The inhibitory suppression of reflex discharges from motoneurones, *J. Physiol.*, **130**, 396–413.

DAVIS, L., JR., and R. LORENTE DE Nó, 1947. Contribution to the mathematical theory of the electrotonus, *Studies from the Rockefeller Institute for Medical Research*, vol. 131, 442–96.

ECCLES, J. C., 1957. *The Physiology of Nerve Cells*, Baltimore, Md.: Johns Hopkins Press.

ECCLES, J. C., 1960. The properties of the dendrites, in *Structure and Function of the Cerebral Cortex*, D. B. Tower and J. P. Schadé, eds., Amsterdam: Elsevier.

FADIGA, E., and J. M. BROOKHART, 1960. Monosynaptic activation of different portions of the motor neuron membrane, *Am. J. Physiol.*, **198**, 693–703.

FATT, P., and B. KATZ, 1951. An analysis of the end-plate potential recorded with an intracellular electrode, *J. Physiol.*, **115**, 320–70.

FATT, P., and B. KATZ, 1953. The effect of inhibitory nerve impulses on a crustacean muscle fibre, *J. Physiol.*, **121**, 374–89.

FOX, C. A., and J. W. BARNARD, 1957. A quantitative study of the Purkinje cell dendritic branchlets and their relationship to afferent fibres, *J. Anat.*, London, **91**, 299–313.

GRUNDFEST, H., 1957. Electrical inexcitability of synapses and some consequences in the central nervous system, *Physiol. Rev.*, **37**, 337–61.

HEARON, J. Z., 1963. Theorems on linear systems, *Ann. N.Y. Acad. Sci.*, **108**, 36–68.

HODGKIN, A. L., and A. F. HUXLEY, 1952. A quantitative description of membrane current and its application to conduction and excitation in nerve, *J. Physiol.*, **117**, 500–44.

HODGKIN, A. L., and B. KATZ, 1949. The effect of sodium ions on the electrical activity of the giant axon of the squid, *J. Physiol.*, **108**, 37–77.

HODGKIN, A. L., and W. A. H. RUSHTON, 1946. The electrical constants of a crustacean nerve fibre, *Proc. Roy. Soc. (London)*, B-133, 444–79.

KUFFLER, S. W., and C. EYZAGUIRRE, 1955. Synaptic inhibition in an isolated nerve cell, *J. Gen. Physiol.*, **39**, 155–84.

LLOYD, D. P. C., 1941. The spinal mechanism of the pyramidal system in cats, *J. Neurophysiol.*, **4**, 525–46.

LORENTE DE NÓ, R., 1938a. Synaptic stimulation as a local process, *J. Neurophysiol.*, **1**, 194–206.

LORENTE DE NÓ, R., 1938b. Analysis of the activity of the chains of internucial neurons, *J. Neurophysiol.*, **1**, 207–44.

LORENTE DE NÓ, R., and G. A. CONDOURIS, 1959. Decremental conduction in peripheral nerve; integration of stimuli in the neuron. *Proc. Nat. Acad. Sci.*, **45**, 592–617.

MASON, S. J., and H. J. ZIMMERMAN, 1960. *Electronic Circuits, Signals and Systems*, New York: Wiley.

MCCULLOCH, W. S., and W. PITTS, 1943. A logical calculus of the ideas immanent in nervous activity, *Bull. Math. Biophys.*, **5**, 115–33.

RALL, W., 1957. Membrane time constant of motoneurons, *Science*, **126**, 454.

RALL, W., 1959. Branching dendritic trees and motoneuron membrane resistivity, *Exptl. Neurol.*, **1**, 491–527.

RALL, W., 1960. Membrane potential transients and membrane time constant of motoneurons, *Exptl. Neurol.*, **2**, 503–32.

RALL, W., 1962a. Theory of physiological properties of dendrites, *Ann. N.Y. Acad. Sci.*, **96**, 1071–92.

RALL, W., 1962b. Electrophysiology of a dendritic neuron model, *Biophys. J.*, **2**, 145–67.

RAMON-MOLINER, E., 1962. An attempt at classifying nerve cells on the basis of their dendritic patterns, *J. Comp. Neurol.*, **119**, 211–27.

RAMÓN Y CAJAL, S., 1909. *Histologie du système nerveux de l'homme et des vertébrés*, vol. 1, Paris: Maloine.

RASMUSSEN, G. L., 1957. Selective silver impregnation of synaptic endings, in *New Research Techniques of Neuroanatomy*, W. F. Windle, ed., Springfield, Ill.: C. C Thomas.

SCHADÉ, J. P., and C. F. BAXTER, 1960. Changes during growth in the volume and surface area of cortical neurons in the rabbit, *Exptl. Neurol.*, **2**, 158–78.

SHOLL, D. A., 1955. The surface area of cortical neurons, *J. Anat. (London)*, **89**, 571–72.

SPENCER, W. A., and E. R. KANDEL, 1961. Electrophysiology of hippocampal neurons: IV. Fast prepotentials, *J. Neurophysiol.*, **24**, 272–85.

WYCKOFF, R. W. G., and J. Z. YOUNG, 1956. The motorneuron surface, *Proc. Roy. Soc. (London)*, **B-144**, 440–50.

YOUNG, J. Z., 1958. Anatomical considerations, *EEG Clin. Neurophysiol.*, Suppl. No. 10, 9–11.

5 MODELS OF OLFACTORY BULB NEURONS AND DENDRODENDRITIC SYNAPTIC INTERACTIONS

5.1 Introduction by Gordon M. Shepherd with Supplemental Comments by Milton Brightman

Rall, W., Shepherd, G. M., Reese, T. S., and Brightman, M. W. (1966). Dendro-dendritic synaptic pathway for inhibition in the olfactory bulb. *Exp. Neurol.* 14:44–56.

Rall, W., and Shepherd, G. M. (1968). Theoretical reconstruction of field potentials and dendrodendritic synaptic interactions in olfactory bulb. *J. Neurophysiol.* 31:884–915.

My part in this study grew out of my work on the physiology of olfactory bulb neurons, carried out under Charles Phillips at Oxford from 1959 to 1962. At that time, the main model for the electrophysiological analysis of neuronal properties and synaptic circuits in the central nervous system was the spinal motoneuron, based on the pioneering work of John Eccles in Canberra and of Kay Frank and Michael Fuortes at NIH. In order to extend this approach, we decided to develop the olfactory bulb as a simple cortical system within the mammalian forebrain, based on several attractive features: its clear separation of afferent and efferent fibers, sharp lamination, near-symmetrical arrangement of layers, and distinct neuron types with well-developed dendritic trees and axonal branching patterns. We found in anesthetized rabbits that the large output cells, the mitral cells, can easily be driven directly by antidromic invasion or synaptically by olfactory nerve volleys, and that the impulse response is followed by profound and long-lasting inhibition (Phillips et al. 1961, 1963; Shepherd 1963a), results that were reported independently by two other laboratories (Green et al. 1962; Yamamoto et al. 1963). We also recorded from the other cell types and worked out one of the early local circuit diagrams in which the mitral cells are subject to feedback and lateral inhibition by the granule cells acting as inhibitory interneurons (Shepherd 1963b). We noted the analogy with Renshaw inhibition in the spinal cord, but with two differences: first, the granule cell lacks an axon, so that the inhibitory output is presumably mediated by its long superficial spine-covered process, and second, impulse firing by the granule cell is limited to brief bursts, so that there must be "sustained transmitter actions outlasting the initial impulse activity."

As the end of my time in Oxford grew near, I wrote to several investigators back in the United States about postdoctoral positions. Among them, because of his early papers on dendrites, was Wilfrid Rall. He wrote back that he was interested not only in our evidence about dendrites but also in the large extracellular field potentials we had discovered in the olfactory bulb. He therefore invited me to join him in a theoretical analysis of the generation of the field potentials in the olfactory bulb by the bulbar neurons. Although he had no position to offer himself, he was able to arrange a joint position for me under Wade Marshall and Kay Frank in the Laboratory of Neurophysiology, then in the west wing of Building 10. This was a result of his close collaboration with Kay and his group on the analysis of dendritic integration in motoneurons.

The prospect of working with Wil was exciting for me for several reasons. Although I had little mathematical background, I had been interested in applying computers to the analysis of neurophysiological data since spending the summer of 1956 running one of the earliest analog computers in Walter Rosenblith's laboratory at MIT. I had also been inspired by the idea of modeling neurons after hearing a talk by Francis Crick at Oxford on the modeling of DNA around 1961. So it seemed like an ideal opportunity to do the kind of multidisciplinary study that people were beginning to talk about as desirable in biology.

Nonetheless, the collaboration was a gamble for both of us. The idea of interrupting my experimental career by taking off two years from the laboratory to do a theoretical study was met with skepticism by most of my colleagues. There was no clear precedent for that kind of career path in the neurophysiology of the central nervous system. On Wil's part, he was obviously taking a risk on someone he had never met, and who lacked any obvious mathematical qualifications to be in NIH's Office of Mathematical Research. Moreover, Wil's work on the motoneuron had encountered stiff opposition from his former mentor, Eccles, and there was deeply rooted disbelief among nearly all neuroanatomists and neurophysiologists (there were not yet "neuroscientists") that theoretical studies had any relevance whatsoever to the complexities of central neurons. However, Wil and I hit it off from the start, and we never had any doubts that we were doing a potentially important project that required our close collaboration.

By the time I arrived in Bethesda, Wil had already settled on the basic approach to the problem. With regard to the field potentials, the key idea was that they are generated by synchronous action of the active cells, and that because of the near radial symmetry of the bulb, the potentials result from a potential divider effect of the recording electrodes along the external current pathway. This reduced the three-dimensional field-potential distribution to a one-dimensional problem, which in turn enabled the active populations to be represented by single representative neurons, so that we could draw on his previous work on field potentials around single neurons.

With regard to simulating the action potentials and synaptic potentials that give rise to the field potentials, the timing was propitious because Wil was just finishing the first stage of developing the compartmental method for neuronal modeling. During the fall after I arrived, he was preparing to deliver his seminal paper launching these methods at the Ojai Symposium on Neural Modeling, held in November of 1962 (Rall 1964). In that paper (see part 4 of this book) he adapted the compartmental program (SAAM) developed by his colleague Mones Berman for kinetic analysis and applied it to the analysis of synaptic integration in an extended dendritic tree.

In our study we extended these methods from the motoneuron to olfactory bulb neurons. We determined early that the field potentials generated by an antidromic volley in the mitral cell axons were likely to be associated with a sequence of antidromic invasion of the mitral cells followed by synaptic excitation of the granule cells, so that simulating these potentials would require representative models of each type of neuron. Since no one had modeled whole neurons before, incorporating the structural diversity of axon, soma, and dendrite as well as the functional properties of synaptic potentials and action potentials, we had to make some hard decisions about the amount of detail to include. Hence the rather long Methods section in the ultimate paper (Rall and Shepherd 1968), explaining at some length the rationale for representing the critical components of each type of neuron. The action-potential model was a particular challenge in this regard. Our first choice was to use the Hodgkin-Huxley model of the impulse in the squid axon, but the parameter values had not yet been determined for mammalian neurons, and given the already considerable computational load imposed by the multicompartmental representation of the neurons and their synaptic properties, the additional load of the full Hodgkin-Huxley equations would have made the models too cumbersome. Wil therefore wrote a Fortran program for the compartmental simulation that included a simplified impulse model as well as the field-potential calculations using the potential divider concept. The impulse model consisted of a pair of nonlinear differential equations representing an activating conductance followed by a quenching conductance. We carried out several voltage clamp simulations showing that these equations behaved in general agreement with the equations describing the sodium and potassium conductances of the Hodgkin-Huxley impulse model. We mention in the paper that a more detailed exploration of this model was in preparation; although this was never realized, the model was used further in Goldstein and Rall 1974.

Modeling the mitral cells required more accurate estimates of the sizes of mitral cell somas and dendrites, and modeling the relation between intracellular and extracellular potentials required estimates of the packing densities of mitral and granule cells. Paul Maclean made his laboratory in Building 10 available so that I could prepare some histological material of the rabbit olfactory bulb for this purpose. Tom Powell had driven home to me the importance of good quality perfusion and fixation and attention to tissue shrinkage, so I used a balanced fixative (Bouin's fluid) and took extra care with these steps. Grant Rasmussen generously gave me some space in Building 9 to work with this material. There I became acquainted with Jan Cammermeyer, who had made it his life's work to battle the infamous "dark neurons," which he showed were caused by too early removal of perfused brain tissue. Because these would interfere with our measurements, I religiously waited several hours after perfusion before starting cautiously to remove the bulbs. Sections were made in all three planes in the bulb, and with the excellent fixation and cresyl violet staining I was able to carry out the cell measurements.

An even more fortunate result of working in Building 9 was that I met Tom Reese and Milton Brightman, who were working down the hall. Tom was finishing his electron-microscopical study of the cellular organization of the olfactory epithelium, and by early 1964 he and Milton started their study of the olfactory bulb. Up to that time there had been no study of the fine structure or synaptic organization of the olfactory bulb. It soon became apparent to us that we had the opportunity for a collaborative study combining electrophysiology, electron microscopy, and biophysical modeling, which must have been the first to involve all three approaches (the combined structural and functional studies of the cerebellum by Eccles, Ito, and Szentagothai and of the retina by Dowling, Boycott, and Werblin were also getting under way about this time). The perfusions for the electron microscopy were difficult, so the study went slowly (at least it seemed to me).

Meanwhile there was plenty to do with Wil. When I arrived, he was working on some camera lucida drawings of Golgi-impregnated motoneurons of cats that had been obtained by Aitken and Bridger as a part of a larger study of motoneuron morphology. Wil was interested in seeing whether the equivalent cylinders for the dendritic trees were different for different size trees. We spent many months on that data but in the end gave it up because we were unsure about how many dendritic branches were hidden or cut off. During this time the mathematical research office moved from Building 10 to Building 31. As an experimentalist I enjoyed the rare privilege of rubbing elbows with mathematicians on a daily basis, and I came quickly to appreciate the unique role the office was playing in bringing theory to bear on modern experimental biology. I also made many new colleagues through Wade Marshall's neurophysiology laboratory and the active Friday noon seminars there in his conference room in Building 10.

Through most of 1964 Wil and I developed a rhythm for doing the work. In the morning we would collect the printout at the computer center of the results of the overnight run of the model. We would spend the morning pouring over the results and the afternoon determining which parameters to add or change. Then it was punching them into the IBM cards and leaving them at the computer center where the Honeywell 800 would grind away overnight. When you only get one or two runs per night, it puts great pressure on your intuition to sense what are the constraining variables and which parameter change will give the most insight into how the model is functioning. That economy is behind the strong feelings Wil and those of us who have worked with him have about the importance of constructing models that are adequately constrained.

By the summer of 1964 we had the models for antidromic impulse invasion of the mitral cells and synaptic excitation of the granule cells pretty well worked out. That left just a couple of months in the fall to wrap up the study before I had to leave for a visiting position at the Karolinska Institute in Stockholm. Our writing mode was to sit together with Wil writing things down in a bound protocol book as we arrived at an interpretation and conclusion. Things seemed to be coming together except for one unsolved problem. After mitral cell antidromic invasion, how are the granule cells excited so that they can then inhibit the mitral cells? The assumption in our Oxford circuit diagram was that this excitation came by way of axon collaterals of the mitral cells. However, the localization of the field potentials in our computational model showed that there was an intense depolarization of the peripheral process of the granule cells in a relatively thin layer at the level of the mitral cell secondary dendrites, which was difficult to reconcile with the different distributions of axon collaterals. The more we struggled with this problem, the more the constraints of the model indicated that the excitation of the granule cell processes must occur at the same narrow level as the subsequent inhibition of the mitral cell dendrites. But how? In a moment, one afternoon, the idea hit us that the excitation of the granule cells must come from the same dendrites that the granule cells then inhibit; in other words, synaptic excitation in one direction and synaptic inhibition in the other must occur between the same two processes. I knew from the classical literature that there was no precedent for this kind of interaction between dendrites, and Wil knew from his knowledge of synaptic mechanisms that there was no precedent for this in the physiological literature. However, the model indicated strongly that some kind of two-way synaptic mechanism must be present.

When I left NIH in November 1964, the project fell into limbo. Most of the analysis was complete, but there were still figures to finalize and much of the text to write. Anyone who knows Wil knows that writing does not come easily for him. Furthermore, the work on the olfactory bulb had taken time away from the major study of synaptic integration in motoneurons that he was continuing to pursue with Kay Frank and his colleagues, and he felt, quite rightly, that that study had the highest priority in order to establish the credibility of the model for dendritic integration. We also needed to know from Tom and Milton whether there was any electron-microscopical evidence for the kind of bidirectional synaptic interactions we were postulating.

Fortunately, the evidence was not long in coming. In a few months Wil wrote me in Stockholm that Tom and Milton had indeed found synapses between mitral and granule cell dendrites. When he heard that these were ordinary synaptic contacts situated side by side with opposite polarities, Wil immediately told them that these were precisely the kinds of connections to mediate the interactions we had postulated. Soon we heard that synapses between dendrites in the olfactory bulb had also been seen by Hirata (1964), who referred to them as the "atypical configuration," and by Andres (1965), but the identification of the synaptic processes was not clear, and without the physiology and model it was difficult to infer a function for the synapses because they seemed to be opposing each other. The convergence of our prediction with the identified synapses was not only an exciting result but Tom's and Milton's electron micrographs and serial reconstructions were stunningly clear, so we agreed to write a short paper together on the dendrodendritic synapses and their interactions and send it to *Science*. The result? Rejection, with the comment by the referee "not of general interest."

This setback occurred while there was continuing skepticism toward Wil's studies of the motoneuron. That period was the low point in Wil's fight for the functional importance of the dendrites, and for the place of theory in the study of neuronal function. I think it was only his stubborn belief in himself that carried him through those difficult years between 1959 and 1966. I was too naive to have any doubts myself. The support of Kay Frank, Bob Burke, Phil Nelson, Tom Smith, and their colleagues was especially important in seeing Wil through this period. I mention these things to give the reader an appreciation of how much opposition Wil had to overcome, and how far things have progressed between then and now. Fortunately, it was the dark before the dawn.

In June I was back in the United States to attend a meeting on sensory receptors at Cold Spring Harbor, where John Dowling reported the studies showing similar reciprocal synapses in the retina. After the meeting I came to Bethesda so that we could decide what to do about getting our paper published. Wil contacted William Windle, the editor of *Experimental Neurology*, who invited us to submit it there. We submitted it in July; it was accepted but not published until January 1966 (Rall et al. 1966). The results on reciprocal synapses in the retina came out independently during this same time period.

By the end of 1966 I was back in the United States, and Wil had finished the study of synaptic integration in motoneurons. The publication of the five motoneuron papers in collaboration with Kay Frank's group in 1967 in the *Journal of Neurophysiology* (see chapter 6.2 in this volume) finally brought vindication for Rall's approach to the analysis of dendrites. It also meant that we could turn to writing the full manuscript of our olfactory bulb study. During 1967, while at MIT and finally Yale, I made periodic trips to Bethesda to get the manuscript done. We would sit together and discuss each sentence and often each word as he would write it out in longhand, for later typing by a secretary. It was slow, but it was a marvelous intellectual experience. I have often taken up pencil and paper (or more recently, sat at the computer) and done the same with a student or colleague if the subject is something I really care about. The paper was finally submitted in March 1968 and published in the last issue of the *Journal of Neurophysiology* that year. It was just over six years since I had arrived in Bethesda.

Epilogue

In considering the significance of this work, the 1966 paper emphasizes the fine-structural evidence for the reciprocal synapses. The beautiful electron micrographs of Reese and Brightman showed these clearly, and their serial reconstruction was so definitive that there never was any doubt about the identity of the participating dendrites. This further left no doubt about the presence, identity, and prevalence of dendrodendritic synapses, which was significant at the time in providing a kind of benchmark for others as they encountered less clearly identifiable presynaptic dendrites in other parts of the nervous system. The physiology section describes how successive phases of the field potentials reflect a sequence of mitral cell invasion, granule cell excitation, and mitral cell inhibition that is mediated in the model by the reciprocal dendrodendritic interactions. It was a satisfying case in which a theoretical model predicted anatomical connections, and in addition provided an explanation for how they would constitute a functional circuit.

In Rall and Shepherd 1968 the emphasis was on the independent evidence from the physiology and the biophysical model that led to the postulate of the reciprocal interactions. Several points in the results reflect key steps in constructing the model that, although not often mentioned, occupied much of our effort. These included (1) the potential divider model for the recording of the field potentials; (2) the contrasting ratios of intracellular and extracellular current paths for mitral versus granule cells (which became crucial in driving us to the postulate of the mitral-to-granule cell connection); (3) the evidence that intracellular conduction velocity cannot in general be inferred from extracellular field potentials; and (4) the exploration of active versus passive dendritic properties (this was the first attempt to combine both into a model of a single neuron, and was the start of our later interest in active properties of dendrites and dendritic spines). All of these points were crucial in putting constraints on the model. Modern-day neuronal models of course bring much more computational power to bear, enabling more extensive simulations of geometry and membrane properties, but few incorporate both extracellular and intracellular data and are as tightly constrained as this original model.

The discussion in the 1968 paper went into some detail regarding the implications of the results. Wil was very much the driving force behind this. The confluence of anatomy, physiology, and biophysical models provided insights into types of neuronal organization not known before, and he wanted to follow these implications to their logical conclusion in order to point out the new principles that were implied. Among these implications were (1) presynaptic dendrites can have either synaptic excitatory or inhibitory outputs; (2) cells without axons, such as the amacrine or granule cell, have synaptic outputs like other neurons; (3) neurons can have local input-output functions not involving the entire neuron; and (4) action potentials are not needed for synaptic activation or neuronal output. There were also implications regarding dendritic spine functions that would be pursued by both Wil and myself in later work. The results specifically supported our previous idea that the granule cells are the general inhibitory interneuron in the olfactory bulb and that they mediate a kind of Renshaw inhibition, but by a different type of local synaptic pathway. I would not have had the temerity myself to stick my neck out in so many directions, but as each point came up in our discussions, Wil assessed it on its merits. We did have the advantage that between us we had a good grasp of the relevant biophysical and physiological literature; my training at Oxford had emphasized the classical antomical literature as well, and Tom and Milton gave us the current coverage of the relevant fine structure. The discussion therefore attempted to place the new findings within a synthesis of these overlapping fields.

It is fair to say that the two papers had a mixed reception. Eccles, despite his opposition to the Rall model of the motoneuron, was characteristically enthusiastic about new data, and he organized a symposium for the 1968 FASEB meeting in Atlantic City on the new evidence regarding synaptic organization, at which Dowling and I spoke. Frank Schmitt included talks by both Wil and myself at the NRP meeting in Boulder in

1969. Roger Nicoll's paper in 1969 on the electrophysiology of the olfactory bulb provided important early support for the model. But physiologists have generally been slow to assimilate the results because of the difficulties of analyzing dendritic properties; for example, after almost 30 years there is not yet clear evidence regarding the functions of the reciprocal synapses in the retina.

Wil and I had intended to pursue further studies together to test the reciprocal model, but the problem with his cataracts made this impossible. In the middle 1970s I therefore began a collaboration with Robert Brayton, a mathematician then at the IBM Watson Research Center, that resulted in a more detailed simulation of the reciprocal dendrodendritic synaptic circuit (Shepherd and Brayton 1979). The significance of this work for subsequent studies of active properties of dendrites and dendritic spines is discussed later in this volume. In 1978 we introduced the isolated turtle brain preparation and applied it to analysis of the synaptic circuits in the olfactory bulb (Nowycky et al. 1978; Mori and Shepherd 1979). This led to direct physiological testing for the reciprocal circuit (Mori et al. 1981); the results of Jahr and Nicoll (1982) were especially convincing in providing evidence from intracellular recordings and pharmacological manipulations for both reciprocal and lateral inhibition.

It was the anatomists who were most immediately influenced by the work. The anatomical findings gave a clear image of the new type of dendritic synaptic organization and served as the model, along with the similar findings in the retina, for the studies just opening up on the synaptic organization of many brain regions. Famiglietti and Peters (1971), Morest (1971), and Ralston (1971) were among the pioneers who showed that presynaptic dendrites are not peculiar to the olfactory bulb and retina but are components of normal circuits in different thalamic relay nuclei. The generality of the findings and interpretations here and in other regions of the nervous system stimulated me to gather the new evidence into a book on the new field of synaptic organization (Shepherd 1974). The term *local circuit* was introduced by Pasko Rakic (1976) to apply to neural organization at this regional level, and the dendrodendritic connections and interactions were the prototype covered by the term *microcircuit*, which was introduced to apply to the most confined and specific of the local circuits (Shepherd 1978).

Although the confirmation of our findings and the general acceptance of the interpretation were gratifying, there is a sense in which Wil, as senior author on this work, has never received the credit that was due. It was a pioneering study, using methods largely developed by him, that, together with the work on the motoneuron, laid the foundations for the field of computational neuroscience. It led to the discovery of a new type of function of neuronal dendrites. And the findings required revision in fundamental concepts, dating from Cajal, of how neurons are organized. The lack of recognition may be due in part to the fact that the new findings introduced new complexities into understanding the rules of neuronal organization, and the time was simply not yet ripe for a new synthesis that could be readily grasped by experimental neuroscientists. It may also reflect the general tendency of theoretical neuroscientists to ignore the importance of dendritic functions. And it may be because Wil Rall is a modest person who feels the evidence should speak for itself.

References

Andres, K. H. (1965). Der Feinbau des Bulbus Olfactorius der Ratte unter besonderer Berucksichtigung der synaptischen Verbindungen. *Z. Zellforsch.* 65:530–561.

Famiglietti, E. V. Jr., and Peters, A. (1971). The synaptic glomerulus and the intrinsic neuron in the dorsal lateral geniculate nucleus of the cat. *J. Comp. Neurol.* 144:285–334.

Goldstein, S. S., and Rall, W. (1974). Changes of action potential shape and velocity for changing core conductor geometry. *Biophys. J.* 14: 731–757.

Green, J. D., Mancia, M., and Baumgarten, R. (1962). Recurrent inhibition in the olfactory bulb. 1. Effects of antidromic stimulation of the lateral olfactory tract. *J. Neurophysiol.* 25:467–488.

Hirata, Y. (1964). Some observations on the fine structure of the synapses in the olfactory bulb of the mouse, with particular reference to the atypical configuration. *Arch. Histol. Japan* 24:293–162.

Jahr, C. E., and Nicoll, R. A. (1982). An intracellular analysis of dendrodendritic inhibition in the turtle in vitro olfactory bulb. *J. Physiol.* (*London*) 326:213–234.

Morest, D. K. (1971). Dendrodendritic synapses of cells that have axons: The fine structure of the Golgi type II cell in the medial geniculate body of the cat. *Z. Anat. Entwickl.-Gesch.* 133:216–246.

Mori, K., Nowycky, M. C., and Shepherd, G. M. (1981). Analysis of synaptic potentials in mitral cells in the isolated turtle olfactory bulb. *J. Physiol.* 314:295–309.

Mori, K., and Shepherd, G. M. (1979). Synaptic excitation and long-lasting inhibition of mitral cells in the *in vitro* turtle olfactory bulb. *Brain Res.* 172:155–159.

Nicoll, R. A. (1969). Inhibitory mechanisms in the rabbit olfactory bulb: Dendrodendritic mechanisms. *Brain Res.* 14:157–172.

Nowycky, M. C., Waldow, U., and Shepherd, G. M. (1978). Electrophysiological studies in the isolated turtle brain. *Soc. Neurosci. Absts.* 4:583.

Phillips, C. G., Powell, T. P. S., and Shepherd, G. M. (1961). The mitral cells of the rabbit's olfactory bulb. *J. Physiol.* 156:26–27.

Phillips, C. C., Powell, T. S., and Shepherd, G. M. (1963). Response of mitral cells to stimulation of the lateral olfactory tract in the rabbit. *J. Physiol.* 168:65–88.

Rakic, P. (1976). *Local Circuit Neurons.* Cambridge, Mass: MIT Press.

Rall, W. (1964). Theoretical significance of dendritic trees for neuronal input-output relations. In *Neural Theory and Modeling* ed. R. F. Reiss. Palo Alto: Stanford University Press.

Rall, W., and Shepherd, G. M. (1968). Theoretical reconstruction of field potentials and dendrodendritic synaptic interactions in olfactory bulb. *J. Neurophysiol.* 31:884–915.

Rall, W., Shepherd, G. M., Reese, T. S., and Brightman, M. W. (1966). Dendrodendritic synaptic pathway for inhibition in the olfactory bulb. *Exp. Neurol.* 14:44–56.

Ralston, H. J. III (1971). Evidence for presynaptic dendrites and a proposal for their mechanisms of action. *Nature* 230:585–587.

Shepherd, G. M. (1963a). Responses of mitral cells to olfactory nerve volleys in the rabbit. *J. Physiol.* 168:89–100.

Shepherd, G. M. (1963b). Neuronal systems controlling mitral cell excitability. *J. Physiol.* 168:101–117.

Shepherd, G. M. (1974). *The Synaptic Organization of the Brain.* Oxford: Oxford University Press.

Shepherd, G. M. (1978). Microcircuits in the nervous system. *Scientific American.* 238:92–103.

Shepherd, G. M., and Brayton, R. K. (1979). Computer simulation of a dendrodendritic synaptic circuit for self- and lateral inhibition in the olfactory bulb. *Brain Res.* 175:377–382.

Yamamoto, C., Yamamoto, T., and Iwama, K. (1963). The inhibitory system in the olfactory bulb studied by intracellular recording. *J. Neurophysiol.* 26:403–415.

Supplemental Comments by Milton Brightman

Our first meeting with Wil, about 30 years ago, here at the NIH, was prompted by Tom Reese's superb electron micrographs of the rat olfactory bulb. The microscopy lab was situated in the basement of Building 9 in what had originally been a plumbing shop. The light was not always adequate and the micrographs were still being rinsed, but I was struck by the image of a single neuronal process that, according to the location of synaptic vesicles, was postsynaptic at one point and presynaptic at another. We were both excited about this unique arrangement.

A short time later, Tom told me that we were to meet with two physiologists who were keenly interested in the finding. It was then that I first met Wil Rall and Gordon Shepherd. Their enthusiasm about what we had seen was very evident as they explained the functional significance of these peculiarly arranged synaptic contacts and how they could account for lateral inhibition in the olfactory cortex. It was the joy with which Wil told us of the implications, as much as anything, that encouraged us to look further.

Dendrodendritic Synaptic Pathway for Inhibition in the Olfactory Bulb (1966), *Exptl. Neurol.* **14:44–56**

Wilfrid Rall, G. M. Shepherd, T. S. Reese, and M. W. Brightman

Anatomical and physiological evidence based on independent studies of the mammalian olfactory bulb points to synaptic interactions between dendrites. A theoretical analysis of electric potentials in the rabbit olfactory bulb led originally to the conclusion that mitral dendrites synaptically excite granule dendrites and granule dendrites then synaptically inhibit mitral dendrites. In an independent electron micrographic study of the rat olfactory bulb, synaptic contacts were found between granule and mitral dendrites. An unusual feature was the occurrence of more than one synaptic contact per single granule ending on a mitral dendrite; as inferred from the morphology of these synaptic contacts, a single granule ending was often presynaptic at one point and postsynaptic at an adjacent point with respect to the contiguous mitral dendrite. We postulate that these synaptic contacts mediate mitral-to-granule excitation and granule-to-mitral inhibition. These dendrodendritic synapses could provide a pathway for both lateral and self inhibition.

Introduction

The purpose of this paper is to bring together two recent but independent lines of evidence which suggest that there is synaptic interaction, in both directions, between the dendrites of mitral cells and the dendrites of granule cells in the mammalian olfactory bulb. By means of these synapses, mitral cell dendrites would excite granule cell dendrites, and granule cell dendrites would then inhibit mitral cell dendrites. The morphological evidence is from an electron micrographic study of the olfactory bulb (Reese and Brightman), while the physiological argument arose originally from a theoretical analysis (Rall and Shepherd) of electric potentials obtained from recent physiological studies on the olfactory bulb (15, 16).

Anatomy

Figure 1 emphasizes, for our purposes, the form and relations of the large mitral cells as seen in Golgi preparations (19). Each mitral cell has

Figures 1 and 3 were drawn by Mrs. G. Turner.

a radial, primary dendrite which receives the incoming fibers from the olfactory epithelium, and several tangential, secondary dendrites which form an external plexiform layer. Into this layer come also many branches of radial dendrites from numerous deeper lying granule cells. These

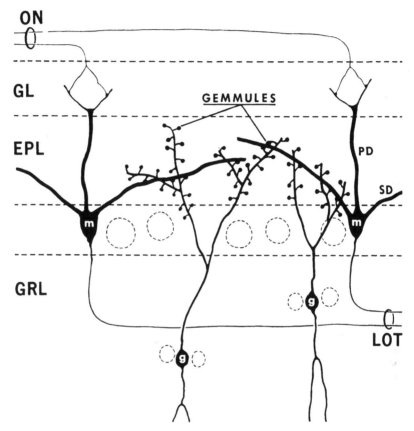

FIG. 1. Layers and connections in the olfactory bulb (adapted from Cajal, 19). GL, glomerular layer; EPL, external plexiform layer; GRL, granular layer; ON, olfactory nerve; LOT, lateral olfactory tract; g, granule cell; m, mitral cell; PD, primary mitral dendrite; SD, secondary mitral dendrite.

branches are studded with gemmules (Golgi spines) which make many contacts with the mitral secondary dendrites. Mitral dendrites resemble dendrites of other multipolar neurons in being distinctly wider than the axon, and in emerging as multiple trunks, whereas the axon is single.

Granule cell dendrites resemble certain other dendrites in bearing gem-mules and being profusely branched.

Methods. Rats weighing 200-250 g were perfused through the heart with a solution of 1% OsO_4 in isotonic sodium phosphate at pH 7.0, and the olfactory bulbs were prepared for electron microscopy by conventional techniques. In order to identify cell processes, it was important to know both the region of the bulb and its orientation in each electron micrograph. This was achieved by embedding large coronal slices of olfactory bulb and sectioning them for electron microscopy only after they were ex-amined with the light microscope. The electron microscopic results are here limited to the deeper regions of the external plexiform layer where most of the large tangential dendrites are from mitral cells. A few of these dendrites, however, are from deep lying tufted cells.

Results. Mitral and granule cell dendrites were easily identified in elec-tron micrographs by comparing their appearance with that in previously available Golgi preparations (19). The mitral secondary dendrites were the only large processes in the external plexiform layer with a tangential and a rostral-caudal orientation (22), while the granule cell dendrites were smaller and had a radial orientation, perpendicular to the mitral dendrites. The mitral secondary dendrites were studded with numerous synaptic endings which were thought to be mostly gemmules from granule cells because their ubiquity corresponded to that of the gemmules in Golgi preparations. Also, in favorable sections (Fig. 2) and in an accurate re-construction of one series of sections (Fig. 3) these endings were shaped like gemmules and arose from a radially oriented granule cell dendrite.

Each granule ending made one or more typical synaptic contacts with a single mitral dendrite and each synaptic contact consisted of a region of increased density and separation of the apposed cell membranes form-ing a cleft filled with a fibrillar dense material. Also part of each synaptic contact was a cluster of vesicles closely applied to the cytoplasmic side of either the mitral or granule cell membrane. These synaptic contacts there-

FIG. 2. Electron micrograph showing many synaptic endings on mitral secondary dendrites (large circular outlines) in the external plexiform layer of the rat olfactory bulb. One of the endings, a gemmule containing many vesicles, is in the center. A fortuitous plane of section along the axis of a granule cell dendrite (photographically darkened) demonstrates the continuity of this dendrite with the gemmule. Although this gemmule contains synaptic vesicles, no synaptic contacts are shown clearly in this plane of section. Lead citrate; $\times$ 20 000.

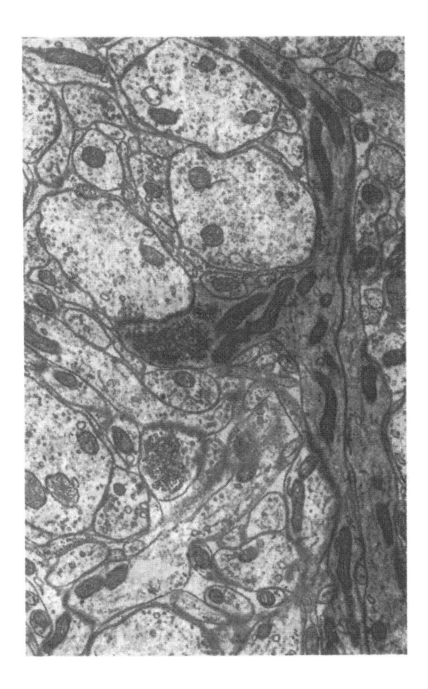

fore closely resembled synaptic contacts in other parts of the central nervous system (6, 14). However, the granule endings on mitral dendrites differed from typical synaptic endings in that two separate synaptic contacts with *opposite* polarities were often found side by side in the same

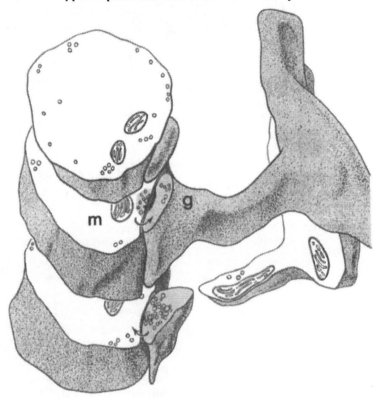

FIG. 3.   Graphical reconstruction (12) of a granule synaptic ending (g) on a mitral secondary dendrite (m). The granule ending is shaped like a gemmule and arises from a granule dendrite lying approximately perpendicular to the mitral dendrite. Within a single ending are two synaptic contacts with opposite polarities (indicated by arrows). The reconstruction was made directly from a series of tracings of twenty-three consecutive electron micrographs; no sections are omitted in showing cut surfaces. Microtubules and endoplasmic reticulum are not shown. × 20 000.

ending (arrows, Fig. 3 and 4). This interpretation of polarity was made by analogy with synapses in other regions of the central nervous system where polarity depends on a grouping of vesicles at the dense segment of the presynaptic membrane (14); this interpretation implies that there is both mitral-to-granule and granule-to-mitral synaptic transmission. That many of the granule endings appeared to make only one synaptic contact with a mitral dendrite could depend on the part of the ending sectioned (Fig. 3).

Another consistent difference in structure which correlated with the polarity of a synaptic region was a dense, filamentous material typically

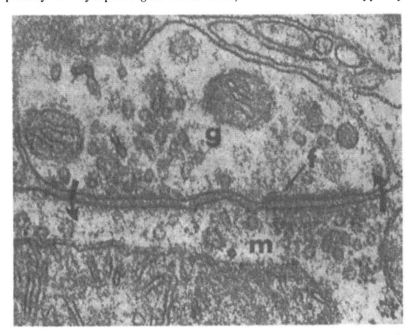

Fɪɢ. 4. A mitral secondary dendrite (m) and one of the many synaptic endings (g), presumed to be gemmules from granule cells. There are two synaptic contacts with opposite polarities (indicated by arrows). Where the polarity is from the mitral dendrite to the granule dendrite (as judged by the grouping of vesicles), a dense filamentous material (f) is attached to the postsynaptic cell membrane. Lead citrate; × 90 000.

attached to the postsynaptic cell membrane at the mitral-to-granule synaptic contacts (Fig. 4, f). In this respect, these synaptic contacts are analogous to those in axodendritic synapses in cortical areas, while the absence of a postsynaptic dense material at the granule-to-mitral synaptic contacts makes them more analogous to those in axosomatic synapses (6). Mitral-to-granule synaptic contacts also differed from granule-to-mitral contacts in having fewer vesicles near the presynaptic membrane and in having a wider synaptic cleft. These structural differences suggest that a different function is associated with each of the two kinds of synaptic contact.

Physiology

Independent evidence for the existence and nature of connections between mitral and granule dendrites has come from electrophysiological studies of the rabbit's olfactory bulb. A weak electric shock to the lateral olfactory tract sets up an impulse volley in some axons of the mitral cells, and these mitral cells are then invaded antidromically. The mitral cells which have not been invaded may nonetheless be inhibited for 100 msec or more following the volley, and during this period, the mitral cell membrane is hyperpolarized. The variable latency of onset of the inhibition in individual mitral cells, together with its prolonged duration, suggested an interneuronal pathway between the stimulated mitral cells and their inhibited neighbors. In view of the anatomical data available at that time, it was proposed that the granule cells function as inhibitory interneurons. It was assumed that mitral axon collaterals would excite the granule cells (presumably at their deep lying dendrites and cell bodies), and that granule cell activity would then deliver synaptic inhibition to the mitral dendrites (16, 21, 26).

The new concept, that mitral secondary dendrites deliver synaptic excitation directly to granule dendrites, arose from a theoretical study in which mathematical computations were adapted specifically to a reconstruction of the electric potential distribution in the olfactory bulb following a strong shock to the mitral axons in the lateral olfactory tract. The potential pattern, as a function of both time and depth in the bulb, is very clear and reproducible (13, 16, 24) (Fig. 5).

Methods. Extensive computations were performed on a Honeywell 800 digital computer. These were based upon the mathematical neuron models presented elsewhere (17, 18). In adapting these models to the present problem, special attention was given to the concentric laminar arrangement of the mitral and granule cell populations in the olfactory bulb. Also, computations were used to assess the theoretical parameters corresponding to

---

Fig. 5. Tracings of experimental recordings from rabbit's olfactory bulb following a strong shock to the mitral axons in the lateral olfactory tract (16). Periods I, II and III are indicated at top; the time from stimulus is shown at bottom. The depth of microelectrode penetration into the bulb is given at left, for each tracing; GL, glomerular layer; EPL, external plexiform layer; MBL, mitral body layer; GRL, granule

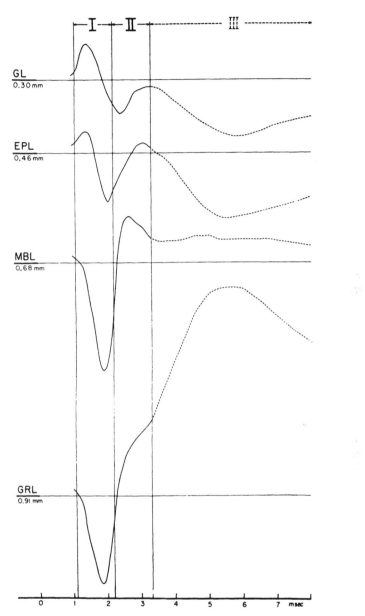

layer. Positivity of microelectrode, relative to a distant reference electrode, is upwards. Dashes distinguish period III, which we attribute primarily to granule cells, from periods I and II, which we attribute primarily to mitral cell activity.

dendritic electrotonic length, dendritic facilitation, active and passive membrane properties, axon-soma-dendritic safety factor, and the effective location of the reference electrode along a potential divider which bridges across the bulbar layers.

Results and Interpretations. To facilitate a brief description of these potentials and the interpretation derived from the reconstructions, we designate three successive time periods in Fig. 5. During period I, there is a brief negativity deep in the bulb, coupled with a positivity at its surface. This can be attributed primarily to flow of extracellular current from mitral dendrites to mitral cell bodies during the active depolarizing phase of synchronous action potentials in the mitral cell bodies. During period II, there is a brief deep positivity coupled with a brief surface negativity; this can be attributed primarily to flow of extracellular current from repolarizing mitral cell bodies to mitral dendrites which have been depolarized, either by passive electrotonic spread, or by active impulse invasion from the cell bodies.

During period III, there is a large positivity centered deep in the granule layer of the bulb, together with a large negativity centered in the external plexiform layer. This implies a substantial flow of extracellular current from the depths of the granule layer radially outward into the external plexiform layer. The population of cells which generates this electric current must possess a substantial intracellular pathway for the return flow of current from the external plexiform layer, through the mitral body layer, into the depths of the granule layer. This requirement is satisfied by the large population of granule cells, but not by the mitral cells. Furthermore, the potential distribution during period III could be reconstructed by assuming that there is a strong membrane depolarization of the granule dendrites in the external plexiform layer, coupled with essentially passive membrane in their deeper processes and cell bodies.

Because this depolarization of granule dendrites would occur in the region of contact with many mitral dendrites, and at a time just after the mitral dendrites were depolarized, it was logical to postulate that the mitral secondary dendrites provide synaptic excitatory input which depolarizes granule dendrites. Furthermore, because period III corresponds with the onset of mitral cell inhibition, the granule dendritic depolarization is both well timed and well placed to initiate synaptic inhibitory input to the mitral dendrites. Thus, the theoretical study led us to expect that dendro-dendritic synaptic contacts would subsequently be found that could mediate both mitral-to-granule excitation and granule-to-mitral inhibition.

These have been discovered independently in electron micrographs of the mitral-granule endings as presented here. These findings also appear to be supported by other authors (1, 9).

Discussion

In summary, the sequence of events following impulse discharge in mitral cells is viewed as follows: Depolarization spreads from the mitral cell bodies into the mitral secondary dendrites; this membrane depolarization activates excitatory synapses which depolarize granule cell dendrites; the synaptic depolarization of granule dendritic membrane then activates granule-to-mitral inhibitory synapses. The resulting hyperpolarization and inhibitory effect in the mitral dendrites might be prolonged by sustained action of inhibitory transmitter.[2]

This schema suggests a pathway in which inhibition is mediated by nonpropagated depolarization of dendritic trees rather than by conduction, in the usual manner, through axons. Because these granule cells have no typical axons, it seems likely that they may function without generating an action potential. Computations with the theoretical model indicate that synaptic depolarization of the granule dendritic membrane can account for the observed potentials. However, we do not exclude the possibility that this depolarization could be augmented by a weak, active, local response. Neither can we completely exclude the possibility that the synaptic potential in the dendrites might cause occasional firing of impulses at the granule cell bodies. A nonpropagated depolarization of the deep-lying granule dendrites should produce a potential distribution opposite to that of period III; this situation has been previously reported and so interpreted (25). That graded amounts of granule dendritic depolarization could be responsible for graded release of inhibitory synaptic transmitter seems reasonable in view of experimental results obtained with presynaptic polarization at neuromuscular junctions (2, 11).

The granule cells can serve as inhibitory interneurons in a more general sense than in the schema proposed above, because their deeper lying processes receive input from several sources (19). Our emphasis upon the synaptic input in the external plexiform layer is not meant to exclude the importance of these other inputs in other situations. In fact, the granule

---

[2] Under conditions such as those in period III in Fig. 5, there is an additional inhibitory effect exerted upon the mitral cells. The extracellular current and potential gradient generated by the granule cells would have an anodal (hyperpolarizing) effect at the mitral cell bodies, coupled with a cathodal effect at the dendritic periphery.

cell is strategically situated to enable its inhibitory activity to represent an integration of several inputs.

It has generally been assumed that dendrites do not occupy presynaptic positions. However, in the olfactory bulb, both granule and mitral dendrites have pre- as well as postsynaptic relationships to each other. This feature is also found in the glomeruli of the olfactory bulb where dendrites, which are postynaptic to palisades of incoming axons, are presynaptic to other structures (20). Expanding the concept of dendrites to include pre- as well as postsynaptic functions adds new possibilities in the interpretation of sequences of synaptic contacts found elsewhere in the nervous system where an ending which is presynaptic to one process is postsynaptic to another (3, 7, 10, 23). For example, such a sequence of synaptic contacts might include a dendrodendritic rather than an axoaxonic contact. Because the morphological evidence for presynaptic inhibition has depended on the identification of axoaxonic synaptic contacts, some of this evidence may need re-examination.

It has long been recognized that the retinal amacrine cell and the olfactory granule cell are very similar with respect to external morphology (19). Recent findings in the retina indicate that arrangements of synaptic contacts there are similar to those in the olfactory bulb and involve the amacrine cells which, like the granule cells, lack an axon (5, 10). It will be interesting, therefore, to see whether the amacrine cells provide a similar dendrodendritic inhibitory pathway.

Because of the importance of adaptation and lateral inhibition in sensory systems (8), it is noteworthy that the mitral-granule dendrodendritic synapses provide an anatomical pathway for such inhibitory effects. From the Golgi preparations, it appears that the secondary dendrites of each mitral cell must contact the dendrites of many granule cells, and that each granule dendritic tree must contact the dendrites of many mitral cells. Thus, each time a mitral cell discharges an impulse, its dendrites deliver synaptic excitation to many neighboring granule dendritic trees, and these in turn, deliver graded inhibition to that mitral cell and many neighboring mitral cells. Such lateral inhibition can contribute to sensory discrimination by decreasing the level of *noisy* activity in mitral cells neighboring the activated mitral cells; also, the self-inhibition would limit the output of the activated mitral cells. When there is a widespread, intense sensory input, the entire granule cell population can exert an adaptive kind of inhibitory effect upon the entire mitral cell population. Such features are in accord with physiological findings (4). Interaction between the mitral and granule cell populations can also provide a basis for rhythmic phenomena; as the granule cell population begins to inhibit the mitral cell population, this begins to cut off a source of synaptic excitatory input to the granule cell population; later, as the level of granule cell activity subsides, this reduces the amount of inhibition delivered to the mitral cells, and permits the mitral cells to respond sooner to the excitatory input they receive.

References

1. ANDRES, K. H. 1965. Der Feinbau des Bulbus olfactorius der Ratte unter besonderer Berücksichtigung der synaptischen Verbindindungen. *Z. Zellforsch. Mikroskop. Anat.* **65**: 530-561.

2. CASTILLO, J., and B. KATZ. 1954. Changes in end-plate activity produced by pre-synaptic polarization. *J. Physiol. London* **124**: 586-604.

3. COLONNIER, M., and R. W. GUILLERY. 1965. Synaptic organization in the lateral geniculate nucleus of the monkey. *Z. Zellforsch. Mikroskop. Anat.* **62**: 333-355.

4. DOVING, K. B. 1964. Studies of the relation between the frog's electro-olfactogram (EOG) and single unit activity in the olfactory bulb. *Acta Physiol. Scand.* **60**: 150-163.

5. DOWLING, J., and B. B. BOYCOTT. 1966. Organization of the primate retina. *Cold Spring Harbor Symp. Quant. Biol.* (p. 38 in 1965 Abstracts).

6. GRAY, E. G. 1959. Axo-somatic and axo-dendritic synapses of the central cortex; an electron microscopic study. *J. Anat.* **93**: 420-432.

7. GRAY, E. G. 1962. A morphological basis for pre-synaptic inhibition? *Nature* **193**: 82-83.

8. HARTLINE, H. K., H. G. WAGNER, and F. RATLIFF. 1956. Inhibition in the eye of Limulus. *J. Gen. Physiol.* **39**: 651-673.

9. HIRATA, Y. 1964. Some observations on the fine structure of the synapses in the olfactory bulb of the mouse, with particular reference to the atypical synaptic configuration. *Arch. Histol. Okayama* [*Saibo Kaku Byorigaku Zasshi*] **24**: 293-302.

10. KIDD, M. 1962. Electron microscopy of the inner plexiform layer of the retina in the cat and pigeon. *J. Anat.* **96**: 179-187.

11. LILEY, A. W. 1956. The effects of presynaptic polarization on the spontaneous activity at the mammalian neuromuscular junction. *J. Physiol. London* **134**: 427-443.

12. MITCHELL, H., and J. THAEMERT. 1965. Three dimensions in fine structure. *Science* **148**: 1480-1482.

13. OCHI, J. 1963. Olfactory bulb response to antidromic olfactory tract stimulation in the rabbit. *Japan. J. Physiol.* **13**: 113-128.

14. PALAY, S. L. 1958. The morphology of synapses in the central nervous system. *Exptl. Cell Res., Suppl.* **5**: 275-293.

15. PHILLIPS, C. G., T. P. S. POWELL, and G. M. SHEPHERD. 1961. The mitral cell of the rabbit's olfactory bulb. *J. Physiol. London* **156**: 26P-27P.

16. PHILLIPS, C. G., T. P. S. POWELL, and G. M. SHEPHERD. 1963. Responses of

mitral cells to stimulation of the lateral olfactory tract in the rabbit. *J. Physiol. London* **168**: 65-88.

17. RALL, W. 1962. Electrophysiology of a dendritic neuron model. *Biophys. J.* **2**: (No. 2, Part 2) 145-167.

18. RALL, W. 1964. Theoretical significance of dendritic trees for neuronal input-output relations, pp. 73-97. *In* "Neural Theory and Modeling." R. F. Reiss [ed.]. Stanford Univ. Press, Stanford, California.

19. RAMÓN Y CAJAL, S. 1911. "Histologie du Systéme Nerveux de l'Homme et des Vertébrés," L. Asoulay [trans.]. Maloine, Paris.

20. REESE, T. S., and M. W. BRIGHTMAN. 1965. Electron microscopic studies on the rat olfactory bulb. *Anat. Record* **151**: 492.

21. SHEPHERD, G. M. 1963. Neuronal systems controlling mitral cell excitability. *J. Physiol. London* **168**: 101-117.

22. SHEPHERD, G. M. 1966. The orientation of mitral cell dendrites. *Exp. Neurol.* **14**: (*in press*).

23. SZENTAGOTHAI, J. 1963. Anatomical aspects of junctional transformation, pp. 119-139. *In* "Information Processing in the Nervous System." R. W. Gerard [ed.]. Excerpta Medica, Amsterdam.

24. VON BAUMGARTEN, R., J. D. GREEN, and M. MANCIA. 1962. Slow waves in the olfactory bulb and their relation to unitary discharges. *Electroencephalog. Clin. Neurophysiol.* **14**: 621-634.

25. WALSH, R. R. 1959. Olfactory bulb potentials evoked by electrical stimulation of the contralateral bulb. *Am. J. Physiol.* **196**: 327-329.

26. YAMAMOTO, C., T. YAMAMOTO, and K. IWAMA. 1963. The inhibitory systems in the olfactory bulb studied by intracellular recording. *J. Neurophysiol.* **26**: 403-415.

5.3 Theoretical Reconstruction of Field Potentials and Dendrodendritic Synaptic Interactions in Olfactory Bulb (1968), *J. Neurophysiol.* 31:884–915

Wilfrid Rall and Gordon M. Shepherd

THE ORIGINAL OBJECTIVE of this research was to apply a mathematical theory of generalized dendritic neurons (36–39) to the interpretation and reconstruction of field potentials observed in the olfactory bulb of rabbit (32, 33). In the course of pursuing this objective, we were led to postulate dendrodendritic synaptic interactions which probably play an important role in sensory discrimination and adaptation in the olfactory system (40). More specifically, our initial aim was to develop a computational model, based on the known anatomical organization of the olfactory bulb and on generally accepted properties of nerve membrane, that could reconstruct the distribution of electric potential as a function of two variables, time and depth in the bulbar layers, following a synchronous antidromic volley in the lateral olfactory tract. The experimental studies of Phillips, Powell, and Shepherd (32, 33) had previously established that the recorded potentials at successive bulbar depths are highly reproducible and correlated with the histological layers of the bulb. These authors recognized the importance of this finding in relation to the symmetry and synchrony of activity in the mitral cell population; they deferred the interpretation of these potentials, in terms of specific neuronal activity, with a view to the present theoretical study.

METHODS

Physiological

The experiments were performed on young rabbits under urethan-chloralose or Nembutal anesthesia. The surgical procedures for exposing the olfactory bulb and lateral olfactory tract, and the details of the stimulating and recording techniques, have been previously described (33).

As illustrated in Fig. 1B, differences in extracellular potential were recorded between a focal penetrating microelectrode tip and a reference chlorided silver plate. The pipette tip was inserted through the successive layers of the olfactory bulb, whereas the silver plate was usually placed under the skin at the back of the head. Moving this reference electrode forward to the position indicated diagrammatically in Fig. 1B, or to the Ringer fluid in the craniotomy over the bulb, had little effect on the general pattern of the potentials recorded when the focal tip was well within the bulb. The pattern was also little affected when mineral oil replaced the Ringer fluid on the exposed dorsal surface of the bulb. The potential amplitudes were smaller with the Ringer fluid, and the amplitudes decreased predictably to zero if the interelectrode distance also decreased to zero.

The tract shocks were somewhat submaximal for the bulbar response in order to minimize the spread of stimulating current. As the shock strength was increased from threshold to maximal the responses changed in amplitude but not in general pattern. The recordings from neighboring electrode penetrations often varied in the relative amplitudes of different components of the responses but not in the general pattern. This variation appeared to be due in part to contributions from single units picked up by the microelectrode; a small back-and-forth adjustment of the microelectrode often reduced these contributions to negligible magnitudes.

Experiments in which the recording pipette penetrated first the dorsal hemisphere of the bulb and then continued on through the ventral hemisphere usually showed responses which were similar in pattern and magnitude, and the same held for recordings from the medial and lateral hemispheres of the bulb (cf. ref. 33, Plates 2 and 3). We conclude that roughly the same proportion of mitral cells per unit area of mitral body layer was invaded antidromically throughout most of the bulb. The synchrony of antidromic invasion in a given region of the bulb was indicated by the brevity and sharpness of the response. The great majority of unitary spikes recorded from the mitral cell layer during antidromic invasion occurred during the first millisecond of the evoked response, i.e., during period I of Fig. 4 below (33, 46).

The input from the recording electrodes was capacitor-coupled with a time constant of about 1 sec. This was long enough to ensure that there was negligible distortion of the relatively rapid potential responses in the period of a few milliseconds which was under study; it was short enough, on the other hand, to provide for accurate superimposition of successive responses on the oscilloscope screen. Tracings such as those in Figs. 3 and 4 were made from records in which 10 responses were superimposed at a rate of 1/sec.

Anatomical

The method for correlating the sequence of summed potential transients with the successive laminae of the bulb is fully described by Phillips et al. (33). Further studies of bulbar structure were carried out with material fixed in Bouin's fluid, embedded in paraffin, and stained with cresyl violet (49). The aim of these studies was to characterize the over-all symmetry of the bulb and to make quantitative estimates of the density and dimensions of the mitral cells for use in the computations, as described below.

The olfactory bulb, as its name implies, approximates in form to a sphere. Figure 1B shows that the bulbar cortex departs from spherical symmetry in being elongated in the anteroposterior axis and open at its posterior connection to the telencephalon; also at its posterodorsal surface it is replaced by the accessory olfactory bulb. Within the bulb the mitral axons converge toward the ventral posterolateral surface to form the lateral olfactory tract, so that a volley of antidromic impulses fans out within the bulb to invade the spherical sheet of mitral cells roughly simultaneously. This applies particularly to the anterior and dorsal regions of the bulb, where our recordings were taken. The retrobulbar area is continuous with the deep granular layer of the bulb, and is more or less synonymous with the anterior olfactory nucleus. In mammals, the lateral part of this nucleus is considered to receive collaterals from mitral axons (27), and would therefore be invaded by an antidromic tract volley. The same would be true of the accessory olfactory bulb, which appears to project to the lateral olfactory tract (2). To the extent that the orientation and timing of current flows in these structures resembled those in the bulb the functional symmetry of the bulb would tend to be preserved.

The diameter of the bulb in young rabbits of the

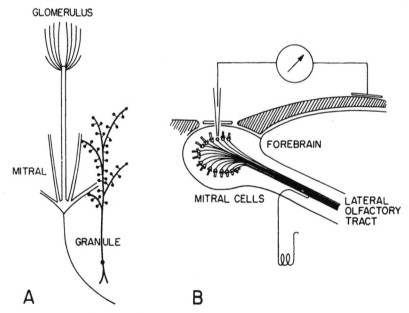

FIG. 1. *A:* schematic diagram of one mitral cell and one granule cell. The mitral primary dendrite ends in a dendritic tuft at the glomerulus; several mitral secondary dendrites extend away from the primary axis and are shown truncated. Granule dendrites are studded with gemmules (Golgi spines) which make contact with the dendrites of many neighboring mitral cells (not shown). *B:* experimental setup for electrical stimulation of lateral olfactory tract and microelectrode recording from the bulb; diagram indicates approximately spherical arrangement of the mitral cell layer, projection of mitral axons to lateral olfactory tract, and relation of the olfactory bulb to telencephalon.

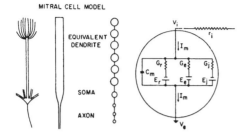

FIG. 2. Successive abstractions of mitral cell. From left: schematic primary and secondary dendrites; dendrites lumped as an equivalent cylinder (36–38); chain of compartments used to represent axon, soma, and dendrites. Enlarged single compartment at right shows the electrical equivalent circuit used to represent the lumped electric parameters of nerve membrane belonging to one compartment. Symbols designate: C_m = membrane capacity; G_r = resting membrane conductance; G_e = excitatory membrane conductance with E_e as the excitatory emf; G_j = inhibitory membrane conductance with E_j as the inhibitory emf; V_i = intracellular potential; V_e = extracellular potential; I_m = net membrane current; r_i designates intracellular core resistance between neighboring compartments.

size used in the physiological experiments was 3 to 4 mm in the transverse axis; a value of 2 mm for the bulbar radius provides a reasonable approximation. Along this radius the inner glomerular boundary lay at 0.3 mm and the mitral cell bodies at 0.7 mm from the outer surface, for the experiment depicted in Figs. 3 and 4. These were typical figures, and imply lengths of primary (or radial) mitral dendrites of some 400 μ. The diameters of the primary dendrites ranged from 2 to 10 μ, with an average of around 6 μ. The trunks of the mitral secondary dendrites are somewhat smaller, around 4 μ, in diameter; according to Cajal (41) they are ". . . two, three or more in number." From Cajal's diagrams of Golgi-stained sections one can see that these secondary dendrites divide several times, and that they often exceed the primary dendrite in over-all length. The secondary dendrites tend to run in the anteroposterior axis of the bulb (49). We are assuming that during antidromic invasion the radial component of extracellular current around the secondary dendrites summates approximately with the current around the primary dendrite, so that the whole mitral dendritic tree can be lumped together as a single equivalent cylinder (see Fig. 2).

From the classical work with the Golgi stain it has been known that the other main constituent of the external plexiform layer consists of branching dendritic processes from the granule cells; one of these is depicted schematically in Fig. 1A. There are many granule cells relative to mitral cells (cf. Fig. 3), and each granule cell branches profusely in the external plexiform layer. It could be assumed

therefore that most of the external plexiform layer is taken up by the granule cell dendritic branches and their dendritic spines; this has recently been borne out by electron micrographs (44, 45; also T. S. Reese, unpublished observations). Quantitative estimates related to the cell densities of both mitral and granule cell populations are presented in the section on RELATIVE RADIAL RESISTANCE ESTIMATES, below.

The existence of synapses between the mitral cell dendrites and the granule cell dendrites in the external plexiform layer was not known when we began this study, although the existence of many gemmules (Golgi spines) on the granule cell processes was known (41). Our theoretical computations and interpretations, as presented in RESULTS, led us to postulate unusual synaptic interactions between these dendrites in the external plexiform layer; we postulated mitral-to-granule synaptic excitation followed by granule-to-mitral synaptic inhibition. Subsequent to these computations and interpretations, the existence of pairs of oppositely oriented synaptic contacts between granule cell gemmules and mitral dendrites became known from independent electron microscopic studies (40, 44, 45; also 3, 18, and K. Hama, personal communication). Electron microscopy of serial sections (44 and Reese, personal communication) shows that granule cell processes account for the major part of the neuropil in the deep third of the external plexiform layer; glia is relatively rare; most synaptic endings (gemmules) contain granule-mitral synaptic contacts of opposite polarity; there are a few unidentified endings present on granule dendrites.

Besides the mitral and granule cells shown in Fig. 1A, the bulb contains two other main cell types: short-axon cells around the glomeruli, and tufted cells in the external plexiform layer just deep to the glomeruli. There is no clear anatomical evidence about the projection of tufted cell axons, whether to the telencephalon or confined within the bulb (51). In microelectrode experiments (32, 47) presumed tufted cells were activated synaptically after stimulation to the tract; these spikes occurred at variable latencies early in period III (see Fig. 4) of the evoked response. In view of their relatively asynchronous firing, and their short dendrites, we assume that the summed current flows around the tufted cells will be small enough so that they can be neglected for the purposes of the present reconstruction. Glomerular cells can similarly be neglected; their dendrites are short and bushy and haphazardly arranged; the main effect on them of tract stimulation was inhibition (47, 48).

It remains to be noted that in experiments like the present ones, employing shocks to the lateral olfactory tract, the possibility exists that centrifugal fibers in or near the tract might contribute to the bulbar response. Anatomical studies (6, 34), involving transection of the tract and the tracing of degenerating fibers into the bulb in Nauta preparations, have suggested that in the rat there is a small projection to the bulb from the olfactory tubercle or rostral part of the pyriform cortex. However in the present experiments the stimulating site was well out on the olfactory tract, lateral and caudal to these regions. Green et al. (15) made similar chronic transections of the tract just behind the bulb in cats and, using electric shocks to the tract on the bulbar side of the lesion, were unable to find any differences in the bulbar responses ascribable to a loss of centrifugal fibers. In view of the uncertainty about the centrifugal fibers, our analysis is based first on the known features of bulbar anatomy, and the obvious physiological consequences of these features. A possible small contribution for centrifugal fibers is discussed in connection with Figs. 13 and 14.

Relative radial resistance estimates

The precise dimensions and densities of the mitral cells and granule cells in the olfactory bulb are less important for our theoretical calculations than are certain order of magnitude estimates of relative resistance values for radial electric current flow in the olfactory bulb. Our original estimates of these relative resistance values were based upon a knowledge of the gross anatomy obtained from Golgi preparations; the most recent electron micrographs provide more detailed information, but do not change the orders of magnitude of these estimates.

For the mitral cell dendrites, we have estimated the ratio of extracellular to intracellular radial resistance to be of the order 1/20, while, for the mitral cell axon, we have estimated this ratio to be about 25 times smaller, or of the order 1/500; in contrast with these estimates, our estimate of this ratio for the granule cell dendrites is of the order 4/1. These estimates are so different from each other that a factor of 2 in uncertainty does not change their relative orders of magnitude. Here we shall attempt to give only a rough anatomical justification for such estimates.

If we treat the mitral body layer as a spherical surface of radius 1.3 mm, it has a surface area of about 20 mm^2. If the number of active mitral cells per bulb is between 20,000 and 40,000 (i.e., approximately 50–100% of the mitral cell population, cf. ref. 2) the amount of this spherical surface area per active mitral cell is between 500 and 1000 μ^2. For a spherical surface in the middle of the external plexiform layer (radius ca. 1.5 mm) these surface areas per active mitral cell become increased to almost 750 and 1,500 μ^2. A mitral primary dendrite, 6 μ in diameter, has a cross-sectional area of about 28 μ^2. Four secondary dendritic trunks having 4-μ diameters would have a

combined cross-sectional area of about 50 μ^2, but these trunks do not extend radially in the bulb. If, for simplicity, we assume that these secondary dendrites are oriented about 60° away from the radially oriented primary dendritic axis, the effective cross section for radial electric current must be reduced by the factor, cos (60°) = 1/2. When the reduced estimate of 25 μ^2 for these secondary dendritic trunks is added to the 28-μ^2 estimate for the primary dendrite, we obtain an estimated effective combined dendritic cross section for radially oriented intracellular electric current of 53 μ^2 for this mitral cell; values ranging from 25 μ^2 to 100 μ^2 seem reasonable, and a value of 50 μ^2 can be regarded as a reasonable order of magnitude estimate for the radial intracellular dendritic cross section per mitral cell. Compared with the values of 500–1,000 μ^2/mitral cell estimated above (second sentence of this paragraph), we obtain ratios for the intracellular to total radial cross section of 1/10–1/20 near the mitral body layer; for the larger radius at the middle of the external plexiform layer, the corresponding ratios are about 1/15–1/30.

Most of the cross-sectional area not occupied by mitral dendrites is occupied by granule dendrites; this is not truly extracellular, but it is available to conduct transient extracellular current generated by the mitral cells. This transient corresponds to a frequency of about 50 cycles/sec; for a granule cell membrane time constant of around 10 msec, this would imply a $\tau\omega$ value of about 30, which means that the capacitative membrane current would be about 30 times that across the membrane resistance. Thus, it can be calculated that the granule dendritic membrane adds relatively little to the impedance for this transient current (generated by mitral cells) that flows radially inside the granule cells; this impedance is primarily due to the resistivity of the granule cell intracellular medium. Because the granule cell processes are radially oriented, it is not necessary to increase the radial (longitudinal) impedance estimate by the factor of 3 derived by Ranck (42) for randomly oriented cylinders. It is not unreasonable to suppose that the intracellular to extracellular radial conductance ratio (for mitral cells) is approximately equal to the ratio of intracellular to total cross-sectional area estimated at the end of the preceding paragraph. From this it follows that a ratio 1/20 provides a reasonable order of magnitude estimate for the extracellular to intracellular resistance ratio for transient radial current generated by the mitral cells.

The mitral cell axon has a diameter of the order of 1 μ (2), and hence a cross-sectional area of about 1–2 μ^2. Compared with the combined dendritic effective radial cross section of around 50 μ^2/mitral cell, the axonal estimate is at least 25 times smaller. Near the mitral body layer, this implies an extracellular to intracellular radial resistance ratio of the order of 1/500.

We knew that granule cells are much more numerous than mitral cells (e.g., Fig. 3), and assumed that granule dendrites would be the most numerous processes in the external plexiform layer; thus, we had guessed that the ratio of extracellular to intracellular radial resistance is probably greater than unity, for granule cells. Electron microscopy of serial sections (44 and Reese, personal communication) shows, indeed, that the granule processes account for the major part of the neuropil in the deep third of the external plexiform layer. When seen in cross section, near the mitral body layer, the tightly packed granule dendrites have individual cross-sectional areas of from 0.1 to 1 μ^2, and the width of the extracellular space between neighbors is around 0.02 μ (approximate figures based on electron micrographs). If one simplifies this to a square lattice, one obtains a ratio for intracellular to extracellular cross-sectional area of $l^2/(2lw) = l/(2w)$, where l is the length of a side and w is the width of extracellular space. The values above thus give a range from 8/1 to 25/1 for this ratio of areas. These granule cell processes and spaces occupy a portion of the total cross section for radial current flow that we estimate to be of the order of 75% (based on examination of a few electron micrographs from the deep third of the external plexiform layer). How much of the remaining 25% is available to the radial extracellular current generated by the granule cell population is not known; presumably somewhere between 5 and 25% of total cross section is available. Thus the ratio of intracellular granule cell cross section to the effectively extracellular cross section probably lies between a low estimate of

$$(75 - 8)/(8 + 25) = 63/33 \simeq 2/1$$

and a high estimate of

$$(75 - 3)/(3 + 5) = 72/8 = 9/1$$

In the absence of specific knowledge of the resistivities of these media, we estimate the ratio of extracellular to intracellular radial resistance for the granule cell population as lying in this same range; this ratio can be expressed as having the order of magnitude 4/1.

Theoretical

The computational reconstructions are based on a theoretical model which actually consists of several component mathematical models. In previous publications (36–39) we have described and reviewed the development of these component models and have also provided several examples of computed results approximating experimental observations on cat motoneurons. The present computations differ from and go beyond the previous examples in several respects. *1*) Here the

specific values of the theoretical parameters of the general model are chosen to approximate mitral cells or granule cells instead of motoneurons. *2*) The compartmental model that was previously used to represent the electrotonic extent of the dendritic trees (38, 39) is here generalized to provide for geometrical and functional differences between the axonal, somatic, and dendritic regions of a neuron. *3*) In addition to the previously used mathematical model of passive nerve membrane and of synaptic excitation and inhibition, the present computations also incorporate a mathematical model which generates action potentials. This new component model is somewhat related to the well-known model of Hodgkin and Huxley (19), but it is computationally less expensive. The use of an active membrane model makes it possible to simulate impulse propagation in the axonal compartments and to simulate invasion of an impulse from axon to soma; it also makes it possible to compare theoretical predictions for the case of active as well as passive dendritic membrane. *4*) The computation of radially symmetrical extracellular field potentials for the olfactory bulb is quite similar, in several respects, to the computation of radially symmetrical extracellular potentials for a single multipolar motoneuron model (37); however, there is a very important new feature, discussed later (with Figs. 5, 6, and 7), which results from what is there described as the punctured spherical symmetry of the bulb.

Compartmental representation of neuron

The diagrams in Fig. 2 provide a schematic summary of three levels of abstraction of a mitral cell. The axon, soma, both primary and secondary dendrites, and the terminal dendritic tuft are shown schematically at far left. The next diagram shows all of the dendrites lumped into an equivalent cylinder with a transition at one end through soma to axon. The third diagram shows the equivalent dendrite represented as a chain of six equal compartments, linked to a smaller somatic compartment, which is itself linked to three still smaller axonal compartments. In most of the actual computations, the number of dendritic compartments was either 5 or 10. Each compartment represents a region of membrane surface for which the membrane capacity and the several parallel membrane conductances are treated as lumped electric parameters, as shown at right in Fig. 2; see (5, 9, 10, 19, 20, 36–39).

Mathematical representation of neuron

The chain of compartments in Fig. 2 is simply a diagram for what is actually a system of ordinary differential equations of first order (38, p. 84–87). For passive membrane, the equations are linear, with constant coefficients. For changing synaptic conductances that are voltage independent, the equations are still linear, but with some time-varying coefficients. For active membrane, the system is augmented by nonlinear differential equations. The basic first order differential equation for the ith compartment can be expressed in the following two alternative forms,

$$(dv_i/dt) = \mu_{ii}v_i + \sum_{j \neq i} \mu_{ij}v_j + f_i \qquad (1A)$$

or

$$(dv_i/dT) = -v_i + (1 - v_i)\mathcal{E}_i - (v_i - \beta_i)\mathcal{J}_i$$
$$+ \chi_i + \tau \sum_{j \neq i} \mu_{ij}(v_j - v_i) \qquad (1B)$$

where these symbols have been precisely defined previously (38), and will therefore be identified more descriptively here. The time derivatives, at left, are proportional to the rate of change of membrane potential in the ith compartment. The first equation distinguishes explicitly between the coefficients, μ_{ii} and μ_{ij}; in the coefficient matrix for this system of equations, the diagonal elements, μ_{ii}, all have negative values which yield the total rate of loss from the ith compartment; the off-diagonal elements, μ_{ij}, all have positive values which yield the rate of gain in the ith compartment due to flow of current from the jth compartment; also, f_i represents the forcing function for the ith compartment. The second equation shows the explicit dependence of this time derivative (where T $=t/\tau$) upon the variables $\mathcal{E}$, $\mathcal{J}$, and χ in the ith compartment, where

$$\mathcal{E} = G_e/G_r$$

expresses membrane excitation as the ratio of excitatory membrane conductance to the resting conductance (see Fig. 2), and

$$\mathcal{J} = G_i/G_r$$

expresses membrane inhibition as the ratio of inhibitory membrane conductance to the resting conductance (see Fig. 2); also χ represents any current that is applied directly to this compartment by means of electrodes, while the summation term represents net current flow to the ith compartment from its immediate neighbors. For passive membrane, $\mathcal{E}$ and $\mathcal{J}$ are both zero; for synaptic input to any compartment, the values of $\mathcal{E}$ and $\mathcal{J}$ are prescribed to express this input. For active membrane, the values of $\mathcal{E}$ and $\mathcal{J}$ have been determined by the following pair of nonlinear differential equations

$$d\mathcal{E}/dT = k_1v^2 + k_2v^4 - k_3\mathcal{E} - k_4\mathcal{E}\mathcal{J} \qquad (2)$$
$$d\mathcal{J}/dT = k_5\mathcal{E} + k_6\mathcal{E}\mathcal{J} - k_7\mathcal{J} \qquad (3)$$

where $\mathcal{E}$, $\mathcal{J}$, v, and T are all dimensionless variables, and the coefficients, k_1 through k_7, are all dimensionless constants. One of many possible sets of values for these seven coefficients found suitable for generating action potentials is the following: $k_1 = 500$; $k_2 = 20,000$; $k_3 = 25$; $k_4 = 0.2$; $k_5 = 5$; $k_6 = 0.05$; and $k_7 = 10$.

Active membrane models

The above equations have been found to generate a wide selection of well-shaped action potentials, and to display such basic properties as a sharp threshold, the expected relation of spike latency to stimulus strength, a refractory period, and at least a qualitative agreement with voltage clamp behavior. This model is conceptually related to the Hodgkin and Huxley (19) model in the general sense that an action potential results from a sequence of two transient changes in membrane conductance: a brief excitatory conductance increase, overlapped by a slightly later and longer lasting increase of an inhibitory or quenching conductance. Although the equations which generate these conductance transients differ significantly from the Hodgkin-Huxley equations, they do define a system which shares the general mathematical properties discussed by FitzHugh (11). The present model is defined in the domain of equivalent electric circuits of nerve membrane; it makes no explicit reference to ionic permeabilities and ionic concentration ratios. The following considerations indicate why this new model was used in preference to the well-established model of Hodgkin and Huxley: the numerical values of the Hodgkin-Huxley parameters have not been determined for mammalian nerve membrane, and would have to be guessed; the present computations are not concerned with manipulation of ionic media; the present computations explore complications of neuronal geometry and spatio-temporal pattern which themselves impose a significant computational load; and use of this simpler model makes it possible to avoid the heavy computational load that use of the Hodgkin-Huxley model would have imposed. A more detailed presentation and exploration of this new model will be presented elsewhere.

Computations

Computations were carried out on a Honeywell 800 computer (during 1963 and 1964) at the National Institutes of Health. The computer program was organized into two major divisions: A) The intracellular sequence of neuronal events, and B) the extracellular field potentials.

A. The sequence of neuronal events was generated by means of *equations 1–3*, above, for a compartmental neuron model of the type indicated by Fig. 2. Any particular computation requires that one assign numbers that specify the following: the number of compartments of each kind (usually three axonal, one somatic, and five or ten dendritic); the kinetic parameters (k_1 through k_7) for active membrane; the ratios representing the geometric hurdles (i.e., changes in safety factor) for propagation from axon-to-soma-to-dendrites; the amount of dendritic facilitation, which could be either in the form of synaptic excitation, $\mathcal{E}$, in the dendritic compartments, or as residual depolarization of the dendritic membrane; and the electrotonic length of the dendritic chain (usually between one-half and twice the characteristic length, λ, of the equivalent cylinder). The geometric relations between axon, soma, and dendrites determine the relative values chosen for the various coefficients, μ_{ij}, of *equation 1*. These coefficients can be defined

$$\mu_{ij} = g_{ij}/c_i$$

where g_{ij} represents the core conductance between adjacent compartments, i and j, and c_i represents the capacitance of the ith compartment. It is helpful to note that $g_{ij}(v_j - v_i)$ defines (by Ohm's law) the net current to compartment i from its neighbor, j, and that dividing this quantity by c_i gives the contribution to the rate of change, (dv_i/dt), due to this net current flow. For most of the mitral cell calculations the value of μ_{ij} between dendritic compartments was four times that between axonal compartments. The important hurdle ratio, $\mu_{sd}/\mu_{sa} = g_{sd}/g_{sa}$, where subscript, sd, means to soma from the nearest dendritic compartment, and subscript, sa, means to soma from the nearest axonal compartment, can be understood as the ratio of combined dendritic core conductance to axonal core conductance. A value of 40/1 was used in many of the calculations; values from 25/1 to 50/1 are implied by the radial resistance estimates of the preceding section.

An impulse once initiated in the most distal of the three axonal compartments would propagate successively to the second and third axonal compartments and then fail to invade the soma compartment, when a hurdle ratio (40/1) was used without any dendritic facilitation. Most of the computations overcame such antidromic block by adding some dendritic facilitation; a few computations were also done with a smaller hurdle ratio. Further details of this will be presented elsewhere.

B. The calculation of the extracellular field potentials from the sequence of intracellular and membrane potential transients generated in all compartments depends on the assumptions of bulbar symmetry and synchrony stated and discussed explicitly in PART II of the RESULTS. In the idealized spherical bulbar model we regard both the intracellular potential, V_i, and the extracellular potential, V_e, as functions of time and radial position, and we have the basic relation

$$\frac{\partial V_e}{\partial \rho} = - (r_e/r_i) \frac{\partial V_i}{\partial \rho}$$

where ρ represents radial position and r_e/r_i gives the ratio of extracellular to intracellular resistance per unit length in the radial direction. It should be noted that this ratio is not constant because r_e decreases with the increase in conical cross

section for increasing radial distance from the center, while r_i remains constant for an equivalent cylindrical dendrite. However, the extracellular field calculation was done in four stages, and during the first stage, this resistance ratio was treated as a constant, usually with a value around 0.05 for mitral dendrites, a value around 0.002 for mitral axons, and a value around 4 for granule cells; (cf. preceding section of METHODS for a justification of these values). The four stages of the extracellular field calculations will now be summarized for the case of the mitral cells.

B-1: First stage. For each time value, we computed

$$\Delta V_e = - 0.05 \Delta V_i$$

for the potential differences between dendritic compartments, from the terminal dendritic compartment up to and including the soma compartment, and we computed

$$\Delta V_e = - 0.002 \Delta V_i$$

from the soma compartment to successive axonal compartments. Using these ΔV_e, the value of V_e at each compartmental depth, relative to $V_e = 0$ at the dendritic terminals, was easily obtained.

B-2: Shunt current correction. When the secondary extracellular current (extra path shown in Figs. 5 and 6) was assumed to be a significant fraction of the total extracellular current, all of the ΔV_e were reduced by this fraction. This correction was omitted in most cases.

B-3: Cone correction. When it was decided to include the correction for the dependence of r_e upon radial position, this correction was introduced at this stage of the calculation.

B-4: Potential divider effect. For each time value and each compartment, V_e was reexpressed relative to the distant reference electrode. This correction is discussed in PART II of RESULTS in association with Fig. 5, and illustrated in PART III of RESULTS in association with Figs. 6 and 7. With the 1/4 potential divider ratio assumed for mitral cell extracellular current, this meant that for each time value an amount equal to one-fifth of the potential difference (V_e at the dendritic terminals, minus V_e at the soma) was added to the values of V_e obtained for each compartment by the previous stages (*B-1* through *B-3*).

Assumption of radial extracellular current

Even with the idealized symmetry and synchrony presented in PART II of RESULTS, it would not be strictly correct to assert that all of the extracellular current in the spherical bulb is radially oriented and that the isopotential surfaces are concentric spherical surfaces. This is because the extracellular current generated by each mitral cell must flow away from its principal axis out into the conical cross section before it can flow along radii of the spherical bulb. However, a good case can be made for neglect of this complication as unimportant to our main purpose; similar neglect is customary for considerations of the intracellular current flow in axons. If there were as few as 10 active mitral cells, symmetrically spaced in the bulb, the true isopotential surfaces would be expected to deviate significantly from spherical surfaces in the manner illustrated elsewhere (Fig. 9 of ref. 37); however, with many thousands of active mitral cells, it has been estimated that the almost spherical isopotential surfaces would be distorted only very slightly by many very small "dimples," one such dimple being centered upon each mitral cell axis; also, this dimpling would be smoothed by the effects of the secondary dendrites. Thus one can regard the departure of the bulb from simple spherical shells and radial extracellular current flow as unimportant to the present study, where the experimental data themselves suggest the radial dependence of the field potentials. All of the computations have been based upon this simplifying assumption.[1]

RESULTS

I. *Electrophysiological recordings to be interpreted*

A shock delivered to the lateral olfactory tract sets up a synchronous volley of impulses in the mitral cell axons. The impulses travel antidromically in the axons into the olfactory bulb, where they invade the bodies of the mitral cells (see Fig. 1). This activity generates extracellular current, and the microelectrode records the potential changes, relative to the reference electrode, caused by the summed current flow generated by the whole population of active mitral cells. Other cells within the bulb are also activated, of course, but the mitral cells are of first interest because they are the main cells in the bulb known to send their axons into the lateral olfactory tract, where electrical stimulation is applied. In the following reconstruction, therefore, current flow around other active elements will be discussed only after the mitral cells have been accounted for.

A typical sequence of recordings from the surface to the depth of an olfactory bulb is shown on the right in Fig. 3. On the left is

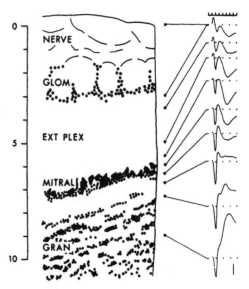

FIG. 3. Tracing of histological section of olfactory bulb, at left. Recorded extracellular potential responses to single volleys in the lateral olfactory tract are shown at right; each is connected to a dot showing position along electrode tract from which recording was obtained. Time scale for responses in msec; small dots show base line at 2-msec intervals. Depth scale at left in 100-μ divisions. Histological layers: olfactory nerve, glomeruli, external plexiform, mitral cell body, granule cell, after Phillips et al. (33). Vertical bar at lower right is 1 mv.

juxtaposed a tracing of a histological section containing the microelectrode path over which these records were obtained. The records are shown connected to the depths at which they were recorded, due allowance being made for distortions during the histological procedures (33). Each record begins with a short base line, followed by a gap indicating the artifact associated with the shock delivered to the lateral olfactory tract, and then a sequence of positive or negative potential deflections. Both the temporal and the spatial sequences are highly reproducible, and were used routinely, at the time of recording, to locate the depth of the recording pipette tip (32, 33, 46). Recordings similar to those in Fig. 3 have also been reported by von Baumgarten et al. (52) and by Ochi (30).

We now wish to focus attention on four recording depths which are most important for reconstructing with a theoretical model the sequence shown in Fig. 3. The critical depths are the layer of mitral cell bodies (MBL)

---

[1] In his analysis of the potential field in squid retina, Hagins (16) recognized and exploited the notion that the potential field becomes effectively one-dimensional when a population of suitably oriented cells is activated synchronously by a suitable stimulus.

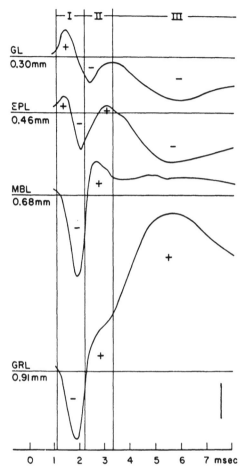

FIG. 4. Enlarged tracings, with faster sweep speed, of the most important potential transients of Fig. 3. Four depths are: GL = glomerular layer; EPL = external plexiform layer; MBL = mitral body layer; GRL = granule layer. Time scale is in msec; vertical lines divide these transient responses into time periods I, II, and III, as shown at top. Polarity, microelectrode potential relative to reference electrode potential, is indicated by + and − symbols. Vertical bar at lower right is 1 mv.

followed by a positive deflection, while the response at GL is similar but of opposite polarity; the response at an intermediate depth (EPL) is a triphasic (+ − +) sequence. From these features we designate three time periods which are crucial for the analysis of the mitral cell activity responsible for these potential transients. During period I there is in general a positive peak at GL and a negative peak at MBL. During period II there is a reversal to a negative peak at GL and a positive peak at MBL. These first two periods each last about 1 msec, and cover most of the duration of mitral cell activity. Period III then follows, from about 3.5–8 msec and beyond; during this period we infer (see PART IV of RESULTS) a dominance of granule cell potentials.

We wish to draw attention to the fact that, to a first approximation, the records at the origin and termination of the mitral dendrites (MBL and GL, respectively) are of similar time course but of opposite sign. In the theoretical treatment below a precise proportionality (with opposite sign) is predicted for that part of the response due to activity in the mitral cell bodies and dendrites. Deviations from a precise proportionality will be attributed to activity in other bulbar elements and in granule cells. This theoretical treatment thus avoids the common neurophysiological practice of treating the negative spike in Fig. 4 as an entity, to be followed through the successive layers and then assigned a conduction velocity. We will show instead that the GL negativity of period II can be regarded as a sign of soma membrane repolarization rather than a sign of arrival of depolarization at the dendritic periphery.

II. Importance of bulbar symmetry and synchrony

An attempt at understanding field potentials in the central nervous system should take full advantage of whatever geometric symmetry is provided by the anatomical structures and whatever synchrony of activity in the neuronal population can be obtained experimentally. Both the degree of symmetry in the rabbit olfactory bulb and the degree of synchrony in the above experiments provide one of the most favorable situations available for study in the mammalian central nervous system. Given these favorable conditions, one can entertain the notion of an idealized system

where the mitral dendrites arise; the glomerular layer (GL) where the primary dendrites terminate; an intermediate depth in the external plexiform layer (EPL) along the dendritic shafts; and also a deeper location in the granule layer (GRL). The records taken at these depths (in Fig. 3) are shown on a more expanded time base in Fig. 4, labeled accordingly. With this time resolution it can be seen that the initial part of the response at the MBL consists of a negative deflection having perfect symmetry and synchrony. Some of the general theoretical consequences of such an idealized system can then be explored and compared with general features of the experimental observations.

First, we imagine an idealized bulb with perfect spherical symmetry, in which the antidromic activation of the mitral cells is assumed to be perfectly synchronous. In this idealized bulb all of the mitral cells are equal in size; all have their cell bodies at the same distance from the center of the spherical bulb; and all have their primary dendritic axes oriented radially outward. The mitral cell bodies are equally spaced throughout the thin spherical shell (mitral body layer) which contains them. A two-dimensional schematic diagram of such radial symmetry is shown in Fig. 5A. The puncture of this spherical symmetry (corresponding to the connection of the olfactory bulb to the telencephalon) is indicated by Fig. 5B. In both diagrams a cone has been sketched in as a reminder of the three-dimensional aspect of our problem. Also, this cone suggests the element of bulbar volume associated with each active mitral cell. For N synchronously active mitral cells, we think of the entire spherical volume as divided into N equal volume elements. The axis of each volume element coincides with the radially oriented primary dendrite of one of the N mitral cells. These volume elements will sometimes be referred to as cones, and sometimes more

correctly as pyramids. Because the number. N, of active mitral cells is large, these cones should be thought of as mere slivers; e.g., $N = 25{,}000$ implies a solid angle of Ω $(4\pi/N)$ $\simeq 5 \times 10^{-4}$/cone; this implies an angle of less than $1°$ between the axis and the surface elements of the cone or pyramid.

FLOW OF CURRENT CONFINED WITHIN CONES. For the idealized bulb (with perfect spherical symmetry) we assume that each active mitral cell produces exactly the same flow of electric current into its associated volume element. Then an appreciation of the spherical symmetry and synchrony can lead one to an intuitive grasp of the consequence that the current produced by each of these cells must remain confined within its own volume element. At the surface of contact between neighboring (pyramidal) volume elements, the gradient of potential and hence the current flow are completely radial. The current is confined within each cone just as effectively as if we could dissect out a single volume element and place it in mineral oil; that is to say, the neurophysiological lore concerning the recording from axons in oil is more relevant to the present case than is the lore concerning the recording from axons in a volume conductor. This simplification, it should be emphasized, depends on both the symmetry and synchrony of this idealized case. For the purpose of the present computations, we have made the further simplifying

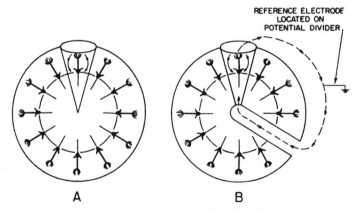

FIG. 5. A: schematic representation of idealized olfactory bulb, with perfect spherical symmetry and perfect synchronization of mitral activity. Radial current around one mitral cell is shown within its associated conic volume. B: puncture of ideal symmetry by connection of bulb to telencephalon; the small component of mitral-generated current which leaks out of the bulb and through the puncture is indicated by dashed line, along with position of reference electrode.

assumption that the extracellular current in the conical slivers can be regarded as uniformly radial (see METHODS).

PUNCTURE OF SPHERICAL SYMMETRY: EXTERNAL CURRENT PATH. We have two good reasons for considering the puncture of spherical symmetry. One is the simple anatomical fact that the olfactory bulb does not have a closed histological structure; the spheroidal cortical layers are punctured by the olfactory tract and by the retrobulbar area. However, this anatomical fact might conceivably have been of negligible importance to the over-all problem.

Our other reason for considering this puncture is that we have electrophysiological evidence for its significance. If the bulb were completely closed, with perfect spherical symmetry and synchrony as outlined above, mitral cell activity should cause no net flow of current outside the glomerular layer; in other words, the electric potential in the outer bulb (from the glomerular layer to the bulb surface) would remain constant and be isopotential with that at the distant reference electrode. This would be an example of the "closed field" characterized by Lorente de Nó (28, 29, 37). However, experimentally, we find that the recorded response at the bulb surface is not negligible, and is almost the same as at the glomerular layer (see outer two records of Fig. 3). In fact this surface record is roughly one-fourth as large (with opposite sign) as that obtained at the mitral body layer during periods I and II (see Fig. 4, and compare GL with MBL record). This is clearly not a closed field; the puncture and/or departures from perfect symmetry and synchrony have significantly changed the recording situation.

Stated briefly, the fact of puncture provides an extra path for electric current to flow between the depth of the bulb and the bulb surface; this path is in addition to and lies in parallel (electrically) with all of the conical slivers (see Fig. 5B). This extra path has a finite electrical resistance that can be viewed as part of a "potential divider." The electric potential difference between the bulb surface and the bulb depth is distributed along the resistance of this extra path, and the distant reference electrode is effectively located somewhere along this resistance; thus, the reference electrode divides the over-all potential difference into two parts.

POTENTIAL DIVIDER. We are concerned with current generated by each mitral cell body and its dendrites; the primary flow of current occurs between the GL and MBL levels of each cone; a relatively small amount of current flows through the extra path (Fig. 5B) that is part of the potential divider. The outer arm of this potential divider consists of a series combination of the following component resistances: the radial resistance (per cone) from outer glomerular layer through the olfactory nerve layer and the pia-arachnoid of the bulb; then the resistance (per cone) from the bulb surface through the cranial tissues which lie between the pia and the nearest point that is isopotential with the distant reference electrode. The inner arm of this potential divider consists of a different series combination of resistances: the radial resistance (per cone) from the mitral body layer inward to where the axons turn to join the lateral tract; then N times the resistance outward through the bulb puncture; then N times the resistance to the distant reference electrode. We have found it useful to think of the outer arm as having one-fourth the resistance of the inner arm.

EXAMPLE OF POTENTIAL DIVIDER EFFECT. Suppose that extracellular currents flowing between GL and MBL have caused the electric potential at MBL to be 2.5 mv negative relative to the potential at GL. This puts a potential difference of 2.5 mv across the potential divider. For a potential divider ratio of 1:4, there would be a potential drop of 0.5 mv over the outer arm and a potential drop of 2.0 mv over the inner arm. Relative to the distant reference point, the potential at GL must be 0.5 mv positive and the potential at MBL must be 2.0 mv negative. Once this example is understood it seems reasonable to interpret the opposite sign and the relative amplitudes of the experimental records at MBL and GL (during period I and II of Fig. 4) largely as consequences of this potential divider effect. This effect has been incorporated in the computations (stage B-4 of THEORETICAL METHODS).

COMMENT ON EXTRACELLULAR POSITIVITY. In answer to a possible objection that the 0.5 mv positivity at the glomerular layer can be understood simply as the familiar positivity recorded near an axonal source of current in a volume conductor, we would draw attention again to the significance of the spherical symmetry of the population in Fig. 5*A*; for this closed field (28, 29, 37) every mitral dendrite would be a source of current and yet the extracellular potential (relative to a distant electrode) would be zero at the GL depth, and it would be negative, not positive, among the dendrites in the EPL. For punctured symmetry, the distant electrode is no longer isopotential with the bulb surface; it lies on the extra path for current flow from the bulb surface to the depths of the bulb. The fact that there is no path for current flow directly from the distant electrode to points along the conical volume elements provides the essential distinction between this case and the familiar case of an axon in a volume conductor.

COMMENT ON SMALLER REGIONS OF SYNCHRONOUS ACTIVITY. If one were to increase the size of the puncture, or to decrease the portion of the spherical layer in which synchronous activation takes place, the direction of change in the potential divider ratio is easily predicted: the resistance of the inner arm of the potential divider would be decreased; hence the ratio of the outer to inner arm resistance would be increased. To at least a first approximation, this approach could be applied to cortical regions substantially smaller than hemispheric shells; the principal requirement would be reasonable synchrony and reasonably uniform density of many active units over the region in question. Then, except for the units near the boundary of this region, it is still approximately true that there is a conical volume element associated with each active unit and that there is no path for current flow directly from the distant electrode to points along the conical volume elements. Thus, we expect that this approach is applicable to cases of partial activation of the olfactory bulb, and that it will also be useful in the study of other cortical populations of neurons in the central nervous system.

III. *Computations for synchronous antidromic activation of mitral cell population*

NEUROPHYSIOLOGICAL SEQUENCE OF MEMBRANE POTENTIAL TRANSIENTS. The computations are designed to represent the following sequence of neurophysiological activity in each of the synchronously active mitral cells: an impulse propagates antidromically along each mitral cell axon to the axon-hillock region; although

the mitral soma membrane depolarization is slowed by the dendritic load, it finally does reach threshold and fire an action potential; this is followed by a spread of membrane depolarization out into the dendrites either rapidly and without decrement in the case of active dendritic membrane, or more slowly and with some electrotonic decrement in the case of passive dendritic membrane.

This sequence of events is generated by a mathematical model that is based on well-known electrical properties of nerve membrane and on available anatomical and physiological knowledge of the relation between axon, soma, and dendrites. Although more details are given below (and in METHODS), a point to be emphasized here is that the mathematical model begins with a representation of basic neurophysiological properties and generates a sequence of events that would reasonably be expected to occur in a representative mitral cell.

DISTINCTION BETWEEN MEMBRANE POTENTIAL AND EXTRACELLULAR POTENTIAL. Because some neurophysiological literature fails to distinguish clearly between membrane potential transients and extracellular potential transients, it seems wise to emphasize the distinction here. A membrane potential transient that takes place uniformly over the entire membrane surface of a neuron would generate no extracellular current flow and would therefore generate no extracellular potential transient. A nonuniformity of membrane potential, as between soma and dendrites, generates a loop of current flow that is partly intracellular and partly extracellular; thus, if the soma membrane is more depolarized than the dendritic membrane, intracellular current flows from soma to dendrites, whereas extracellular current flows from dendrites to soma. The recorded extracellular potential represents the difference, ΔV_e, measured between two recording electrodes placed in a field of extracellular current flow. With various special recording arrangements, this ΔV_e can bear various relations to the transient nerve membrane potential, V_m, at the region of interest; ΔV_e can be made essentially proportional either to V_m itself, to its first time derivative, or to its first or second derivative with respect to distance along the nerve axis; in general, ΔV_e is proportional to none of these. The essential logic is this: nonuniform membrane activity

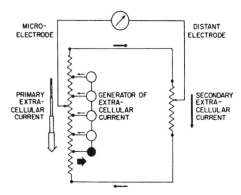

MICRO-
ELECTRODE

DISTANT
ELECTRODE

PRIMARY
EXTRA-
CELLULAR
CURRENT

GENERATOR OF
EXTRA-
CELLULAR
CURRENT

SECONDARY
EXTRA-
CELLULAR
CURRENT

FIG. 6. Diagram showing the relation of the recording electrodes to the extracellular current generated by a mitral cell at moment of active inward soma membrane current (heavy black arrow); dendritic membrane current is outward. The primary extracellular current flows radially from dendrites to soma. The smaller, secondary extracellular current flows out through surrounding structures and back through the bulbar puncture. Distant electrode acts as potential divider along external resistance path; microelectrode acts as potential divider along internal radial resistance path.

of a neuron generates extracellular current; this extracellular current, together with that generated by other neurons, sets up a field of extracellular current flow; the details of this field depend on the geometric arrangement of the cells, their degree of synchrony or asynchrony, and the shape and possible inhomogeneity of the volume conductor; finally, the recorded extracellular potential transient depends on the location of both electrodes in this field.

COMPUTATION OF EXTRACELLULAR TRANSIENTS. The computational sequence has been outlined in METHODS. A general understanding of the computed results can be obtained by a study of Figs. 6 and 7. In Fig. 6 the chain of compartments represents the soma and dendrites of a mitral cell; the open circles represent dendritic compartments, while the filled circle represents the soma compartment at the time (period I) of active inward membrane current. The black arrows show the direction of membrane current at each compartment: inward at the soma, outward from the dendrites. The open arrows show the direction of extracellular current flow. The primary extracellular current flows from dendrites to soma (radially inward in the bulb). The secondary extracellular current

flows outward along the external resistance path and back through the bulbar puncture. As shown in Fig. 6, the distant reference electrode taps the potential drop along the secondary pathway, whereas the microelectrode taps the potential drop along the primary (radial) pathway. With the help of this diagram we can now explain the relation between the three columns of computed results shown in Fig. 7.

The transients shown in Fig. 7 provide an overview of a complete set of computed results. The transient at lower left is the intracellular action potential at the soma, following antidromic propagation through the axonal compartments. The dendrites are here assumed to be passive and are represented by compartment numbers 5 through 9. The intracellular transients at two dendritic locations, 6 and 9, illustrate the delay and attenuation of passive electrotonic spread from the soma into the dendrites, primarily during periods I and II.

As outlined in METHODS, the radial gradient of intracellular potential is used to compute the radial gradient of extracellular potential. If the reference electrode were placed near the dendritic terminals, the computed distribution of extracellular potential would result in the transients illustrated in the middle column of Fig. 7. It may be noted that the extracellular transient at the soma level is proportional to the difference between the intracellular transients at soma, 4, and dendritic terminals, 9. The soma extracellular negativity of period I reflects that soma membrane depolarization exceeded dendritic terminal membrane depolarization throughout this time; the soma extracellular positivity of period II reflects that the actively repolarizing soma has become less depolarized than the passive dendritic terminals.

When this distribution of extracellular potential was expressed relative to the different reference potential found at the distant electrode (see Figs. 5 and 6), the computed transients became changed to those shown in the third column of Fig. 7. A potential divider ratio of 1:4 was used with the result that the terminal extracellular transient has an amplitude exactly minus one-fourth that of the soma extracellular transient in the third column. If the potential divider effect were the only consideration, the soma extracellular amplitude would become exactly four-fifths that of the middle column. However, this particular computation provided a 20% reduction of the extracellular amplitudes at all depths, to allow for the possibility that the ratio of secondary to primary extracellular current might be this large (see Fig. 6); compare also shunt current correction (*B-2* of COMPUTATIONS, METHODS). It also included a cone correction (*B-3* of METHODS) providing for the change of extracellular resistance, r_e, per unit radial distance in the bulb; this correction amounted to a 10% increase of amplitude at the soma depth.

FOUR SETS OF EXTRACELLULAR TRANSIENTS. The transients in Fig. 8 were all computed relative to a distant reference, as just described for Fig. 7. Comparison of sets *A* and *B* shows the effect of dendritic electrotonic length when the dendritic membrane is assumed to be passive; sets *C* and *D* display two results obtained by assuming active dendritic membrane.

A striking feature of these comparisons is that during period I, all four sets show a very

similar sequence (along the dendrites) from a positive peak at the dendritic terminals to a negative peak at the soma, and this sequence is also similar to that of period I in the experimental transients in Figs. 3 and 4. Thus period I can be seen to provide support for this class of theoretical models, but no basis for deciding between active and passive dendrites.

During period II, significant differences can be seen between these four theoretical sets of transients. Thus, comparing sets *A* and *B* (Fig. 8) both the negativity at the dendritic terminals and the positivity at the soma are smaller and less well peaked in *A* than in *B*. This can be attributed to the greater electrotonic length of *A*; passive electrotonic attenuation and slowing of the intracellular transient in compartment 14 of *A* is much greater than in compartment 9 of *B*.

The results for the active dendrites of *C* and *D* (Fig. 8) differ distinctly from those for the passive dendrites of *A* and *B* during period II in two respects. First, the active dendrites

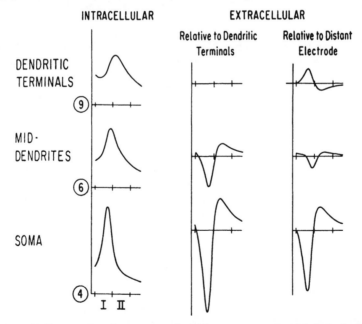

FIG. 7. Computed voltage transients for axon-soma-dendritic compartmental model of mitral cell during antidromic invasion. Left-hand column: intracellular transients in soma, 4; dendritic shafts, 6; and dendritic terminals, 9. Soma is active, dendrites are passive; dendritic electrotonic length equals λ/2. Extracellular transients at these compartments are shown in the middle column computed relative to the dendritic terminals, and in right-hand column computed relative to distant reference electrode. Time scales divided into periods I and II. Amplitude of intracellular soma peak about 86% of axonal spike amplitude potential; amplitude of negative extracellular soma peak, relative to distant electrode, about 1.5 mv.

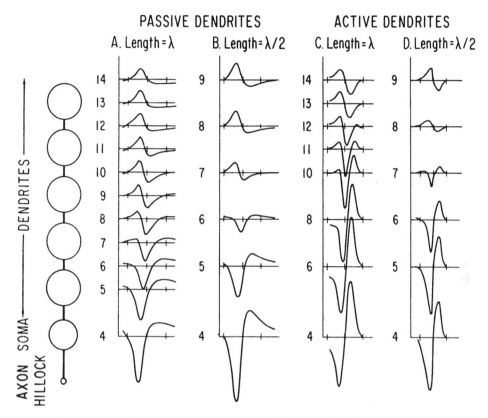

FIG. 8. Computed extracellular voltage transients for four different sets of membrane properties in compartmental model of mitral cell during antidromic impulse invasion. Potential is expressed relative to the distant reference electrode. Length of chain of dendritic compartments indicated at top; 5-compartment chain, 5–9, represents λ/2; 10-compartment chain, 5–14, represents λ. Compartmental location is indicated by number beside each transient. Transients for compartment 4 correspond to soma in schematic model at left; other transients are from dendritic chain. Time marks indicate periods I and II.

are associated with a period II positive peak at the soma that is approximately as large as the negative peak of period I; similarly, the period II negative peak at the terminals is approximately as large as the positive peak of period I. In other words, these are almost symmetrical diphasic transients; this can be attributed to the fact that a full-sized action potential propagates to the dendritic terminals. Second, there is a sharper triphasic transient at the middendritic locations in the case of active dendrites. In this case the active dendrites of short electrotonic length tend to fire in synchrony with the soma; this makes the extracellular current flows smaller, and a larger factor (r_e/r_i) for converting from the intracellular to extracellular potentials is necessary, especially in D of Fig. 8. Of in-

terest in this connection is the finding that with a little background facilitation the dendritic terminals can actually fire before the soma which is slowed by the axon-soma delay and the loading effect of the dendrites. In such cases the polarities of the computed transients in periods I and II are reversed, in disagreement with experiment.

When the computed transients during period II are considered in relation to the experimental transients of Figs. 3 and 4, certain similarities may be noted. At the level of the mitral cell bodies the experimental transient agrees best with the case of the electrotonically short passive dendrites (Fig. 8, series B), whereas at the dendritic terminals (GL) the agreement is best with the case of the active dendrites (series C and D). In the midplexiform region (EPL) the experimental transient agrees approximately with the computed transient for location 6 of the electronically short passive dendrites (series B), and also with the transients of locations 11 and 12 of the electrotonically long active dendrites (series C). The computations thus suggest that the experimental records were from a population of mitral cells which had electrotonically short passive dendrites or electrotonically long active dendrites, or perhaps both types were present in the experimental population. We shall pursue this point below in the DISCUSSION.

All of the computed transients differ from the experimental transients in two important respects. During period I the computed transients at soma and dendritic terminals are strictly inversely proportional, whereas in the experimental recordings the transient at the dendritic terminals leads that at the mitral cell bodies (see Fig. 4). Also, in the experimental records the activity in period II and period III appears to overlap. These points suggest the possibility of at least two additional generators of sufficient extracellular current to modify the extracellular potentials produced by the current from the mitral cells alone. Later we shall show how this additional current is most probably generated.

AMBIGUITY OF CONDUCTION VELOCITY. In this presentation of the extracellular transients, we have emphasized time periods I and II; we have not treated the negative peak as though it were an entity which propagates from the soma to the dendritic terminals. The four sets of computed results in Fig. 8 show a progressive delay of the negative peak that is quite similar to that observed experimentally. An experimental assessment of how well this progressive delay corresponds to the soma-dendritic progression of the intracellular peak would require reliable intracellular recording from several sites along the dendrites; such observations are beyond the reach of present techniques. However, the theoretical computations can provide detailed numerical results, with good resolution for both time and distance, which are relevant to this question.

Figure 9 summarizes the apparent velocities of 4 features of the computed transients,

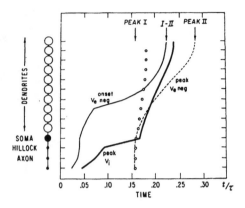

FIG. 9. Apparent progression of computed transients through compartmental model of mitral cell. *Heavy line:* peak of intracellular transient. *Light line:* onset of negativity in extracellular transient, expressed relative to distant electrode. *Dashed line:* peak of extracellular negativity. *Open circles:* peaks of extracellular negativity, expressed relative to dendritic terminals. Time expressed as t/τ.

with a time resolution of approximately 10 μsec, and a distance resolution in terms of compartmental lumping of approximately 50 μ. These 10 dendritic compartments were passive; the electrotonic decrement of the intracellular transient was essentially the same as shown in the first column of Fig. 7. The heavy line in Fig. 9 plots the peak of the intracellular transient as a function of compartment location and time. For the three axonal compartments, this line represents propagation of the active axonal action potential; the same line with smaller slope from axon hillock to soma shows the delay of the soma action potential resulting from unfavorable geometric safety factor; from soma into dendrites the heavy line indicates the apparent velocity of the intracellular transient peak associated with electrotonic spread into the passive dendrites. This slope is approximately constant, and its magnitude is of the order of 1 mm/msec for a membrane time constant of the order of 5 msec.

We now ask whether any feature of the extracellular transients can provide a reliable guide to this apparent intracellular velocity. It is a familiar neurophysiological practice to plot, against distance, the time of onset or the time of peak of an assumed entity such as a negative wave in a set of experimental extracellular transients. Thus in Fig. 9, the thin line represents a plot of the time when the computed extracellular transient begins its negative excursion, while the dashed line represents a plot of the time of peak negativity. It is apparent that these extracellular features do not provide a reliable guide to the intracellular apparent velocity.[2] Plots have also been carried out for several cases of active dendrites as well as several cases of passive dendrites; all of these have shown significant discrepancies rather similar to those in Fig. 9.

Both extracellular plots show a large shift (or slowing of apparent velocity) in the mid-dendritic region. This can be understood as a consequence of the potential divider effect (see METHODS and Figs. 5, 6, and 7); the open circles in Fig. 9 show the absence of this large shift for a plot of the extracellular negative peak, when this is referred to the extracellular potential at the dendritic terminals as in the middle column of Fig. 7.

It is important to note that the extracellular plots in Fig. 9 all agree with experiment in showing no appreciable axon-soma delay. Because the axonal core resistance per unit length is estimated to be at least 25 times that of the combined dendritic intracellular pathway for radial current flow (see section on RELATIVE RADIAL RESISTANCE ESTIMATES in METHODS), the extracellular potential gradients computed between axonal compartments are much smaller than those computed between dendritic compartments. This explains why the computed extracellular potentials associated with the axonal compartments differ little from that at the soma compart-

ment, and hence, why the computed extracellular potentials do not reveal the significant axon-soma delay that occurs intracellularly. This agreement with experiment thus provides additional support for the order of magnitude estimate made for these relative radial resistances; furthermore, this provides important indirect support for a major conclusion[3] reached in a later section of RESULTS, on the basis of very similar quantitative considerations.

MITRAL EXTRACELLULAR POTENTIAL GRADIENTS. The theoretical results provide extracellular potential as a function of both depth and time. Figures 7 and 8 have displayed potential as a function of time at several depths; however, our understanding of these results has depended also upon thinking of the potential as a function of depth at several points in time. To make this point of view more explicit, Fig. 10 provides this type of plotting for the same computed results that were plotted as transients in Fig. 8. The points in time on the left refer to periods I and II of the previous figures.

The changing slope of these plots corresponds to the changing gradient of extracellular potential in the bulb; the direction of extracellular current flow must be everywhere downhill in these plots. The over-all result common to all four sets is that the extracellular potential falls steadily from the dendritic periphery to the soma for the early and peak times of period I, and that the reverse is seen for the peak and late times of period II. This is in general agreement with the experimental plots shown in Fig. 11. At the time of transition from period I to period II the computed extracellular potential must (by definition) be zero at both the soma and the dendritic terminals; minor deviation from this in Fig. 10 is due merely to the fact that the printed output of these computations was given in time steps that were too large to provide the precise transitional plot. Thus, it is useful to examine the plots for late I and

[2] A careful consideration of Fig. 9 suggests that a more reliable estimate of intracellular apparent velocity can be obtained from the MBL extracellular transient alone. One way to see this is that the peripheral negative peak really corresponds to the soma positive peak (i.e., the period II peak) and that the intracellular peripheral peak occurs at a time between I–II transition and II peak. For an almost instantaneous invasion, the period II peak corresponds to inflection of intracellular fall, whereas with electrotonic delay, period II peak may be very close to intracellular peripheral peak. Therefore, the time from soma intracellular peak to peripheral intracellular peak can be estimated to lie in the range of values greater than the time from period I peak to I–II transition and less than the time from period I peak to period II peak. An approximate rule of thumb for choosing a suitable value in this range is to take the time from period I peak to the time when the increasing period II peak reaches half its maximum amplitude.

[3] An important conclusion (in PART IV of RESULTS), that the mitral cell population could not generate the potential distribution observed during period III, is a consequence of these same quantitative considerations. Because of these relative radial resistance values, the mitral axons can be ruled out as the source of the large potential gradient generated in the depths of the granule layer during period III. This forced our attention upon the granule cell population.

early II together with that for I-II transition. Then it can be seen that in every case we find a transitional distribution of potential which has a minimum in the proximal or mid-dendritic region. Thus, whether the dendrites are assumed to be active or passive, there is a time when the extracellular current flows from the dendritic periphery and from the (repolarizing) soma toward the middendritic region.

The experimental plots in Fig. 11 do not show a prominent minimum of this kind in the dendritic region. In addition, the potential gradients for current flow are much less steep than they are for the computed plots illustrated in Fig. 10. These differences would appear to be due in large part to several simplifications required by the computational model. Thus in the experimental situation there is a degree of asynchrony in the activity of neighboring mitral cells. In a given cell the secondary dendrites do not reach as far radially as does the primary dendrite. The mitral cells and their dendrites differ in size,

and they may differ in active or passive membrane properties. It can be intuitively appreciated that all these features would have the effect of smearing and/or partial canceling of the individual extracellular current flows of the population of mitral cells, and thereby lessening the extracellular potential gradients.

Comparison of the plots of Figs. 10 and 11 also shows clearly that other generators of extracellular current must be active in the experimental situation. The experimental values at the mitral cell body and dendritic terminals are not proportional nor are they both zero during the I-II transition period. This point will be dealt with below, in PART V. In addition, the steep gradients deep to MBL late in period II are not found with the computed model of the mitral cell. We shall next inquire into the possible source of this current flow.

IV. *Granule cell computations and period III*

The potential transients from the mitra

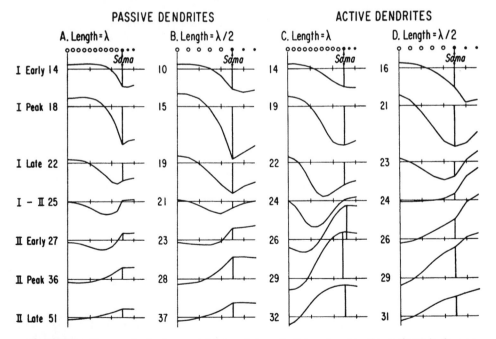

FIG. 10. Dependence on depth of computed extracellular potentials, referred to distant electrode, for compartmental model of mitral cell during antidromic impulse invasion. Same four sets of membrane properties as in Fig. 8. Distributions of extracellular potentials along compartmental chains are shown at instants of time specified at left in terms of an arbitrary computational index, and in terms of the transients in periods I and II. In each figure the horizontal base line indicates 0 potential, the vertical line relates the base line to the potential recorded at the soma.

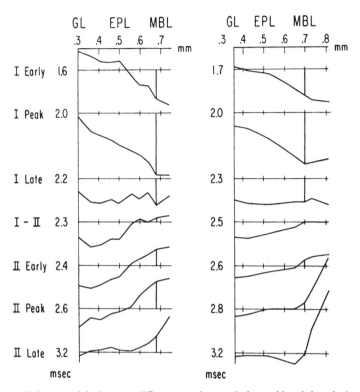

FIG. 11. Extracellular potentials, from two different experiments, during antidromic impulse invasion. Distributions of extracellular potentials with respect to radial depth, as indicated on abscissas above, for different instants of time as specified at left (in terms of periods I and II, and as instant of time in msec). Horizontal base line indicates 0 potential; vertical line relates base line to potential recorded at soma.

cell model are nearly completed by the time of period III (cf. Fig. 8). In the experimental records, on the other hand, a large positivity develops deep in the granule layer late in period II and during the initial few milliseconds of period III. Roughly simultaneously with this a large negativity develops in the deeper half of the external plexiform layer. This distribution of potential implies a substantial flow of extracellular current from the depths of the granule layer radially outward into the plexiform layer. The population of cells which generates this current must possess a substantial intracellular pathway for the return flow of current from the external plexiform layer through the mitral body layer to the granule layer. The mitral cells cannot provide this intracellular pathway because their axons (in the granule layer) have a core resistance per unit length estimated as at least 25 times the effective radial intracellular resistance of their combined dendrites in the external plexiform layer.[4] There is however a large population of granule cells with appropriate location and orientation and in sufficient size and number (see Figs. 1, 3, and ANATOMICAL METHODS) to provide this pathway. We therefore attempted to determine whether a reconstruction of granule cell activity could account for the experimental transients in period III.

Although the computation illustrated in Fig. 12 was designed for this granule cell problem, it can also be viewed simply as a chain of twelve equal compartments. We have computed the consequence of synaptic excitation in compartments 7 through 12, while compartments 1 through 6 simulate passive membrane properties. For simplicity the in-

---

[4] See the relative radial resistance estimates in METHODS. Also, an earlier footnote (no. 3) near Fig. 9 draws attention to an important supporting observation, namely, the fact that extracellular records do not reveal significant axon-soma delay.

tensity and temporal distribution of synaptic excitation was assumed to be the same in each of the six outer compartments; this intensity had the stepwise temporal pattern shown at the bottom of Fig. 12; these steps provide a crude approximation to a temporally dispersed synaptic input. The seven transients displayed in the first column of Fig. 12 sample transient membrane depolarization that is produced in the outer six compartments and spreads electrotonically to the inner six compartments. The delay and attenuation of peak that occur with this electrotonic spread are similar to that computed elsewhere for synaptic potentials (38) and for end-plate potentials (9).

The middle column of Fig. 12 shows the extracellular potential transients, relative to compartment 12, that were computed from the intracellular transients. The computation consists merely of taking the compartmental differences, ΔV_i, multiplying by $(-r_e/r_i)$, and then multiplying by cone factor, as outlined in METHODS. Cone conductance correction for the granule model is greater than for the

mitral model because the deep granule dendrites extend to smaller values of bulbar radius (i.e., the total range of radius values is greater for the granule cells than for the mitral cell bodies and dendrites).

It should be emphasized that this column shows only extracellular positivity, and that this results without assuming membrane hyperpolarization anywhere in this neuron model. Obviously, if the extracellular potential were referred to compartment 1 instead of to compartment 12, the resulting transients would all assume negative polarity; this would correspond to placing an experimental reference electrode at the center of the olfactory bulb. However, since experimental recordings are referred to a distant electrode, the transients in the third column of Fig. 12 show the computed results for a potential divider factor of 1/2 (i.e., the resistance from the distant reference electrode to the outer dendritic terminals of the granule cells is assumed to be half that of the resistance to the deep dendritic terminals of the granule cells). It can be seen that these these transients are basically

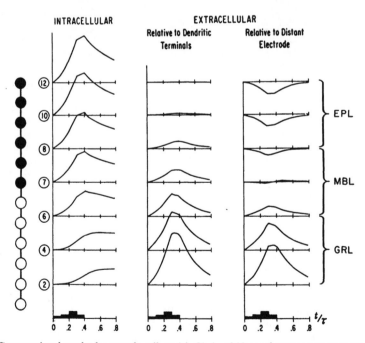

FIG. 12. Computational results for granule cell model. Chain of 12 equal compartments corresponds to an electrotonic length of 1.7 λ. Filled circles indicate loci of membrane depolarization, stepwise time course of synaptic excitatory conductance, $\mathcal{E}$, shown below. Time in t/τ; each of the four depolarizing ($\mathcal{E}$) steps had a time duration of 0.1 τ. Computed potential transients, intracellular and extracellular, as shown, refer to compartment number at left, and corresponding olfactory bulb layer at right.

similar to those recorded during period III (Figs. 3, 4). Here we can view the six outer compartments as representing the extension of the granule dendrites into the external plexiform layer. Compartment 1 represents the deep dendritic terminals. The location of the granule cell body need not be specified for present purposes; this location can be anywhere in the range from compartment 2 to 6 in the granule layer. The level of the mitral cell bodies corresponds approximately to compartment 7 of this granule cell model.

Under these assumptions the computed granule transients show a negativity in the external plexiform layer, a positivity in the granule layer which grows with increasing depth, and a relatively flat response at the mitral body layer. There is an approximate temporal coincidence of the positive and negative peaks, and a steep potential gradient across the mitral body layer. In these basic features there is good agreement between the computed transients and the experimental records during period III. Also, it should be added that there was no difficulty in accounting for the magnitude of the extracellular potential gradient observed during period III in spite of the fact that the intracellular potential gradient is expected to be much smaller during granule cell synaptic activity than during a mitral cell action potential. The compensating factor is the relatively large r_e/r_i ratio (see METHODS), estimated for the granule cell population. For example, the intracellular synaptic potential amplitude could be as little as 3 mv, with an intracellular difference of only about 1 mv between compartments 4 and 8 (in Fig. 12) because an r_e/r_i ratio of 9:1 would result in an extracellular potential difference of 9 mv between these EPL and GRL locations; this is even a little more than is usually observed. Alternatively, the intracellular synaptic potential could be as large as 15 mv if the r_e/r_i ratio were as small as 2:1. The present experimental evidence does not permit us to determine the most probable values in this range.

V. Superposition to reconstruct field potentials

The four sets of transients in Fig. 13 provide an illustrative example of how a theoretical model system composed of three sets of neurons which generate overlapping extracellular currents would be sufficient to account for the experimental observations dur-

ing the first 8 msec or so of the bulbar response. The column on the right can be seen to agree well with the major features of the experimental series of Figs. 3 and 4; this column actually represents the superposition of the other three columns. The mitral column presents transients identical with those of B in Fig. 8; i.e., the case of passive dendrites with electrotonic length $= \lambda/2$. The granule column displays transients very similar to those computed according to the granule cell model presented with Fig. 12. The hypothetical transients shown as dashed lines in the column labeled "other" are presumed to result from deeper lying neuronal structures (see fine print below for explanation).

The three component columns of Fig. 13 are meant to represent neither a unique fit nor an exhaustive representation of components in the resultant field potential. For example, we expect that a further small contribution to periods I and II would be provided by activity in those axon collaterals and centrifugal fibers which extend into the external plexiform layer; this contribution would be small because of the same quantitative considerations that apply to the mitral axons (see section on RELATIVE RADIAL RESISTANCE ESTIMATES in METHODS; see also previous footnotes 3 and 4).

The need for introducing a third generator of extracellular current in Fig. 13 can be appreciated most easily by reexamining the transition from period I to period II. The computed mitral transients provide a sharply defined instant of I-II transition at which both the GL transient and the MBL and GRL transients cross the base line. The experimental transients of Fig. 3 do not show such close proportionality between GL, as compared with MBL and GRL; in fact, the vertical line marking I-II transition was chosen as a compromise between the earlier time for GL and the later time for MBL and GRL, when the transient crossed the base line. The same discrepancy is evident also in Fig. 11, where it can be seen that the GL potential is negative when the MBL potential is close to zero.

There are two reasons for concluding that superposition of granule and mitral computed transients would not account for this observed shift in base line crossover. One is that the granule transient must arise later because of synaptic delay. The other reason is that the potential divider effect is similar for the granule and the mitral computations. Indeed, if the two potential divider factors were identical, it would be impossible to obtain any discrepancy between the

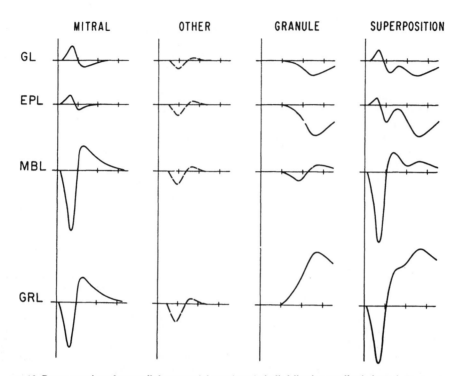

FIG. 13. Reconstruction of extracellular potential transients in bulb following a volley in lateral olfactory tract. Computed transients for mitral and granule cells at four levels in bulb are shown, with presumed contribution by other deeper lying elements (labeled "other"). Superposition at right from simple addition of the three separate transients at each level. Time markers along 0 potential base lines are approximately 2 msec per division. Polarity, positivity upward, negativity downward, as before. The relative amplitudes of the component transients were chosen to satisfy this superposition; factors that determine the voltage amplitude of the granule component are discussed in the final paragraph of SECTION IV.

base-line crossovers at GL and GRL, although shifts could of course occur at intermediate depths, EPL and MBL. Actually the potential divider factor is similar, but not quite the same, because the granule cells generate significant extracellular current at deeper levels than do the mitral cells. It was such considerations that led to the suggestion that other elements which end in the depth of the bulb and do not extend into the EPL might have their endings activated at the time of I-II transition. Such a generator of extracellular current would have the important feature that the voltage transients at GL and GRL would have the same polarity and should differ only somewhat in amplitude. This is because the potential divider situation differs significantly from both the mitral case and the granule case; this is illustrated diagrammatically in Fig. 14. The essential point is that for the granule cells (or mitral cells), the primary extracellular current (open arrow of Fig. 14*A*, and battery of Fig. 14*B*) flows through the same (radial) resistance along which the microelectrode picks up its potential, while for the "other" deep-lying elements the primary extracellular current (open arrow of Fig. 14*C*, and

battery of Fig. 14*D*) does not flow through that same radial resistance.

An example of a series of transients due to other nervous elements in the bulb is shown tentatively as dashed lines in Fig. 13, where the negative peak could be due to one set of elements and the positive peak might be due to another set of elements. Thus, for example, the negative peak could be ascribed to deep terminals that are invaded by an impulse, whereas the positive peak, if needed, could be ascribed to deep terminals which impulses fail to invade. In the experimental situation it has been stressed (33) that there are centrifugal fibers as well as collaterals from mitral axons which may be activated by a shock to the lateral olfactory tract. These elements could generate the potentials ascribed to "other" in Fig. 13.

VI. *Postulated mitral-granule synaptic interactions*

The reconstruction of the observed field potentials during period III depended on the assumption of granule cell activity and, in particular, on the assumption of substantial

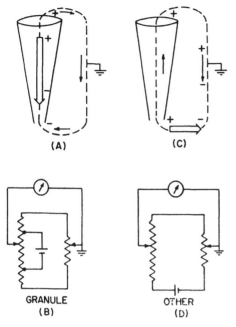

(A)   (C)

GRANULE   OTHER
(B)   (D)

FIG. 14. Diagrams (*A* and *B*) show extracellular current for granule cells or mitral cells, in contrast with diagrams (*C* and *D*) for deeper lying other elements. In both *A* and *C*, open arrow indicates the primary extracellular current, and dashed line indicates secondary extracellular current (cf. Figs. 5 and 6). *B* and *D* are simplified equivalent electric circuits for *A* and *C*, respectively; in both cases, the resistance at left represents the radial resistance, and the resistance at right represents the extra pathway which passes through bulb puncture; the battery is a nondistributed representation of the neuronal generator of extracellular current (cf. Fig. 6). The direction of current flow shown in *A* and *B* corresponds to that produced by mitral cells during period I; this is opposite to that produced by granule cells during period III.

synaptic excitation of the granule dendrites in the external plexiform layer. Mitral cells were ruled out as the primary generators of current during period III because their axons could not provide the necessary amount of current in the deep granule layer. Synaptic excitation of deep-lying granule processes was ruled out as the primary cause, because this would produce a field potential of polarity opposite to that observed. Synaptic inhibition of the deep-lying granule processes would produce the correct polarity of field potential, but would be unlikely to account for the observed extracellular amplitudes and would be unable to account for a subsequent granule-to-mitral inhibition; however, we have not ruled out

the possibility that there could be synaptic inhibition of the deep-lying granule processes simultaneous with the postulated synaptic excitation of the outer granule processes in the external plexiform layer.

Once this massive synaptic excitation in the external plexiform layer was recognized as the best explanation of period III, the question arose as to what the source of this synaptic excitation might be. One possibility would be the recurrent collaterals of the mitral cell axons. However, we recognized that the mitral dendrites could provide a more substantial source of synaptic excitation, provided that effective synapses exist between the intimately related dendrites (of granule and mitral cells) in the external plexiform layer. This was an intriguing possibility because the mitral dendrites are themselves depolarized late in period I and during period II, just when the synaptic excitatory activity would have to be initiated. It was already known from unitary studies that many mitral cells undergo inhibition during period III (33), and that the minimal latency for the onset of inhibition occurs early in period III (i.e., 3–5 msec after the tract shock). From these considerations the conclusion was drawn that the granule dendritic depolarization in the EPL is in its turn both well timed and well placed to initiate synaptic inhibitory input to the mitral cell bodies and dendrites.

POSTULATED DENDRODENDRITIC SYNAPSES. This theoretical study thus led us to postulate, prior to any knowledge of electron-microscopic evidence, that there might be dendrodendritic synaptic connections in the external plexiform layer that could mediate mitral-to-granule synaptic excitation followed by granule-to-mitral synaptic inhibition. However, since there was no precedent for this, we did not know whether to expect conventional synaptic contacts with synaptic vesicles or some new kind of contact capable of two different kinds and orientations of synaptic activity. It was thus an exciting experience to learn several months later from Reese and Brightman that their independent electron-micrographic studies (44, 45) revealed two kinds of synaptic contacts, of opposite polarity, between mitral secondary dendrites and gemmules of granule dendrites. The polarity of these synaptic contacts was judged by the same criteria used elsewhere in the mammalian central nervous system (13, 31); i.e., by the grouping of synaptic vesicles close to the presynaptic membrane of the synaptic contacts (40, 44). Then we learned that these two kinds of contacts in the external plexiform layer had been observed independently by others (3, 18; K. Hama, personal communication). The remarkable finding of these pairs of oppositely oriented synaptic contacts fitted the needs of our theoretical postulate so well that we decided to publish jointly a brief statement of the anatomical, physiological, and theoretical considerations supporting the postulation of such dendrodendritic synaptic interactions (40). Further studies in rat, rabbit, and cat (44) have shown that the mitral-granule-dendrodendritic synapses predominate in the inner part of the external plexiform layer; indeed, it has been shown with serial reconstructions made from electron micrographs that the inner third of the external plexiform layer contains mainly granule den-

drites, granule gemmules, mitral primary and secondary dendrites, remarkably little glia, and a few unidentified endings on granule dendrites (44 and Reese, personal communication).

DISCUSSION

Postulated sequence of events

The scheme of these postulated synaptic interactions is illustrated by the diagrams in Fig. 15; the three diagrams at top (*A*) summarize the postulated sequence of events. The first diagram (I–II) indicates that depolarization of the mitral dendritic membrane occurs during the latter part of period I, whether by passive electrotonus or by active impulse invasion, and this causes excitatory synaptic activity (ε) during period II by means of the excitatory synaptic contact (arrow) from the mitral dendrite to the gemmule of a granule cell dendrite. The next diagram (II–III) in-

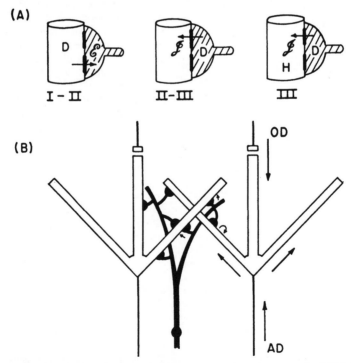

FIG. 15. *A:* postulated mechanism of dendrodendritic synaptic pathway between mitral (light) and granule (shaded) dendrite, during successive time periods (I, II, III) following antidromic volley in mitral cell. I–II, depolarization (D) of mitral dendrites activates excitatory (ε) synapses to granule dendrite. II–III, synaptic depolarization of granule dendrite activates inhibitory (J) synapse to mitral dendrite. III, persisting inhibiting hyperpolarization of mitral dendrite. *B:* diagram illustrating how antidromic (AD) invasion of one mitral cell leads to inhibition of neighboring mitral cell through extensive synaptic contacts with granule dendritic gemmules. Mechanism works similarly during orthodromic (OD) activation via olfactory nerves as indicated above.

dicates the resulting depolarization (D) of the granule gemmule which activates the inhibitory synaptic contact (arrow) thus delivering inhibition ($\mathcal{g}$) to the mitral dendrite. This begins late in period II, when the mitral dendrite is itself repolarizing (see Fig. 7); the rapid process of repolarization would help shut off the ($\mathcal{E}$) synapse, and would move the membrane potential in the same direction as would the developing ($\mathcal{g}$) activity. In the third diagram (III) inhibitory activity continues and produces hyperpolarization (H) of the mitral cell membrane; persisting ($\mathcal{g}$) activity might be due partly to long-lasting depolarization (D) of the granule dendrite, and possibly also to prolonged transmitter release or action.

Dendritic action potentials not required
for synaptic activation

With both kinds of synaptic contacts, we suggest that the synaptic activation would not require a presynaptic action potential in either dendrite; the membrane depolarization itself could activate the synapse, as has been demonstrated experimentally for the nerve-muscle junction (4, 22, 24, 26) and for the squid synapse (3a, 23). The reason for considering this possibility is that this pathway has no apparent need for a propagated action potential in either the mitral dendrites or the granule dendrites; passive electrotonic spread would seem to be sufficient for spread of depolarization over the relatively short dendritic distances involved. Except for gemmules with unusually long and thin stems, membrane depolarizations produced at individual gemmules would spread over the granule dendritic tree and summate with each other, thus activating (in a graded manner) all of the inhibitory synapses belonging to this same granule dendritic tree. Thus, each depolarized granule dendritic tree would deliver graded synaptic inhibition not only to the mitral cells that were previously active, but also to any others with which they have synaptic contacts.

In unitary studies (15, 33, 48, 55) recordings of spikes attributable to activated granule cells have been rare; furthermore, the impulse activity was brief in relation to the long-lasting character of the mitral inhibition. It was therefore suggested (48) that the granule cell might be capable of long-lasting transmitter liberation in the absence of the usual type of impulse activity. The role of the granule dendrites in mediating inhibition from one mitral cell to another implies a certain amount of spread of depolarization from an activated granule gemmule into the contiguous granule dendritic tree. Although this could occur to a considerably extent by passive spread alone, as pointed out above, it would of course be helped by any regenerative or "active" properties of the granule membrane. Since normal impulse activity in granule cells is so rarely elicited, any active spread of depolarization in the granule dendrites would likely be of a decrementing or nonpropagating nature. It is also relevant to note that some of our computations explored the effect of a weakly active granule cell membrane; we found that unless we applied synaptic inhibition to the deep (GRL) portions of the granule cells, the depolarization of the outer dendritic branches (in EPL) would spread to the deeper level too effectively, and result in an unsatisfactory reconstruction of the extracellular potential distribution observed during period III; in other words, the simplest reconstruction of period III was obtained with passive granule cell membrane.

Functional implications of
dendrodendritic synaptic pathway

It is clear from diagram *A* in Fig. 15 that each antidromic impulse in a mitral cell will result in subsequent inhibition back upon itself (a negative feedback). In addition, as diagram *B* illustrates, depolarization of one mitral cell, by antidromic (AD) invasion, leads to inhibition of neighboring mitral cells through their contacts with mutual granule dendrites. The dendrodendritic synapses thus provide a mechanism for the inhibition (self-inhibition and lateral inhibition) which is a prominent feature of mitral cell responses to tract stimulation (15, 33, 46, 48, 54, 55). For neuronal circuits in general, it may be noted that such a dendrodendritic pathway must be regarded as an alternative to the recurrent axon collateral pathway for recurrent inhibition.[5]

During natural orthodromic activation of

---

[5] It was very recently brought to our attention that Tönnies and Jung (50) did suggest and appreciate the importance of the idea of dendritic feedback (Rückmeldung) as an alternative to a recurrent collateral pathway; at that time (1948) they were concerned with motoneurons of spinal cord.

the mitral cells it may be anticipated that the dendrodendritic synaptic mechanisms would function in essentially the same manner as in the case of antidromic invasion. Input from olfactory nerves (indicated diagrammatically at the top of Fig. 15B) depolarizes the primary mitral dendrite; the depolarization spreads, actively or passively, to trigger an impulse at the axon hillock and soma. The secondary dendrites are depolarized by electrotonic spread or an impulse, just as in the case of an antidromic impulse (the difference being the synaptic depolarization of the primary dendrite in the orthodromic case) and the sequence of granule excitation and mitral inhibition ensues as already described. Mitral inhibition elicited by either antidromic or orthodromic volleys should therefore be similar, and this is what has been found in physiological experiments (47, 48, 54). The powerful nature of the inhibition is also in accord with the physiological findings.

Because of the widespread distribution of the dendrodendritic contacts, activity in one mitral cell or group of mitral cells would be accompanied by inhibition of most of the surrounding inactive or less active mitral cells. It may be deduced that during natural activity a mitral cell would exert on its neighbors the kind of lateral inhibition which is a common feature of many sensory systems (17, 43). The inhibitory "surrounds" would be elongated in the anteroposterior axis of the bulb, to correspond with the orientation of the mitral secondary dendrites (49). It is for future research to test the conjecture that such lateral inhibition contributes to sensory discrimination in the olfactory system. There can be little question that both the lateral inhibition and the self-inhibition of the mitral cells must contribute to adaptation in the olfactory system; however, the relative importance of this adaptive mechanism to the total adaptive capacity of the system must be evaluated by future research.

Pathways for granule cell activation

On the basis of unitary studies it has been suggested (33, 48) that the granule cell is the general inhibitory interneuron in the bulbar cortex, mediating inhibition of the mitral cells as well as of tufted and glomerular cells. The present results support and extend that interpretation. With regard to the pathway for granule cell activation, the present evi-

dence suggests that the primary pathway for the case of antidromic mitral invasion is by way of the synaptic connections between mitral secondary dendrites and granule dendrites in the external plexiform layer. It would appear that this is also the main pathway during orthodromic activation via the olfactory nerves. But we should like to emphasize that this does not exclude the possibility, or indeed likelihood, of other inputs to the granule cell, in either these cases or in other cases. For instance, the present evidence does not exclude the possibility that mitral axon collaterals deliver an input to the deep granule cell processes during antidromic mitral invasion; this would be in analogy with Renshaw inhibition in the spinal cord, as was postulated in the early unitary studies (8, 33, 48). The evidence does however suggest that this input, if excitatory, is limited, since it would give rise to extracellular potential gradients the reverse of those which actually occur during the onset of mitral inhibition (in period III).

The mitral axons have another well-developed system of recurrent collaterals which terminate in the external plexiform layer and which might provide thereby an input to either the mitral secondary dendrites or peripheral granule dendrites. A direct connection with the mitral secondary dendrites was, however, ruled out by the long latency of onset of antidromic mitral inhibition, and the polysynaptic character of the inhibition (33, 48). A recurrent collateral input to the granule dendrites (in the EPL), on the other hand, might be expected to have an action similar to the input we have postulated from the mitral secondary dendrites, and is therefore difficult to rule out. If the inhibition were mediated by granule cells activated by mitral recurrent collaterals, it should begin earlier when evoked by the antidromic route than by the orthodromic route. In fact, unitary studies (33, 46, 48) have shown that inhibition begins at approximately the same latency following either an orthodromically or an antidromically evoked spike in the mitral cell body; this would be expected with a dendrodendritic pathway, as described above in relation to Fig. 15 B.

In other studies (55) it has been found that repetitive stimulation of the lateral olfactory tract does not augment the mitral inhibitory potentials. Such observations are consistent with the dendrodendritic pathway, because the antidromic volley is blocked at the mitral cell bodies and therefore cannot activate the mitral to granule synapses. Similarly, alternating periods of mitral cell invasion and bockage at certain frequencies of tract stimulation (15) are consistent with the self-inhibitory feature of the dendrodendritic pathway. It may be concluded that the evidence from several lines of physiological study is consistent with the dendrodendritic inhibitory pathway.

Until now the term "recurrent inhibition" has been used in connection with recurrent axon collaterals which are present in many neurons of the central nervous system. Since the dendrodendritic pathway provides for the same type of negative feedback as that mediated by recurrent collaterals it may be well to use the term "recurrent inhibition" in a general physiological sense without restricting it to one anatomical pathway. It appears that further work is needed to characterize the functions of the mitral axon collaterals. One possibility is that the recurrent collaterals provide for activation of the tufted cells in the external plexiform layer (33, 48).

The other input to the external plexiform layer which needs to be considered is the centrifugal fibers which enter the bulb along with the lateral olfactory tract, and might therefore be excited by a shock to the tract. Anatomical studies show that these fibers ". . . form only a very small proportion of the total number of fibers in the tract" (34, cf. 41); nonetheless, following transection of the tract. ". . . severe terminal degeneration is found throughout the periventricular and granule cell layers, and many fibers extend superficial to the mitral cells to reach the external plexiform and glomerular layers." Recently, Price (35) has obtained electron micrographs of such degenerating terminals making synaptic connection with gemmules of granule cells in the external plexiform layer; the gemmules in turn formed reciprocal synapses of the type described by Rall et al. (40) with presumed mitral dendrites. It appears therefore that the centrifugal fibers would be able to exert an important influence on the granule cells, possibly by raising or lowering the excitability of the gemmules, but the unitary studies to date have given no evidence of what the action of the centrifugal fibers might be. With regard to mitral inhibition following tract volleys it is unlikely that centrifugal fibers

play any major role, since the inhibition is not affected by chronic transection of the tract (which causes the centrifugal fibers to degenerate) (52). In addition, orthodromic volleys in the olfactory nerves do not directly activate the centrifugal fibers, yet the mitral inhibition following these volleys is closely similar to that following tract volleys (47). However, a small input from centrifugal fibers following tract volleys cannot be ruled out, and we have included these fibers among the "other" elements which make a small contribution to the summed extracellular potentials in the bulb (cf. Figs. 13 and 14).

During normal olfactory activation of the bulb, or by other experimental methods of activation, different inputs to the granule cells may predominate. Thus, a volley in the anterior commissure gives rise to extracellular potential gradients of opposite polarity to those in our period III (53), i.e., negativity in the granular layer and positivity in the external plexiform layer. Walsh (53) suggested that this gradient arose from a synaptic depolarization of the deep granule processes by the commissural fiber input. Other possible inputs to the granule cells include the stellate cells in the granule layer and tufted cell collaterals in the inner plexiform layer. Finally, the several types of centrifugal fibers to the bulb from the forebrain terminate in close relation to the granule cells. Thus the granule cell is likely to play a most complex role as a final common path for inhibition in the olfactory bulb.

Amacrine cells

The granule cell is analogous to the amacrine cell of the retina in lacking an axon (41). Thus it is of considerable interest that electron-microscopic studies have revealed further similarities; the retinal amacrine cells have been found to participate in "serial" or "reciprocal" synapses with bipolar cells (7, 7a, 25, 43a). Although there are differences in the structural details, there is some formal similarity in that these retinal amacrine cells appear to be both postsynaptic and presynaptic to the bipolar cells, whereas the olfactory granule cell gemmules appear to be both postsynaptic and presynaptic to the mitral cell dendrites. On the basis of these similarities, we (40) commented that it will be interesting to learn whether the retinal amacrine cells provide a dendrodendritic inhibitory pathway similar to that we have proposed for the olfactory bulb. By this we implied the possibility that such a mechanism for lateral inhibition and adaptive inhibition might be common to several sensory systems. These possibilities must, of course, be tested by future research. It may be noted that the orientation of the amacrine cells in the retina lacks the simple radial orientation which was basic to our analysis of granule cell potentials.

It recently came to our attention that Gray and Young (14, 56) have suggested that the amacrine cells in the optic lobe (VU2) of *Octopus* function as inhibitory interneurons. These amacrine cells have synapses with vesicles on both sides, and both presynaptic and postsynaptic functions were postulated. These cells are very numerous in this lobe and Young (56) regards them as important components of the memory system in *Octopus*.

Rhythmic potentials

The resting activity of the bulb is characterized by spontaneous potential oscillations ("EEG waves") of large amplitude (12). During odorous stimulation of the olfactory mucosa the activity recorded from the surface of the bulb consists of rapid "induced" potential waves (1). Though a discussion of the nature of these types of activity is beyond the scope of this paper, we have previously noted that the dendrodendritic synaptic interactions between mitral and granule cell populations are well suited for the development of rhythmic activity (cf. 40). Impulse discharge in many mitral cells results in synaptic excitation to the processes of a large number of granule cells. These granule cells constitute an internuncial pool that delivers graded inhibition to the mitral cells. As the granule cell pool begins to inhibit the mitral cells, this begins to cut off the source of synaptic excitatory input to the granule cells. As the granule cell activity subsides, the amount of inhibition delivered to the mitral cells is reduced; this permits the mitral cells to respond again to the excitatory input from the glomeruli. In this way a sustained excitatory input to the mitral cells would be converted into a rhythmic sequence of impulse followed by inhibition, locked in timing to a rhythmic activation of the granule cell pool. The amplitude of the resulting extracellular potentials would be enhanced both by the synchrony inherent in the tight synaptic coupling between mitral and granule cell populations, and by the radial alignment of the processes. Further work is needed to test this hypothesis. It will also be interesting to see whether similar mechanisms underlie the development of extracellular potential oscillations in other regions of the central nervous system.

Electric coupling

It should also be noted that the radial potential gradient generated by the granule cell population must have a direct electrical effect on the mitral cells. Under conditions such as those in period III of Fig. 4, the extracellular potential gradient, from GRL to EPL, must have an anodal (hyperpolarizing) effect upon all mitral cell bodies, coupled with a cathodal (depolarizing) effect upon the mitral dendritic terminals; the magnitude of such membrane polarizations could be as much as 1 mv. This would exert a small inhibitory influence upon the impulse trigger zone near the mitral axon-hillock and soma region of all mitral cells. A reversed extracellular potential gradient would, of course, exert a small excitatory effect upon this impulse trigger zone. These effects would be expected also during rhythmic synchronized activity of the granule cell population of the kind described above.

Other studies of tract-evoked potentials

Experimental transients similar to those under study here have been the subject of previous interpretations using the neurophysiological lore of current sources and sinks. Von Baumgarten et al. (40, 52) considered the early part of the evoked response in the rabbit to signal mitral activity, but they could not distinguish between active or passive invasion of the dendrites, or invasion of mitral axon collaterals in the external plexiform layer. These authors concluded that the large negative potential (in the EPL during our period III) was due to tufted cell activation and the large positive potential (in the GRL during our period III) to granule inhibition; in doing so they appear to have overemphasized the minor differences in time course between the two transients. Ochi (30) concluded that the early part of the response represented an antidromically propagated impulse in the mitral dendrites because of the gradual increase in latency. However, as we have indicated above (cf. Fig. 9), this should not be regarded as a reliable guide to intracellular conduction velocity. Ochi noted the similarity in time course between the large negative and positive potentials, and suggested that the negative potential represented a current sink due to synaptic activation of the mitral dendrites via the mitral axon collaterals; the positive potential he regarded as the associated current source, without further identification of the pathway involved. In his interpretation the source would have to include the mitral axons, which we assess to be inadequate for the large current flow generated. In the turtle, according to Iwase and Lisenby (21), there is a " . . . slow negative excursion" (in the external plexiform layer) which is the result of " . . . depolarization of the mitral cell basal dendrites and of the activities of granular cells which synapse with the mitral cell dendrites." No explanation was offered for how this potential distribution might arise, or what the granule cell contribution to this potential might be.

Mitral dendritic membrane properties

Our computations with the mitral model favor the assumption of either electrotonically short passive dendrites or electrotonically longer active dendrites (cf. Fig. 8). We are inclined not to press further in deciding between these alternatives. One reason is that the experimental transients in different microelectrode penetrations vary somewhat in their relative amplitudes. Also the critical time for discriminating between these theoretical alternatives is in period II, at a time when the current flows from other elements, as well as from granule cells, have become significant. A unique fit of theory with experiment is not possible at this time, because either the active or the passive dendritic case can be accommodated by adjustment of the component transients in various superpositions, of which Fig. 13 is only one example. Rather than engage further in these details we should like to point out the possibility that mitral dendrites of both types might be present in the experimental population. Such a mixed population of active and passive mitral dendrites could be interpreted in the following manner. The larger mitral cells have thick dendrites which are correspondingly short electrotonically, so that normal orthodromic activation of the glomeruli (cf. Fig. 1) would

be effective by passive spread alone. The smaller mitral cells with their thin dendrites would be electrotonically more distant from the glomeruli and active impulse propagation might be necessary to transfer the glomerular input to the mitral axon. Another interpretation would be that normally all the mitral dendrites have active properties, but that the conditions of surgery, anesthesia, and experimentation render the dendrites passive, beginning with the larger ones. These possibilities would seem to be open to further study.

SUMMARY

1. A computational neuron model has been developed and tested for its sufficiency in reconstructing field potentials recorded in the olfactory bulb after a volley in the lateral olfactory tract. One set of computations simulates synchronous antidromic invasion of the mitral cell population; another set stimulates synchronous synaptic activation of the granule cell population. The theoretical results establish that the initial brief time periods (I and II) of the recorded field potentials can be attributed primarily to activity of the mitral cell population. The recorded potential distribution during the following longer time period (III) could not be due to extracellular current flow generated by the mitral cell population; it could be due to current generated by the granule cell population. The timing and location of such mitral and granule cell activity led us to postulate that mitral dendrites deliver synaptic excitation to granule dendrites, and that granule dendrites then deliver synaptic inhibition to mitral dendrites. Structures for such a dendro-dendritic synaptic pathway have been demonstrated in electron micrographs by others.

2. Realistic sequences of antidromic and synaptic activity in representative neurons were computed by means of a mathematical model that is based upon known anatomical facts and nerve membrane properties. The functional relations between axonal, somatic, and dendritic membrane were simulated by the mathematical equivalent of a compartmental model. The values assigned to several theoretical parameters of the general model provide for approximations to particular neuron types, such as mitral cells or granule cells. The values of these parameters determine the following: a) the geometric factor for invasion of soma and dendrites by an impulse propa-

gating antidromically along the axon, *b*) the magnitude of background facilitation in the dendritic membrane, *c*) the extent to which the dendritic membrane is assumed "active" or "passive" with respect to impulse propagation, and *d*) the effective electrotonic length of the dendrites. This general model includes also a mathematical model for generating action potentials with adjustable kinetics. Numerous exploratory computations were used to find several different combinations of these theoretical parameters which result in approximations to the experimental data.

3. In developing the theoretical model, the spherical symmetry of the bulbar layers and the synchrony of bulbar activation permit an important simplification: the field potentials become essentially functions of only two variables, time and radial depth in the bulb. The relative values of intracellular and extracellular resistance (per unit distance along bulbar radii) for mitral dendrites, mitral axons, and granule dendrites were found to be of basic importance to these theoretical reconstructions. Although the values used are only approximate, they differ by orders of magnitude; this forced the conclusion that the mitral cells could not generate the potentials of period III, and that the granule cell population provides the only plausible generator of these potentials.

4. The experimental finding of a potential difference between bulbar surface and distant reference electrode implies that the spherical symmetry of the bulb is punctured, thus providing an extra pathway for current flow between the depth and surface of the bulb. The position of the distant reference electrode along this extra pathway gives rise to a potential divider effect in the recordings. This effect is crucial to the interpretation of the recorded transients and is incorporated in the theoretical model. For mitral cell activity, a potential divider ratio of approximately 1:4 in the theoretical model produces a superficial (GL) potential transient that is one-fourth the amplitude of the deep (MBL) potential, and of opposite sign. Similar considerations apply to the interpretation of granule cell potentials, with a ratio (ca. 1:2) reflecting the deeper distribution of the granule cell processes.

5. During period I, both the positivity in the outer bulbar layers (GL to surface) and the negativity at the mitral body layer (MBL

and deeper) of the computed field potentials are produced by the flow of extracellular current from the mitral dendrites radially inward to the actively depolarizing mitral cell bodies. During period II, both the negativity in the outer layers and the associated deep positivity of the computed potentials are produced by the flow of extracellular current radially outward from repolarizing mitral soma membrane to depolarized mitral dendrites. During period III, both the computed negativity in the external plexiform layer and the computed positivity in the granule cell layer are produced by the flow of extracellular current from the deep processes of the granule cells radially outward to the synaptically depolarized granule cell dendrites in the external plexiform layer.

6. Field potentials during periods I and II of antidromic mitral activity are best simulated by assuming either active dendrites of relatively long electrotonic length or passive dendrites of relatively short electrotonic length. Overlap of mitral and granule activity during period II prevents further discrimination between these cases. Usual methods for estimating intracellular conduction velocity from field potentials are shown to be unreliable in the case of a detailed simulation of mitral intracellular potentials and bulbar field potentials.

7. The concept of the granule cell as an inhibitory interneuron acting upon mitral cells is reinforced and extended. The dendrodendritic synaptic pathway we have postulated provides a possible mechanism for adaptive and lateral inhibition of the mitral cells. This pathway contains several novel features which are of general interest in neurophysiology, apart from the olfactory bulb: *a*) dendritic membrane can transmit as well as receive synaptic information, *b*) dendrodendritic synapses provide a mechanism for axonless neurons to interact integratively with other neurons, *c*) such neurons may function without generation of an action potential, and *d*) these synaptic interactions also provide a mechanism for generating rhythmic activity in neuronal populations.

ACKNOWLEDGMENTS

We are grateful to Dr. T. S. Reese and Dr. M. W. Brightman for continuing consultation and advice. Drs. C. G. Phillips, T. P. S. Powell, P. G. Nelson, and T. G. Smith have provided valuable suggestions during revisions of this manuscript.

The principal results of this study were presented briefly at the 23rd International Physiological Congress, Tokyo, September, 1965; also at the Neurophysiology Group Meeting of The American Physiological Society, Atlantic City, April, 1966, and at several subsequent symposia.

Present address of G. M. Shepherd: Dept. of Physiology, Yale University School of Medicine, New Haven, Conn.

REFERENCES

1. ADRIAN, E. D. The electrical activity of the mammalian olfactory bulb. *Electroencephalog. Clin. Neurophysiol.* 2: 377–388, 1950.

2. ALLISON, A. C. The morphology of the olfactory system in the vertebrates. *Biol. Rev.* 28: 195–244, 1953.

3. ANDRES, K. H. Der Feinbau des Bulbus Olfactorius der Ratte unter besonderer Berücksichtigung der synaptischen Verbindungen. *Z. Zellforsch.* 65: 530–561, 1965.

3a. BLOEDEL, J., GAGE, P. W., LLINÁS, R., AND QUASTEL, D. M. J. Transmitter release at the squid giant synapse in the presence of tetrodotoxin. *Nature* 212: 49–50, 1966.

4. CASTILLO, J. AND KATZ, B. Changes in end-plate activity produced by pre-synaptic polarization. *J. Physiol., London* 124: 586–604, 1954.

5. COOMBS, J. S., ECCLES, J. C., AND FATT, P. The inhibitory suppression of reflex discharges from motoneurons. *J. Physiol., London* 130: 396–413, 1955.

6. CRAGG, B. G. Centrifugal fibers of the retina and olfactory bulb, and composition of the supraoptic commisures in the rabbit. *Exptl. Neurol.* 5: 406–427, 1962.

7. DOWLING, J. E. AND BOYCOTT, B. B. Neural connections of the retina: fine structure of the inner plexiform layer. *Cold Spring Harbor Symp. Quant. Biol.* 30: 393–402, 1966.

7a. DOWLING, J. E. AND BOYCOTT, B. B. Organization of the primate retina: electron microscopy. *Proc. Roy. Soc., London, Ser. B* 166: 80–111, 1966.

8. ECCLES, J. C., FATT, P., AND KOKETSU, K. Cholinergic and inhibitory synapses in a pathway from motor-axon collaterals to motoneurons. *J. Physiol., London* 216: 524–562, 1954.

9. FATT, P. AND KATZ, B. An analysis of the end-plate potential recorded with an intracellular electrode. *J. Physiol., London* 115: 320–70, 1951.

10. FATT, P. AND KATZ, B. The effect of inhibitory nerve impulses on a crustacean muscle fibre. *J. Physiol., London* 121: 374–89, 1953.

11. FITZHUGH, R. Impulses and physiological states in theoretical models of nerve membrane. *Biophys. J.* 1: 445–466, 1961.

12. GERARD, R. W. AND YOUNG, J. Z. Electrical activity of the central nervous system of the frog. *Proc. Roy. Soc., London, Ser. B* 122: 343–352, 1937.

13. GRAY, E. G. Axo-somatic and axo-dendritic synapses of the cerebral cortex: an electron microscopic study. *J. Anat.* 93: 420–432, 1959.

14. GRAY, E. G. AND YOUNG, J. Z. Electron microscopy of synaptic structure of octopus brain. *J. Cell. Biol* 21: 87–103, 1964.

15. GREEN, J. D., MANCIA, M., AND BAUMGARTEN, R. VON. Recurrent inhibition in the olfactory bulb. 1. Effects of antidromic stimulation of the lateral olfactory tract. *J. Neurophysiol.* 25: 467–488, 1962.

16. HAGINS, W. A. Electrical signs of information flow in photoreceptors. *Cold Spring Harbor Symp. Quant. Biol.* 30: 403–418, 1966.

17. HARTLINE, H. K., WAGNER, H. G., AND RATLIFF, F. Inhibition in the eye of *Limulus. J. Gen. Physiol.* 39: 651–673, 1956.

18. HIRATA, Y. Some observations on the fine structure of the synapses in the olfactory bulb of the mouse, with particular reference to the atypical synaptic configuration. *Arch. Histol. Japan.* 24: 293–302, 1964.

19. HODGKIN, A. L. AND HUXLEY, A. F. A quantitative description of membrane current and its application to conduction and excitation in nerve. *J. Physiol., London* 117: 500–44, 1952.

20. HODGKIN, A. L. AND KATZ, B. The effect of sodium ions on the electrical activity of the giant axon of the squid. *J. Physiol., London* 108: 37–77, 1949.

21. IWASE, Y. AND LISENBY, D. Olfactory bulb responses in the turtle, with special reference to the deep negative spike. *Japan. J. Physiol.* 15: 331–341, 1965.

22. KATZ, B. AND MILEDI, R. Propagation of electric activity in motor nerve terminals. *Proc. Roy. Soc., London, Ser. B.* 161: 453–482, 1965.

23. KATZ, B. AND MILEDI, R. Input-output relation of a single synapse. *Nature* 212: 1242–1245, 1966.

24. KATZ, B. AND MILEDI, R. The release of acetylcholine from nerve endings by graded electric pulses. *Proc. Roy. Soc., London, Ser. B* 167: 23–38, 1967.

25. KIDD, M. Electron microscopy of the inner plexiform layer of the retina in the cat and pigeon. *J. Anat.* 96: 179–187, 1962.

26. LILEY, A. W. The effects of presynaptic polarization on the spontaneous activity at the mammalian neuromuscular junction. *J. Physiol., London* 134: 427–443, 1956.

27. LOHMAN, A. H. M. The anterior olfactory lobe of the guniea-pig. *Acta Anat., Basel* 53: Suppl. 49, 9–109, 1963.

28. LORENTE DE NÓ, R. Action potential of the motoneurons of the hypoglossus nucleus. *J. Cell. Comp. Physiol.* 29: 207–287, 1947.

29. LORENTE DE NÓ, R. Conduction of impulses in the neurons of the oculomotor nucleus. In: *The Spinal Cord* (Ciba Found. Symposium), edited by J. L. Malcolm and J. A. B. Gray. Boston: Little, Brown, 1953.

30. OCHI, J. Olfactory bulb response to antidromic olfactory tract stimulation in the rabbit. *Japan. J. Physiol.* 13: 113–128, 1963.

31. PALAY, S. L. The morphology of synapses in the central nervous system. *Exptl. Cell. Res., Suppl.* 5: 275–293, 1958.

32. PHILLIPS, C. G., POWELL, T. P. S., AND SHEPHERD,

G. M. The mitral cells of the rabbit's olfactory bulb. *J. Physiol., London* 156: 26p–27p, 1961.

33. PHILLIPS, C. G., POWELL, T. P. S., AND SHEPHERD, G. M. Responses of mitral cells to stimulation of the lateral olfactory tract in the rabbit. *J. Physiol., London* 168: 65–88, 1963.

34. POWELL, T. P. S., COWAN, W. M., AND RAISMAN, G. The central olfactory connexions. *J. Anat.* 99: 791–813, 1965.

35. PRICE, J. L. The termination of centrifugal fibers in the olfactory bulb. *Brain Res.* 7: 483–486, 1968.

36. RALL, W. Theory of physiological properties of dendrites. *Ann. N. Y. Acad. Sci.* 96: 1071–1092, 1962.

37. RALL, W. Electrophysiology of a dendritic neuron model. *Biophys. J.* 2 (No. 2, Part 2): 145–167, 1962.

38. RALL, W. Theoretical significance of dendritic trees for neuronal input-output relations. In: *Neural Theory and Modeling*, edited by R. F. Reiss. Stanford, Calif.: Stanford Univ. Press, pp. 73–97, 1964.

39. RALL, W. Distinguishing theoretical synaptic potentials computed for different soma-dendritic distributions of synaptic input. *J. Neurophysiol.* 30: 1138–1168, 1967.

40. RALL, W., SHEPHERD, G. M., REESE, T. S., AND BRIGHTMAN, M. W. Dendro-dendritic synaptic pathway for inhibition in the olfactory bulb. *Exptl. Neurol.* 14: 44–56, 1966.

41. RAMÓN Y CAJAL, S. *Histologie du Système Nerveux de l'Homme et des Vertébrés* (L. Asoulay, transl.) Paris: Maloine, 1911.

42. RANCK, J. B., JR. Analysis of specific impedance of rabbit cerebral cortex. *Exptl. Neurol.* 7: 153–174, 1963.

43. RATLIFF, F. *Mach Bands: Quantitative Studies on Neural Networks in the Retina*. San Francisco, Calif.: Holden-Day, 1965.

43a. RAVIOLA, G. AND RAVIOLA, E. Light and electron microscopic observations on the inner plexi-

form layer of the rabbit retina. *Am. J. Anat.* 120: 403–426, 1967.

44. REESE, T. S. Further studies on dendro-dendritic synapses in the olfactory bulb. *Anat. Record* 154: 408, 1966.

45. REESE, T. S. AND BRIGHTMAN, M. W. Electron microscopic studies on the rat olfactory bulb. *Anat. Record* 151: 492, 1965.

46. SHEPHERD, G. M. *Transmission in the Olfactory Pathway* (Ph.D. thesis), Oxford University, 1962.

47. SHEPHERD, G. M. Responses of mitral cells to olfactory nerve volleys in the rabbit. *J. Physiol., London* 168: 89–100, 1963.

48. SHEPHERD, G. M. Neuronal systems controlling mitral cell excitability. *J. Physiol., London* 168: 101–117, 1963.

49. SHEPHERD, G. M. The orientation of mitral cell dendrites. *Exptl. Neurol.* 14: 390–395, 1966.

50. TÖNNIES, J. F. AND JUNG, R. Über rasch wiederholte Entladungen der Motoneurone und die Hemmungsphase des Beugereflexes. *Arch. Ges. Physiol.* 250: 667–693, 1948.

51. VALVERDE, F. *Studies on the Piriform Lobe*. Cambridge, Mass.: Harvard Univ. Press, 1965.

52. VON BAUMGARTEN, R., GREEN, J. D., AND MANCIA, M. Slow waves in the olfactory bulb and their relation to unitary discharges. *Electroencephalog. Clin. Neurophysiol.* 14: 621–634, 1962.

53. WALSH, R. R. Olfactory bulb potentials evoked by electrical stimulation of the contralateral bulb. *Am. J. Physiol.* 196: 327–329, 1959.

54. YAMAMOTO, C. AND IWAMA, K. Intracellular potential recording from olfactory bulb neurones of the rabbit. *Proc. Japan Acad.* 38: 63–67, 1962.

55. YAMAMOTO, C., YAMAMOTO, T., AND IWAMA, K. The inhibitory system in the olfactory bulb studied by intracellular recording. *J. Neurophysiol.* 26: 403–415, 1963.

56. YOUNG, J. Z. The organization of a memory system. *Proc. Roy. Soc., London, Ser. B* 163: 285–320, 1965.

6 MOTONEURON MODELS OF DISTRIBUTED DENDRITIC SYNAPSES AND MECHANISMS OF NONLINEAR SYNAPTIC INTERACTIONS

6.1 Introduction by Robert E. Burke

Rall, W. (1967). Distinguishing theoretical synaptic potentials computed for different soma-dendritic distributions of synaptic input. *J. Neurophysiol.* 30:1139–1169.

The paper reprinted in the next chapter, "Distinguishing theoretical synaptic potentials computed for different soma-dendritic distributions of synaptic input," is a landmark paper for several reasons. In many respects, it represented the culmination of Wil Rall's work over the previous decade (much of it included in this volume), in which he developed a mathematical framework for understanding the electrical properties of dendritic neurons and the synapses that contact them. Many of the applications of this elegant cable theory were implicit in rigorous mathematical formulas, where they were protected from the mathematically unwashed, such as myself. In this paper, however, Wil took explicit examples from experimental data and showed how those results were not only explicable but in fact predictable from an understanding of cable theory as applied to dendritic neurons. His exposition was deliberately nonmathematical, using examples of limiting cases that were clearly understandable to nonmathematicians. Even people like myself, whose eyes glaze over when confronted with a differential equation, could see the "why" of our experimental results. Although Wil's earlier work had influenced many people in biophysics, I believe that this 1967 paper revealed the power of applied mathematics for many neurophysiologists.

This is not to say that the paper was purely a didactic explication of things already published. In fact, there is much that was new. For example, Wil introduced the quantitation of postsynaptic potential (PSP) shapes using the notion of "shape indices" and showed how these depended not only on spatial location of the input but also on dendritic electrotonic length and the time course of conductance input (see his "Comment on nonuniqueness" in chapter 6.2). The last fact in particular has often been neglected in later papers by others who took shape index data as generally indicative of electrotonic location, without attention to the important underlying assumptions. In a final sentence, Wil provided the following summation: "A theme common to all of these computations and interpretations is that results, which may appear paradoxical when examined only at the soma, can be understood quite simply when attention is directed to the synaptic input location with special attention to the effective driving potential there."

This paper was the fourth in a series of five that were published in 1967 (Smith et al. 1967; Nelson and Frank 1967; Burke 1967, Rall 1967; Rall et al. 1967). The first three papers reported experimental observations on cat α-motoneurons and the group Ia EPSPs generated in them. They were written by colleagues who had come to NIH in the 1950s and 1960s to work with the late Karl Frank, who was a major pioneer in using intracellular micropipettes to study cellular and synaptic processes. I was one of these people and can give a personal perspective on the genesis of this series, which is still referred to by some of our friends as "the '67 Book." My participation in this effort indelibly influenced my entire scientific career, and I hope that this brief reminiscence will give some idea of the excitement that comes to a young scientist who is lucky enough to work with great mentors.

I came to the NIH in 1964 to learn intracellular recording with Kay Frank (as he was universally known). He suggested that I could start by applying the method to cat motoneurons, in order to see whether or not group Ia EPSPs in motoneurons summated linearly. This question was of interest because Ia EPSPs did not always behave as expected for synaptic potentials that were generated by an increased postsynaptic conductance change. Working in Kay's lab, Tom Smith and Ray Wuerker had earlier found that Ia EPSPs were difficult, and frequently impossible, to invert by applying depolarizing current to the motoneuron soma, despite claims to the contrary (e.g., Eccles 1957). They also found that it was usually impossible to detect postsynaptic conductance changes during Ia EPSPs, even when using a sensitive AC analysis method (Smith et al. 1967). Phil Nelson and Kay had also observed that Ia EPSPs showed great variability in their response to currents injected at the motoneuron soma, which was only partially explainable by the nonlinear rectification behavior of the motoneuron membrane (Nelson and Frank 1967). Nonlinear potential summation would fit with the behavior expected for "chemical" synapses, while exclusively linear summation could have two interpretations: (1) Ia EPSPs are generated in part by electrical transmission (which we felt unlikely); or (2) Ia EPSPs are produced by purely chemical synapses that are widely distributed over the dendritic tree, in relative electrotonic isolation from one another. The latter notion seemed unlikely to me, probably because my earliest inspiration toward neurophysiology had come from John Eccles's classic monograph *The Physiology of Nerve Cells*, in which Eccles took the position that "the dendrites are so long, relative to their diameter, that changes in the membrane potential of more distal regions would make a negligible contribution to potentials recorded by a microelectrode implanted in the soma" (Eccles 1957, p. 6).

After starting experiments with electrically evoked composite Ia EPSPs, I also literally began playing around with the "synaptic noise" produced in motoneurons when their parent muscle was stretched (Granit et al.

1964). Much to my surprise, I found that it was often possible to recognize large-amplitude, rhythmically occurring EPSPs, ticking along within the background synaptic signals at frequencies that varied with levels of stretch, as would be expected for PSPs produced by an individual group Ia afferent (Burke and Nelson 1966). When I showed such records to Kay, he became quite excited and exclaimed, "You've got to stretch these signals out and look at their shapes!" He pointed me to Wil's 1964 paper describing the shape differences to be expected for EPSPs generated at different electrotonic locations. Luckily, my data had been recorded on FM tape, and reanalysis showed that, indeed, the shapes for any given single-fiber EPSP were quite consistent, but those produced by different fibers had very different shapes (Burke 1967). It was immediately obvious to us that we had an experimental validation of Wil's theoretical predictions. The single-fiber EPSP shape differences and the fact that composite Ia EPSPs often exhibited linear summation (Burke 1967) both fit very well with the idea that group Ia synapses were widely, and variably, distributed over the motoneuron surface. Furthermore, the fact that some Ia fibers produced somatic EPSPs with quite prolonged shape indices strongly suggested that synapses located on distal regions of the motoneuron dendrites could indeed produce significant voltages at the motoneuron soma. Needless to say, all this was very satisfying to both Wil and Kay, because it provided direct experimental support for Wil's view of dendritic function as critical to our understanding of neuronal input-output relations. For me, it was a revelation of what science was about!

Although Wil had illustrated the effects on dendritic location of synaptic potential shape in 1964, that paper (Rall 1964) was in a monograph that was not widely available. It seems fair to say that the 1967 paper under discussion here contained the first thorough theoretical exploration of the behavior of dendritic PSPs in the general neurophysiological literature. In it, Wil used compartmental equivalent cylinder models to explore examples of the interactive effects of conductance duration, amplitude, and spatial location on peak depolarization, illustrating important sources of nonlinear dependence between local voltage perturbation and fixed driving potentials at various points in the cylinder. He also looked at interactions between EPSPs and hyperpolarizations produced by injected currents at the soma and by simulated inhibitory conductances in different spatial locations. All of these simulations had immediate relevance for understanding our experimental findings.

A large fraction of this paper was devoted to an analysis of the detectability of dendritically located conductance changes underlying EPSPs when currents are injected into the soma. This section arose directly from Wil's consideration of the largely unsuccessful attempts by Tom Smith and colleagues (Smith et al. 1967) to use AC currents and sensitive phase-detection methods to define the Ia EPSP conductance. Wil recognized that the problem was primarily one of signal-to-noise ratios. The key insight was that, if a major fraction of the Ia conductance were delivered to the dendrites (a view not generally accepted at the time), the electrotonic cable intervening between the soma (the source of current and the site of measurement) and the distant sites of conductance change produces an inevitable decrement to both the local perturbing voltage changes at the synaptic sites and the results of that perturbation as reflected at the soma. Any such detection system thus faces an electrotonic decoupling that is larger than the electrotonic distance involved. Given the relatively small perturbations of local EPSP driving force that were experimentally feasible, Wil concluded that the expected magnitude of signal distortion at the soma, though theoretically present, would be below detection threshold at remarkably short electrotonic distances. Furthermore, the time course of the distorted signal did not match that of the conductance change itself, even when detectable. To all of us involved in this series of papers, these insights came as major surprises. These inconvenient properties of dendrites continue to plague everyone who tries to voltage clamp dendritic neurons (see Rall and Segev 1985; Spruston et al. 1993).

My own favorite aspect of this paper is Wil's remarkable "computational dissection" of the synaptic and redistribution (or "loss") currents that are inherent as synaptic potentials are generated in dendrites (section 2 and figure 4). This brief section presents concise and wonderfully lucid insights into why synaptic potential shapes and amplitudes change in an electrotonic cable. It bears careful and repeated study by anyone interested in how dendritic neurons process synaptic information.

Wil was the senior author on the last paper in the series of five papers of 1967 entitled "Dendritic location of synapses and possible mechanisms for the monosynaptic EPSP in motoneurons" (Rall et al. 1967). This paper was a concerted attempt to discuss the implications of the experimental observations in the first three papers in the light of Wil's theoretical results (paper four of the series). For reasons of economy, the paper has not been reprinted in this volume, but there are several aspects of it that are worth attention. It was in this paper that the first graphs of EPSP shape indices appeared in the form that later became widely used. Figure 1 here (reproduced from figure 5 in the original) encapsulates the central theme of this paper—the comparison of experimental data with modeling results. At the time, this was a rather startling thing to do with respect to neuronal electrophysiology.

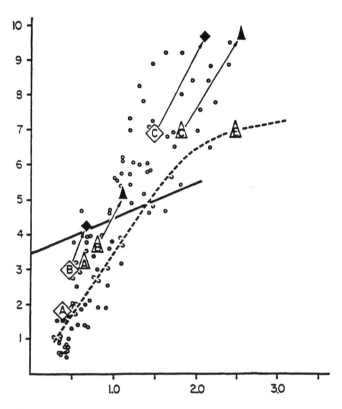

Figure 1

Shape index plot of EPSP half-width (ordinate) versus time to peak (abscissa), with scales in ms (from Rall et al. 1967). Small open circles denote experimentally observed single-fiber EPSPs. Large open symbols show shape indices for simulated EPSPs with "fast" (diamonds; alpha function with peak time of 0.1 ms) and "medium" (triangles; peak time of 0.2 ms) synaptic conductance time courses, recorded in compartment 1 of a 10-compartment cylinder (time constant = 5 ms; $L = 1.8$). Compartmental location of active conductances: $A = 1$, 2, 9, 10; $B = 1, 2, 3, 4, 9, 10$; $C = 3, 4, 9, 10$; $E =$ all 10, weighted to produce equal somatic amplitudes. Arrows and solid symbols show the effects of increasing time constant to 7 ms. The dashed line indicates the locus of shape indices for somatic EPSPs produced by conductances in individual compartments. The solid line shows the locus of shape indices of composite EPSPs produced by conductance changes of different durations applied at equal strength in all 10 compartments. Reproduced from Rall et al. 1967.

Figure 1 illustrates the time to peak and half-width of experimental single-fiber EPSPs from paper three (Burke 1967), with overlays derived from idealized cable models with ten compartments. The membrane time constant and electrotonic length (5 ms and 1.8, respectively) chosen for the model were thought to be representative of cat motoneurons. Subsequent experiments showed that these guesses were quite reasonable. The small open circles denote shape indices of individual EPSPs produced by 11 group Ia afferents in seven cat motoneurons. The dashed line shows the locus of shape indices for EPSPs generated in individual compartments of the model and recorded in the "soma" compartment. The large open symbols denote the shapes of composite EPSPs generated by conductances with "fast" or "medium" time courses, activated simultaneously in multiple compartments. The large filled symbols and arrows indicate changes that were produced when the model time constant was increased from 5 to 7 ms. The point of the figure was to show that a model system with a realistic range of parameters could generate synaptic potentials that fit reasonably well with experimental results. Although the simple compartmental model used for this figure is unrefined by today's standards, it represented a significant step in the evolution of thinking about dendritic function and the importance of synapses that are found on dendrites, because it brought together theoretical and experimental results in a way that was new and compelling.

An important deficiency in the 1967 comparison was the lack of time-constant estimates for the motoneurons; I had not looked at them because I did not anticipate their eventual importance. It was clear that variations in motoneuron time constant could not explain all of the observed shape differences because one notable example showed that two Ia fibers that ended on the same motoneuron generated EPSPs with markedly different shapes (Burke 1967, figure 10). However, figure 1 clearly shows that even a modest variation in time constant can account for a considerable range of shapes. Subsequent work by Jack et al. (1971) addressed this problem by plotting Ia EPSP shape indices that were normalized by motoneuron time constant. In addition, these authors plotted regions on the shape index plot that would account for likely variations in the values of dendritic electrotonic length, dendritic to somatic conductance ratios, and normalized synaptic-current time course. Their results, for a large sample of single-fiber EPSPs, allowed Jack and co-workers to conclude that Ia EPSPs arose from all regions of the dendritic membrane. Other studies soon confirmed and extended these observations (Mendell and Henneman 1971; Iansek and Redman 1973). Later, it became possible to inject horseradish peroxidase into individual group Ia afferents and motoneurons postsynaptic to them, to demonstrate that putative Ia boutons are indeed widely distributed in the dendritic trees (Burke et al. 1979; Brown and Fyffe 1981). In a remarkable experiment, Redman and Walmsley (1983) then combined such histological reconstructions with electrophysiology to show that the two methods produced the same estimates of electrotonic location. More recently, anatomical data on motoneurons and Ia bouton locations have been combined with estimates of motoneuron membrane properties to model the range in size and amplitude of composite group Ia EPSPs that arise from spatially dispersed boutons (Segev et al. 1990). The steady accumulation of evidence that group Ia EPSPs are generated largely in the motoneuron dendrites has been a source of much satisfaction for Wil and for all of us involved in this work.

In 1967, most of us felt that Ia EPSPs were generated by "chemical" synapses despite the existence of some experimental data that seemed incompatible. The wide spatial distribution of group Ia synapses proved to be the factor that brought all of the evidence back into line. It will be obvious to readers of this paper that the linchpin in this effort was Wil Rall. His insights and model results were essential to generating a cohesive and rigorous summation of the experimental results then available. It may be difficult for readers today to imagine that, only 25 years ago, the function of neuronal dendrites was poorly understood, frequently neglected, and even explicitly denied. The fact that dendrites now enter into everyone's thinking about neuronal function is a tribute to the clarity and force of Wil Rall's pioneering contributions to neuroscience.

References

Brown, A. G., and Fyffe, R. E. W. (1981) Direct observations on the contacts made between Ia afferents and α-motoneurones in the cat's lumbosacral spinal cord. *J. Physiol. (Lond)* 313:121–140.

Burke, R. E. (1967) The composite nature of the monosynaptic excitatory postsynaptic potential. *J. Neurophysiol.* 30:1114–1137.

Burke, R. E., and Nelson, P. G. (1966) Synaptic activity in motoneurons during natural stimulation of muscle spindles. *Science* 151:1088–1091.

Burke, R. E., and Walmsley, B., and Hodgson, J. A. (1979) HRP anatomy of group Ia afferent contacts on alpha motoneurones. *Brain Res* 160:347–352.

Eccles, J. C. (1957) *The Physiology of Nerve Cells.* Baltimore: The Johns Hopkins Press.

Granit, R., Kellerth, J.-O., and Williams, T. D. (1964) Intracellular aspects of stimulating motoneurones by muscle stretch. *J. Physiol. (Lond)* 174:435–452.

Iansek, R., Redman, S. J. (1973) The amplitude, time course and charge of unitary excitatory post-synaptic potentials evoked in spinal motoneurone dendrites. *J. Physiol. (Lond)* 234:665–688.

Jack, J. J. B. Miller, S., Porter, R., and Redman, S. J. (1971) The time course of minimal excitatory post-synaptic potentials evoked in spinal motoneurons by group Ia afferent fibres. *J. Physiol. (Lond)* 215:353–380.

Mendell, L. M., and Henneman, E. (1971) Terminals of single Ia fibers: Location, density, and distribution within a pool of 300 homonymous motoneurons. *J. Neurophysiol.* 34:171–187.

Nelson, P. G., and Frank, K. (1967) Anomalous rectification in cat spinal motoneurons and effect of polarizing currents on excitatory postsynaptic potentials. *J. Neurophysiol.* 30:1097–1113.

Rall, W. (1964) Theoretical significance of dendritic trees for neuronal input-output relations. In *Neural Theory and Modeling*, ed. R. F. Reiss. Stanford, CA: Stanford University Press.

Rall, W. (1967) Distinguishing theoretical synaptic potentials computed for different soma-dendritic distributions of synaptic input. *J. Neurophysiol.* 30:1139–1169.

Rall, W, Burke, R. E., Smith, T. G., Nelson, P. G., and Frank, K. (1967) Dendritic location of synapses and possible mechanisms for the monosynaptic EPSP in motoneurons. *J. Neurophysiol.* 30:1169–1193.

Rall, W., and Segev, I. (1985) Space clamp problems when voltage clamping branched neurons with intracellular electrodes. In *Voltage and Patch Clamping with Microelectrodes*, ed. T. G. Smith, H. Lecar, S. J. Redman, and P. Gage. Bethesda, MD: American Physiological Society.

Redman S. J., and Walmsley, B. (1983) The time course of synaptic potentials evoked in cat spinal motoneurones at identified group Ia synapses. *J. Physiol. (Lond)* 343:117–133.

Segev, I., Fleshman, J. W., and Burke, R. E. (1990) Computer simulation of group Ia EPSPs using morphologically-realistic models of cat α-motoneurons. *J. Neurophysiol.* 64:648–660.

Smith, T., Wuerker, R., and Frank, K. (1967) Membrane impedance changes during synaptic transmission in cat spinal motoneurons. *J. Neurophysiol.* 30:1072–1096.

Spruston, N., Jaffe, D. B., Williams, S. H., and Johnston, D. (1993) Voltage- and space-clamp errors associated with the measurement of electrotonically remote synaptic events. *J. Neurophysiol.* 70:781–802.

6.2 Distinguishing Theoretical Synaptic Potentials Computed for Different Soma-Dendritic Distributions of Synaptic Input (1967), *J. Neurophysiol.* 30:1138–1168

Wilfrid Rall

BY MEANS OF COMPUTATIONAL EXPERIMENTS with a mathematical neuron model, it is possible to make many detailed predictions, some of which can be tested by comparison with suitably controlled experimental observations. In particular, a theoretical model which permits a choice of both the time course and the soma-dendritic location of synaptic input, makes it possible to explore the way in which the shape of a synaptic potential can be expected to depend upon these two aspects of synaptic input. It is also possible to explore such related problems as the following: the effect of superimposing various combinations of synaptic input, both excitatory and inhibitory, and at various locations; the effect of applied hyperpolarizing current upon the shape of a synaptic potential; and the detectability at the neuron soma of a synaptic conductance transient located in the dendrites.

Many such computational experiments have been carried out, with two somewhat different objectives in mind. One objective has been to explore and gain insight into the general properties of the theoretical model, while the other objective has been to test the applicability of this theoretical model to the particular case of motoneurons in the cat spinal cord. The experimental observations presented in several companion papers (1, 8, 15) have provided an unusual opportunity for such a comparison of theory and experiment. This comparison has been carried out as a collaborative effort; the implications of this for our understanding of synaptic potentials in cat motoneurons are presented in a separate paper (14). The present paper is not about motoneurons, but about the properties and implications of the more general theoretical model.

There are several positive advantages to separating the consideration of a general model from its application to a particular neuron type. The general model can be tested for applicability to different neuron types; some applications may differ only in the value of the membrane time constant needed to relate a general result to a particular neuron type; other applications may differ in the values of theoretical parameters corresponding to electrotonic length or to the time course of synaptic current; still other applications may require explicit consideration of several sets of dendrites, such as the basal and apical dendrites of pyramidal cells.

Theoretical predictions that canot be tested experimentally are usually regarded as scientifically meaningless; however, it is important to distinguish between predictions that could never be tested, and others that are testable, in principle, but which require greater experimental control or finesse than is currently available. The present research provides several illustrations of the latter. For example, when synaptic input is located in the dendrites, a comprehensive computation can provide not only the synaptic potential time course predicted to occur at the soma, but also the time course of the synaptic current and the transient membrane depolarization at the dendritic location, as well as the details of the electrotonic spread of current and of membrane depolarization from the dendrites to the soma. Such details are not easily tested in neurons; yet these details can have great value in enriching our physical intuitive understanding of such related events. We can build our physical intuition upon the quantitative answers to precise questions obtained for the theoretical model, and this physical intuition can then be helpful in the interpretation of approximately similar experimental observations.

Several examples of the differences between the brief synaptic potential computed when synaptic input is restricted to the neuron soma or proximal dendrites, and the slower rising and longer lasting synaptic potential computed when synaptic input is restricted to distal portions of the dendrites have appeared as illustrations in previous theoretical papers (12, 13). The earliest theoretical results relating the time course of a synaptic potential to the time course of nonuniformly distributed synaptic current appeared in 1959 (9). The fact that passive decay (as seen at the soma) should be fastest when membrane depolarization is greatest at the soma, and slowest when membrane depolarization is greatest in the dendritic periphery was demonstrated theoretically and illustrated graphically in 1960 (11, p. 515–516, 521, 528–529). The theoretical basis for transforming an extensively branched neuron into an equivalent cylinder, and for representing nonuniform distributions of synaptic excitatory and/or synaptic inhibitory membrane conductance, was presented in 1961, and this theory was used to compute an early illustrative comparison of synaptic potential shapes obtained for synaptic input restricted to half of the soma-dendritic surface (12, Fig. 7). The use of a compartmental model of soma-dendritic surface was introduced in 1962 as means of computing the consequences of many spatiotemporal patterns of synaptic input (13). Because of the new quantitative experimental detail now available (1, 8, 14, 15) the present computations have avoided the artificiality of step changes in synaptic conductance value by introducing a smooth transient synaptic conductance time course as the synaptic input.

METHOD

Compartmental model. For most of these computations, the soma-dendritic surface of a neuron has been represented as mathematically equivalent to a chain of 5 or 10 equal compartments. This concept is illustrated schematically in Fig. 1, where the dashed lines divide

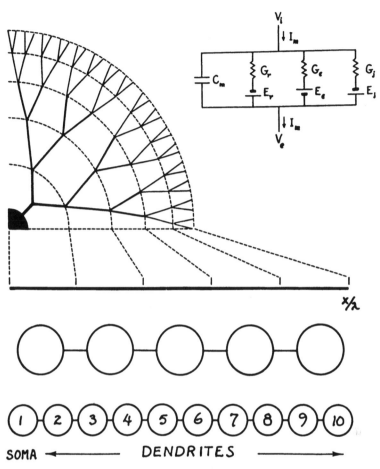

FIG. 1. Schematic diagrams. Electric equivalent circuit model of nerve membrane, at upper right. Branching dendritic tree, at upper left. Diagram indicates the mathematical transformation (12) of a class of dendritic trees into an equivalent cylinder, and into approximately equivalent chains of equal compartments (13). See text and references (12, 13) for details and discussion.

the dendritic branching system into 5 regions of equal membrane surface area. When each such region is approximated as a compartment, in which the membrane capacity and the several parallel membrane conductances (see inset in upper right of Fig. 1) are treated as lumped electric parameters, the essential simplifying assumption is that spatial nonuniformity within each region is completely neglected. Spatial nonuniformity of the whole neuron is represented only by the differences between regions.

Soma and dendritic compartments. With the most commonly used chain of 10 compartments, shown at bottom of Fig. 1, the neuron soma has been identified with compartment 1, while compartment 10 represents a lumping of the most peripheral portions of all dendritic trees belonging to this neuron model. The intermediate compartments represent increments of electrotonic distance, as measured from the dendritic trunks to the dendritic periphery.

Electrotonic distance, Z. In a dendritic tree, the electrotonic distance, Z_1, from the soma to any dendritic point x_1, can be defined by the integral

$$Z_1 = \int_0^{x_1} dx/\lambda$$

where x measures actual distance along the lengths of successive branches from the soma to the point in question, and λ represents the characteristic length (or length constant) which changes with branch diameter at each point of branching. For a branching system that is transformable to an equivalent cylinder (12), or to a chain of equal compartments (13), each dendritic compartment represents not only an equal amount of membrane surface area, but also an equal increment in electrontoic distance (12, 13). Thus, for the 10-compartment chain at the bottom of Fig. 1, the increment per compartment usually had the value, $\Delta Z = 0.2$; then the values, $Z = 1.0$ in compartment 6, and $Z = 1.8$ in compartment 10, express the corresponding electrotonic distances away from the soma compartment. Occasionally, computations were done with $\Delta Z = 0.1$, or with $\Delta Z = 0.4$ as the electrotonic increment per compartment.

Mathematical model. The actual mathematical model is a system of ordinary differential equations which are linear and of first order; some coefficients are constants, but others (those related to synaptic conductance) are functions of time. This system of equations was presented and derived in a previous publication (13).

Dimensionless variables of the model. The state of the system at any time is defined by three variables in each compartment. Two of these are independent variables representing synaptic excitatory and inhibitory conductance, while the dependent variable represents membrane potential. When there is externally applied current, this must be considered as an additional independent input variable. Each of these variables has a very specific definition in the mathematical model. Also, each variable is defined as a dimensionless ratio that has a useful physical intuitive meaning.

Synaptic intensity variables. The synaptic excitatory intensity, $\mathcal{E}$, and the independent synaptic inhibitory intensity, $\mathcal{J}$, must be specified for each compartment. They are defined as the membrane conductance ratios,

$$\mathcal{E} = G_\epsilon / G_r \qquad \mathcal{J} = G_j / G_r$$

where G_r, G_ϵ and G_j are parallel membrane conductances in the electrical equivalent circuit shown as an inset in Fig. 1; G_r represents resting membrane conductance in series with the resting battery, E_r; G_ϵ represents synaptic excitatory conductance in series with the synaptic excitatory battery, E_ϵ; G_j represents synaptic inhibitory conductance in series with the synaptic inhibitory battery, E_j. The values of E_r, E_ϵ, and E_j are assumed to remain constant. This formal model (12, 13) is only a slight generalization of more familiar membrane models (2, 3, 6). The two variables, $\mathcal{E}$ and $\mathcal{J}$, will sometimes be referred to as synaptic input; the time course in each compartment is prescribed and, for all of the present computations, is assumed to be independent of membrane potential and of applied current.

Membrane potential disturbance, v. This variable provides a dimensionless measure of the deviation of membrane potential from its resting value. It is defined

$$v = (V_m - E_r)/(E_\epsilon - E_r)$$

where V_m represents the potential difference across the membrane (inside potential minus outside potential).

The variable, v, is normalized in the sense that

$$v = 1, \quad \text{when} \quad V_m = E_\epsilon$$

Thus, excitatory deviations from the resting potential are represented as positive values on a scale extending from 0 to 1. These positive values of v correspond to membrane depolarization; this is consistent with the experimentally observed positivity of intracellularly recorded excitatory synaptic potentials. The value, $v = 1$, corresponds to the limiting amount of depolarization, for $\mathcal{E}$ very large, and $\mathcal{J}$ small, and in the absence of applied current.

Peak amplitudes of $v = 0.01$ and $v = 0.1$ were obtained in several series of computed synaptic potentials. This means depolarization one-hundredth or one-tenth of the way toward the limiting value. For example, if $(E_\epsilon - E_r) = 70$ mv, then $v = 0.01$ corresponds to 0.7 mv, and $v = 0.1$ corresponds to 7 mv. Negative values of v represent membrane hyperpolarization. For example, if $(E_j - E_r)/(E_\epsilon - E_r) = -0.1$, then this value represents the limiting negative value of v (for $\mathcal{J}$ much larger than $\mathcal{E}$, and in the absence of applied current).

Dimensionless time variable, T. This variable is defined

$$T = t/\tau$$

where t represents time and τ represents the passive membrane time constant. Results expressed in terms of T can be equally valid for neurons which may have different membrane time constants.

Dimensionless slope divided by peak. Although the theoretical slope, dv/dT, is already a dimensionless quantity, the comparison of experimental and theoretical rising slopes of synaptic potentials is facilitated by considering the value of the slope divided by the peak amplitude of the synaptic potential. This dimensionless quantity can be expressed

$$(dv/dT)/v_p = \tau(dV/dt)/V_p$$

where $V = V_m - E_r$, is in millivolts, dV/dt is in millivolts per millisecond (i.e., volts per second), and subscript, p, designates the peak value of v or V. Usually, the slope has been measured at the point where the rising synaptic potential reaches half of its peak amplitude, i.e., the point halfway up; sometimes the slope was also measured at the point halfway down. To compare with experiment, consider, for example, a rising slope of 12 v/sec for a synaptic potential having a peak amplitude of 4 mv, then $(dV/dt)/V_p = 3$ msec^{-1}, and, for a membrane time constant, $\tau = 5$ msec, we obtain a dimensionless value of 15 for the slope over peak defined above.

Depolarizing current density. The dimensionless slope, dv/dT, is also a dimensionless measure of net depolarizing current density. This net current refers to the difference between the actual synaptic current at the region in question, and the loss current composed of electrotonic current spread to neighboring regions and of current that leaks across the local passive membrane resistance. The actual net depolarizing current density can be expressed

$$C_m \frac{dV_m}{dt} = [C_m(E_\epsilon - E_r)/\tau] \frac{dv}{dT}$$

where C_m represents the membrane capacitance. For example, if $C_m = 1$ μf/cm^2, $(E_\epsilon - E_r)$ = 70 mv, and $\tau = 5$ msec, the factor enclosed by the square brackets has a value of 14 μamp /cm^2.

Computation method. The computations were carried out with the computer program SAAM 22, on the IBM 7094 at the National Bureau of Standards. The computer program is the current version of a program developed over a period of years by Berman, Weiss, and Shahn; it is especially suited for computations with compartmental models, and contains many features that contribute to its versatility. One feature is that the computations can be required to adjust the values of one or more parameters to obtain a least-squares fit between the theoretical points and several data points; this feature was used to find, for any given compartmental and temporal distribution of synaptic input, $\mathcal{E}$, the magnitude of $\mathcal{E}$ that produces a synaptic potential having a prescribed peak value (usually $v = 0.01$, or $v = 0.10$). Another feature is that one or more parameters can be required to vary with time in proportion with any prescribed transient function; this feature was used to prescribe smooth time variation of synaptic input, $\mathcal{E}$ and/or $\mathcal{G}$, in one or more compartments.

Synaptic transient function. Most of the computations used a transient of the form de fined by

$$F(T) = (T/T_p) \exp(1 - T/T_p)$$

where T represents dimensionless time as a variable starting from zero, and T_p is a constant to be selected. This transient has the following features, $F(T) = 0$ for $T = 0$, $F(T) = 1.0$, the peak value, at $T = T_p$, and $F(T)$ returns to zero for large values of T. Also $F(T) = 0.5$ at nearly $T = 0.23$ T_p, on the way up, and again at nearly $T = 2.68$ T_p, on the way down; thus the half-width (width at half of peak amplitude) is very nearly 2.45 T_p. The area under the entire curve equals eT_p, where e is the base of the natural logarithms. Graphic examples of this transient are provided by the dotted curves in Figs. 2 and 4. The three particular choices of T_p used most, 0.02, 0.04, and 0.092, provide the transients referred to in the text as "fast," "medium," and "slow" input transients.

Fast input transient. This transient reaches its peak at $T = 0.02$, and has a half-width (duration at half of peak amplitude) of about 0.049 in units of T. For a membrane time constant of $\tau = 5$ msec, this would imply a peak time of 0.1 msec, and a half-width of about 0.245 msec.

Medium input transient. This transient reaches its peak at $T = 0.04$, and has a half-width of about 0.098 in units of T. For a membrane time constant of $\tau = 5$ msec, this would imply a peak time of 0.2 msec, and a half-width of about 0.49 msec.

Slow input transient. This transient reaches its peak at $T = 0.092$, and has a half-width of about 0.225 in units of T. Also, the area under this curve is 0.25 in units of T; this area equals that of a rectangular pulse of unit height and of duration 0.25 in units of T, such as the synaptic input used in numerous earlier computations (cf. 13, Fig. 6).

RESULTS

I. *Different shapes of computed synaptic potentials*

Effect of synaptic input location. Four examples of computed excitatory postsynaptic potentials (EPSP) are illustrated by the solid curves in Fig. 2.

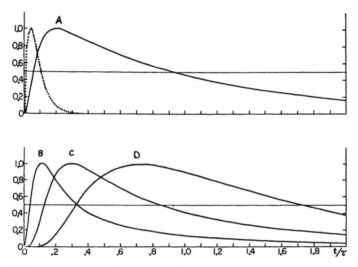

FIG. 2. Comparison of four EPSP shapes computed for a chain of 10 compartments. Dotted curve shows the assumed excitatory conductance transient; it is the medium input time course defined in METHODS. Curve A shows the EPSP for equal input in all compartments. Curves B, C, and D all show an EPSP in compartment 1 for different cases of synaptic input restricted to 1 of the 10 compartments. For curve B, synaptic input was in compartment 1 alone; for curve C, input was in compartment 4 alone; for curve D, input was in compartment 8 alone. Ordinate scale represents amplitudes relative to each peak amplitude. The same EPSP shapes were obtained for peak amplitudes, $v = 0.01$ and $v = 0.10$; the synaptic intensity required for each case can be found (below) in Table 3.

The obvious differences in shape are due to differences in the location of synaptic input assumed for each computation. Exactly the same time course of synaptic excitatory conductance was assumed in each case; this time course, shown as a dotted curve, is the medium input transient defined above (in METHODS). Curve A shows the EPSP computed for the case of synaptic input distributed equally to all compartments. This EPSP reaches peak value at $T = 0.20$ and has a half-width of 0.88 in units of T. Curve A represents not only the EPSP that occurs in the soma compartment, but also the time course of membrane depolarization in every dendritic compartment; there is no electrotonic spread between compartments for this case of equal synaptic input to all compartments. After the synaptic input transient is completed (after $T = 0.3$ for this medium input transient), the decay of such a spatially uniform EPSP is a simple passive exponential decay.

Curves B, C, and D illustrate 3 examples of EPSP shapes computed in the soma compartment of a chain of 10 compartments when the synaptic input was localized to a single compartment. Thus curve B was obtained when synaptic input was restricted to the soma compartment, curve C was obtained with input restricted to compartment 4, while curve D was obtained with input restricted to compartment 8. Although synaptic excitatory conductance had the same (dotted) time course as for case A, larger synaptic intensities were required in cases B, C, and D, in order to obtain an EPSP of the same peak amplitude as curve A.

Curve B rises about 1.65 times as fast as curve A, reaches its peak in about half the time required by curve A, and has a half-width that is only one-third that of curve A. Also, when both curves have decayed to half of peak amplitude, curve B falls three times as fast as curve A; this faster decay can be understood intuitively as the consequence of electrotonic spread from the soma compartment toward the dendritic compartments (cf. 11, p. 515–516, 528–529).

Curve C is somewhat similar to reference curve A; however, there are significant differences. Curve C rises more slowly and falls more rapidly than curve A; the slower rise can be understood intuitively as the consequence of electrotonic spread from the input compartment (no. 4) toward the soma, while the faster fall is the consequence of electrotonic spread away from compartments 1, 2, 3, and 4, toward the peripheral dendritic compartments.

Curve D is more delayed, rises more slowly, has a more rounded peak, and begins to decline more slowly than the other curves. The half-width value of 1.42, in units of T, is nearly five times that of curve B, and is 60% larger than that of curve A. This sluggish rise to a very rounded peak can be understood intuitively as the consequence of electrotonic spread from the distal dendritic input compartment (no. 8) to the soma.

EPSP shape and amplitude. The 4 EPSP shapes in Fig. 2 illustrate equally well the results obtained for several different EPSP amplitudes. In particular, 1 complete set of results having the small EPSP peak, $v_p = 0.01$, was compared with another set having a 10-fold larger peak amplitude. When these results were scaled relative to their peak amplitudes (as in Fig. 2), the 2 sets of EPSP curves differed negligibly (i.e., rarely by more than the thickness of the curve). To understand why shape distortions occur for still larger EPSP amplitudes, and why the agreement is not exact even at small amplitudes, it is necessary to remember that the synaptic input has been treated as an excitatory conductance transient. For small amounts of membrane depolarization, the time course of synaptic current is essentially the same as that of the synaptic conductance. For a large transient membrane depolarization at the synaptic input location, the effective driving potential (for synaptic current) changes enough to cause a significant distortion of synaptic current time course; this can result in a significant change of EPSP shape. In practice, one is usually concerned with small EPSP amplitudes (i.e., less than $v_p = 0.2$). For this range of practical interest, the EPSP shape computed for a given synaptic input location and time course can be regarded as approximately independent of EPSP amplitude.

Quantitative shape indices. The comparison of computed EPSP shapes with experimentally observed EPSP shapes can be facilitated by focusing attention upon a few quantitative measures. Definitions of several shape indices are stated below. These shape indices are used in Table 1 to summarize the computed results obtained for the same medium input transient as in Fig. 2, and for the same chain of 10 compartments having an over-all electrotonic length equal to twice the characteristic length.

Table 1. Quantitative EPSP shape characteristics
(chain of ten compartments: medium & transient)

Location of Synaptic Input	All Cpts	Cpt 1	Cpt 2	Cpt 3	Cpt 4	Cpt 6	Cpt 8	Cpt 10
Time of peak (from T=0)	0.20	0.11	0.16	0.22	0.29	0.47	0.73	0.86
Time to peak (from EPSP foot*)	0.19	0.10	0.14	0.19	0.24	0.38	0.59	0.67
Same, for $\tau = 5$ msec	0.95 msec	0.5 msec	0.7 msec	0.95 msec	1.2 msec	1.9 msec	2.9 msec	3.3 msec
Half-width time	0.88	0.29	0.42	0.57	0.73	1.14	1.42	1.46
Same, for $\tau = 5$ msec	4.4 msec	1.45 msec	2.1 msec	2.8 msec	3.6 msec	5.7 msec	7.1 msec	7.3 msec
Slope/peak: halfway up $(dV/dT)/V_p$	9.4	15.5	11.0	8.4	6.8	4.5	2.9	2.4
$(dv/dt)/v_p$, for $\tau = 5$ msec	1.9 msec^{-1}	3.1 msec^{-1}	2.2 msec^{-1}	1.7 msec^{-1}	1.4 msec^{-1}	0.9 msec^{-1}	0.6 msec^{-1}	0.5 msec^{-1}
Slope/peak: halfway down $(dV/dT)V_p$	−0.5	−1.52	−1.05	−0.81	−0.65	−0.48	−0.47	−0.47

* Time of foot defined as point of intersection with the base line of a line drawn from the point halfway up, through the point one-tenth way up. Except where noted otherwise, time is dimensionless, $T = t/\tau$.

Time and peak. It is useful to distinguish between time of peak, measured from the time of synaptic input initiation (T = 0 in Fig. 2) and time to peak measured from the "foot" of the EPSP. The time, T = 0, is easy to obtain for a computed EPSP, but is usually not known for an experimental EPSP. The foot of the EPSP is sometimes characterized as the point where EPSP rise can first be detected; an alternative, used here is to define the time of the foot operationally as the point of intersection with the base line, of a line drawn through the two points where the rising EPSP attains 10% and 50% of its peak amplitude. When this operational definition is applied to Fig. 2, the time of foot values, T = 0.05 and T = 0.14, are obtained for curves C and D. In Table 1 the values of time to peak (from EPSP foot) range from T = 0.10 to T = 0.67 (or from 0.5 msec to 3.3 msec for $\tau = 5$ msec).

Half-width. This quantity provides a useful measure of the sharpness of an EPSP; it is defined as the width of the EPSP at half of peak amplitude. For the series in Table 1, the half-width is about three times the time to peak, for single compartment locations from 1 to 6; this factor becomes progressively smaller for input locations 8 and 10, but it is more than 4.6 for the case of uniform input to all compartments.

Rising slope divided by peak. The slope, dv/dT, is determined at the point where the rising EPSP attains half of its peak amplitude; this slope is often the maximal rising slope. An amplitude independent quantity is obtained by dividing this slope by the EPSP peak amplitude. The resulting dimensionless shape index values cover a sixfold range, from 2.5 to 15.5 in Table 1. Thus, for a membrane time constant, $\tau = 5$ msec, the quantity, $(dv/dt)/v_p$, ranges from 0.5 msec^{-1} for input to compartment 10 alone, to 3.1 msec^{-1} for input to compartment 1 alone. There is an approximate inverse proportionality between these rising slope/peak values and the time-to-peak values, in other words, the time to peak is approximately 1.6 times the reciprocal of the rising slope/peak value. A similar proportionality was found to apply to many experimental EPSP shapes, and also to theoretical EPSP shapes computed with either the fast or the slow synaptic conductance time course.

Falling slope divided by peak. Here the slope, dv/dT, is determined at the point where the falling EPSP attains half of the EPSP peak amplitude and this slope value is divided by the peak amplitude. A value of -0.5 corresponds to uniform passive decay. The cases where synaptic input was confined to compartments 1, 2, 3, or 4 all fall more rapidly than this because of electrotonic spread out into the peripheral half of the chain, while the cases where synaptic input was confined to compartments 6, 8, or 10 fall slightly more slowly because of electrotonic spread toward the soma from the peripheral half of the chain.

Plot of half-width versus time to peak. In comparing these theoretical EPSP shapes with EPSP shapes observed in motoneurons, it was found useful to represent each shape as a point in a two-dimensional plot: the ordinate of each point is the half-width value, while the abscissa is the corresponding time to peak. Several examples of such shape index plots are illustrated in a companion paper (14). Such plots provide a means of grasping and comparing the variety of EPSP shapes found for different values of the theoretical parameters.

Effects of fast, medium, and slow synaptic input transient. Table 2 provides a summary comparison of EPSP shapes obtained in three different computational series, using the three cases, fast, medium, and slow, of synaptic conductance time course defined in METHODS. The numerical details of Table 2 are presented with the hope that they may be found useful in the examination of experimental results from various neuron types having different membrane time-constant values, and a similar time course of synaptic current or synaptic conductance; one example of this (for cat motoneurons) is provided in a companion paper (14). Here, comments are made about only a few general aspects of these numerical results. Perhaps most striking is the fact that changing the input time course at single compartmental locations has a proportionately much larger effect for proximal input locations than for distal input locations. For example, both the time-to-peak values and the slope/peak values change by a factor of about 3.5 (fast to slow) for input in compartment 1, compared with a factor of 1.3 (fast to slow) for input in compartment 10; the corresponding factors for half-width are somewhat smaller. The increment of change in time-to-peak values remains more nearly constant; this increment has a value of 0.15 (fast to slow) for input in compartment 1 or 10. This can be understood approximately as follows: this common time increment represents primarily the shift of peak depolarization in the input compartment caused by the change in the synaptic input time course. The half-width does not behave in the same way; the increments themselves decrease as input is shifted to more distal locations, so much so that for inputs in compartment 8 or 10, the EPSP

Table 2. EPSP shape index values comparing effects of fast, medium,
and slow synaptic input transients

Location of Synaptic Input	All Cpts	Cpt 1	Cpt 2	Cpt 3	Cpt 4	Cpt 6	Cpt 8	Cpt 10
Time to peak (from foot)								
Fast	0.11	.06	.09	.14	.19	.33	.54	.61
Medium	0.19	.10	.14	.19	.24	.38	.59	.67
Slow	0.35	.21	.25	.31	.37	.51	.68	.76
Half-width								
Fast	0.80	.18	.33	.50	.69	1.12	1.41	1.44
Medium	0.88	.29	.42	.57	.73	1.14	1.42	1.46
Slow	1.07	.53	.63	.75	.89	1.24	1.47	1.52
$(dV/dT)/V_p$, halfway up								
Fast	17.7	27.0	17.6	12.3	8.9	5.2	3.1	2.6
Medium	9.4	15.5	11.0	8.5	6.8	4.5	2.9	2.4
Slow	4.8	7.6	6.1	5.1	4.3	3.2	2.4	2.0

half-width value changes by less than 5% over this range of synaptic input time course. Apparently the EPSP half-width is determined primarily by the slowing and rounding effects of electrotonic spread from these distal input locations. This conclusion receives additional support from the fact that the same half-width values were also obtained with a square synaptic conductance pulse (duration $\Delta T = .25$) at these same distal input locations.

Effect of different electrotonic length. Computations were carried out to discover how the EPSP shape index values change when the chain of 10 compartments is assumed to have a different effective electrotonic length. This is important because of uncertainties about the correct value of the characteristic length constant, λ, even in experimental situations where the actual dimension of the dendritic branches are fairly well known. As defined in METHODS, an electrotonic length increment, $\Delta Z = 0.2$ per dendritic compartment, implies a value, $Z = 1.8$, for the electrotonic length of the 9 dendritic compartments. This length was used in computing the EPSP shapes of Tables 1 and 2. Other computations were carried out with $\Delta Z = 0.1$, implying

$Z = 0.9$ for the 9 dendritic compartments, and with $\Delta Z = 0.4$, implying $Z = 3.6$ for the dendritic chain.

Two useful approximate generalizations can be stated: doubling ΔZ approximately doubles the time-to-peak value obtained for a given input compartment; a smaller factor, between 1.4 and 1.5, of increase was found for the half-width values. More detailed results are summarized in Fig. 3, which uses a common Z scale to plot the dendritic input locations in the 3

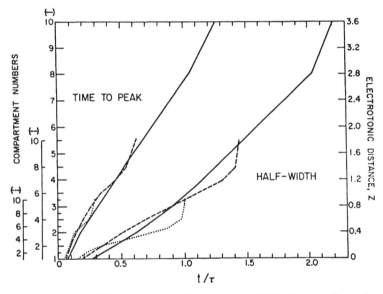

Fɪɢ. 3. Effect of dendritic electrotonic length upon EPSP shape index values. Three cases, $\Delta Z = 0.1$, 0.2, and 0.4 per dendritic compartment, are shown. The three sets of compartment numbers, shown at left, are spaced to fit a common ordinate scale, expressed as electrotonic distance, Z, shown at right. For each input location (as ordinate), both the time-to-peak and the half-width values were plotted (as abscissa). The solid lines connect points plotted for case ($\Delta Z = 0.4$) where compartment 10 is $Z = 3.6$ distant from the soma, implying a value, $Z = 3.6$, for the dendritic electrotonic length. The dashed lines represent the case ($\Delta Z = 0.2$) implying a value, $Z = 1.8$, for dendritic electrotonic length. The dotted curves represent the case ($\Delta Z = 0.1$) implying a value, $Z = 0.9$, for the dendritic electrotonic length. The fast synaptic input transient (see ᴍᴇᴛʜᴏᴅs) was used for all of these cases.

sets of computations; time-to-peak values and half-width values were both plotted (as abscissa), for each of the several input locations (as ordinate). It is instructive to compare two examples of input at the electrotonic distance, $Z = 1.2$, away from the soma. Both compartment 4 with $\Delta Z = 0.4$, and compartment 7 with $\Delta Z = 0.2$ are at this distance from the soma. In both cases, the time-to-peak value was 0.45 in the EPSP computed at the soma; however, the input in compartment 7 resulted in a longer half-width value (1.31) than that (1.15) for the input in compartment 4. Both this particular difference, and the deviations of the shorter curves from the longer curves in Fig. 3, are consistent with earlier generalizations stating that electrotonic spread toward the soma from the distal half of the chain causes the early decay to be slower than a spatially uniform decay, while electrotonic spread from the proximal half to the distal half of the chain causes faster early decay.[1] Figure 3 has the merit of displaying both shape index values plotted versus one Z scale that is common to the three cases. For other purposes it is useful to plot each of these half-width values against its corresponding time-to-peak value; such a plot can be found in a companion paper (14, Fig. 6).

Comment on nonuniqueness. From the preceding figures and tables, it is apparent that one cannot infer the location and time course of synaptic input from EPSP shape alone. Most of these computed EPSP shapes can be at least approximately duplicated by several alternative combinations of synaptic input location and time course; by permitting multiple input locations, the number of possible combinations becomes greatly increased (14). When an EPSP is very brief, this restricts consideration to more proximal locations and to faster input transients, but some reciprocity of choice remains within this range. When an EPSP is very slow, either or both slow input time course and electrotonic distance of input location may be responsible. With slow experimental EPSP shapes one must beware of the possible effects of temporal dispersion of synaptic activity. In any given application to experimental EPSP shapes, it is important to assess the extent to which one can safely assume reasonable ranges of values for these three unknowns: synaptic conductance time course, restricted location of synaptic input, and dendritic electrotonic length.

Comment on 5 or 10 compartments. Because quite a few computations were done with a chain of 5 compartments, the effect of this upon EPSP shape merits a brief statement. In particular, comparisons were made between a 5-compartment chain having $\Delta Z = 0.4$ per compartment, and the 10-compartment chain having $\Delta Z = 0.2$ per compartment. The essential difference is a factor of 2 in the coarseness of lumping. As might be expected intuitively, it was found that the EPSP shape computed for synaptic input restricted to 1 coarse lump (e.g., compartment 2 of the chain of 5) was approximately the mean of the 2 EPSP shapes computed for the same synaptic input time course restricted to one or the other of the 2 corresponding finer lumps (e.g., compartment 3 or 4 of the chain of 10).

Combinations of synaptic input locations. It should be noted that the variety of computed EPSP shapes is greatly increased when the synaptic input is not restricted to a single location. Several examples of this are pro-

---

[1] The mathematical treatment of such equalizing electrotonic spread (12) implies the existence of several equalizing time constants which are smaller than the passive membrane time constant. The relative values of these time constants depend upon the electrotonic length of the equivalent cylinder or chain of compartments. Experimental determination of the first equalizing time constant, relative to the passive membrane time constant provides a means of estimating the underlying electrotonic length of the system. For the particular case of cat motoneuron EPSP's, this experimental determination is complicated by the unknown process that causes EPSP decay to end in an after-hyperpolarization; the response to an applied current pulse appears better suited for this experimental determination, as has recently been verified by P. G. Nelson (personal communication).

vided in a companion paper (14, Fig. 5). Two examples are provided in a later section of the present paper (Fig. 5) in the course of illustrating a more general argument. A brief generalization can summarize the results of many such computations: for any given synaptic excitatory conductance time course, a somatic or proximal dendritic input location contributes especially to the early rising portion of the EPSP, while a distal input location contributes toward a longer half-width and toward a slower rise and fall; the particular time-to-peak value and half-width value depend upon the relative weights of the proximal and distal contributions of the two component EPSP's (see Fig. 5 below for an illustration). It is helpful to note that for EPSP shapes of small amplitude and different input locations, the two component EPSP shapes sum almost linearly. Conditions for nonlinear summation are discussed in a later section of this paper, and (13, 14).

II. *Computational dissection of synaptic and other electric current relating transient excitatory conductance to the resulting EPSP*

Only when synaptic input is uniform over the entire soma-dendritic surface is it correct to deduce the time course of synaptic current from the EPSP by a simple application of the differential equation

$$I = C \frac{dV}{dt} - \frac{V}{R}$$

for a single lumped resistance in parallel with a single lumped capacitance. In cases where synaptic input is distributed nonuniformly, unmodified application of the above procedure would be expected to result in erroneous inferences; such errors would be further compounded if incorrect values of the membrane time constant were used (see 11 for a discussion of such errors).

In an actual physiological case of localized dendritic synaptic input, it would be extremely difficult to measure the true time course of synaptic current at the dendritic location, and to compare this with the time course of the electrotonic spread current which actually depolarizes the soma. Here, advantage is taken of the complete information that can be obtained from computational simulation of such situations.

The example illustrated in the right-hand side of Fig. 4 represents a case of synaptic input that was restricted to compartment 6 of a chain of 10 compartments. The dotted curve at upper right represents the time course of the excitatory conductance transient in compartment 6, while the solid curve at lower right represents the resulting EPSP in compartment 1. All of the dashed curves represent electric currents, each of which plays a role in the complex of events relating the EPSP to the conductance transient. The uppermost dashed curve represents the synaptic current that is generated in compartment 6 by the excitatory conductance transient. Its time course

Fig. 4. Computational dissection comparing transients of conductance, current, and voltage in perturbed compartment and in compartment 1, for 2 cases. Top left shows the $\mathcal{E}$ transient in compartment 2 of a chain of 10 compartments; this was responsible for all of the current and voltage transients shown on the left side of the figure. Top right shows the $\mathcal{E}$ transient in compartment 6 of a chain of 10 compartments; this was responsible for all of the current and voltage transients shown on the right side of the figure. Both $\mathcal{E}$ transients are plotted to a common ordinate scale, expressed as dimensionless $\mathcal{E}$ values. All of the current transients, shown as dashed lines at left and right, have been plotted to a common ordinate scale; the ordinate scale values express the dimensionless slope, dv/dT. All of the voltage transients, shown as solid curves at left and right, have been plotted to a common ordinate scale; however, the dimensionless v values are exactly one-tenth of the numerical scale shown; the EPSP peak amplitude in compartment 1 is $v = 0.10$ in both cases.

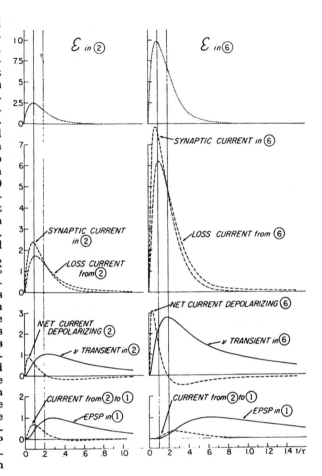

is very similar (but not identical)[2] to that of the conductance transient This synaptic current is not completely available for depolarizing the membrane capacity in compartment 6; it must also supply the "loss current" consisting of current spread from compartment 6 to compartments 5 and 7, as well as a small leak, or self decay, through the resting membrane resistance of compartment 6.

A graph of this loss current is shown superimposed upon that of the synaptic current, and these two currents can be seen to be of quite comparable

[2] This synaptic current reaches its peak value at $T = 0.075$, which is earlier than the time, $T = 0.092$, of peak conductance. This can be understood in terms of the effective driving potential, $(1-v)$, which falls as the membrane becomes more depolarized. The synaptic current is proportional to the product, $(1-v)\mathcal{E}$, in compartment 6. At $T = 0.075$, rounded values are $v = 0.19$ and $\mathcal{E} = 9.7$; thus, the synaptic current is proportional to (0.81) $(9.7) = 7.9$, at this time. At $T = 0.092$, rounded values are $v = 0.22$ and $\mathcal{E} = 9.9$; thus, the synaptic current is smaller, being proportional to (0.78) $(9.9) = 7.7$, at this later time.

magnitude. The loss current has a smaller and later peak, but for times greater than $T = 0.19$, the loss current exceeds the synaptic current. It is the difference between these two currents that must be regarded as the net depolarizing current in compartment 6. This net current is also shown in the figure, together with the voltage transient in compartment 6. This net current peaks earlier and has a peak amplitude that is less than half that of the actual synaptic current; also, this net current is negative for times greater than $T = 0.19$, because this is when the loss current exceeds the synaptic current. For the same reason, the peak depolarization in compartment 6 also occurs at $T = 0.19$, and the decay from peak depolarization is faster than for a purely passive decay of a uniformly distributed depolarization.

But this is not the end of the story. So far, attention has been focused upon the dendritic location designated as compartment 6. What happens at the soma, here represented as compartment 1? One could present, in turn, the current spread from compartment 6 to 5, then 5 to 4, 3 to 2, and finally 2 to 1; only the net current from compartment 2 to compartment 1 is illustrated in Fig. 4. This current has a much smaller and later peak than the synaptic current or any of the other currents illustrated. However, from the perspective of compartment 1, it is this current that generates the EPSP by flowing into the parallel resistance and capacity of compartment 1.

This EPSP reaches its peak amplitude ($v = 0.1$) at $T = 0.62$, and the early part of its decay is slower than for a case of passive decay of a uniformly distributed depolarization. This slower decay can be attributed to the tail of current spreading to the soma from the dendrites; however, one should hasten to add that this entire EPSP must be attributed to current spread from the dendrites.

Further understanding of these results can be obtained by comparing the right and left sides of this figure. The left side represents a similar computation for the case of synaptic input confined to compartment 2, which may be thought of as corresponding to the proximal portions of the dendritic trunks. The left and right sides have been plotted to the same scale, to facilitate visual comparisons of amplitude and time course. Thus, in compartment 2, with the same excitatory conductance time course, the required amplitude is only one-fourth that required in compartment 6. The synaptic current at left is slightly more than one-fourth that at right. The relation of loss current and synaptic current is qualitatively similar at left and right. The net depolarizing current in the perturbed compartment is smaller and slower at left; the peak is one-fourth as great and the reversal to negative values occurs at $T = 0.24$ as compared with 0.19 at right. As before, this necessarily defines the time of peak depolarization in the perturbed compartment, and the decay is more rapid than for passive decay of a uniformly distributed depolarization. The time course of current flowing from compartment 2 to compartment 1 is shown at lower left; this time course is proportional to the difference between the voltage transients in these two compartments, both of which are shown as solid curves at left. This current has negative values for times greater than $T = 0.36$; this means that the spread of current into the dendrites is sufficient to make the depolarization in compartment 2 decay more rapidly than in compartment 1; after $T = 0.36$, there is a flow of current all the way from compartment 1, through compartment 2, into the dendritic periphery.

Perhaps favorable experimental preparations will permit a test of some of these predictions in the near future. At present, it seems fair to say that such computations help to illustrate the importance of synaptic input location to a consideration of the relation between synaptic current, the loss current due to electrotonic spread, and the net depolarizing current in any given compartment.

III. *Synaptic intensity required at different soma-dendritic locations: amount of nonlinearity for different amplitudes and locations*

If the same EPSP amplitude is to be obtained, at the soma compartment, it is intuitively obvious that a greater intensity of synaptic excitatory con-

Table 3. Synaptic intensity (peak ε) dependence upon location, upon conductance time course, and upon prescribed EPSP amplitude at soma

Location of Synaptic Input	All Cpts	Cpt 1	Cpt 2	Cpt 3	Cpt 4	Cpt 6	Cpt 8	Cpt 10
Medium conductance transient								
A. Peak ε for small EPSP, *v*=0.01	.109	0.256	0.406	0.612	0.89	1.7	2.6	3.08
B. (Peak *v* in input compartment)	(0.01)	(0.01)	(0.011)	(0.015)	(0.022)	(0.041)	(0.063)	(0.11)
C. Peak ε for large EPSP, *v*=0.10	1.15	2.74	4.41	6.88	10.5	24.3	49.9	234.
D. (Peak *v* in input compartment)	(0.1)	(0.1)	(0.11)	(0.155)	(0.22)	(0.405)	(0.602)	(0.94)
Slow conductance transient								
E. Peak ε for large EPSP, *v*=0.10	0.58	1.75	2.50	3.55	5.01	9.86	17.1	33.6
F. (Peak *v* in input compartment)	(0.1)	(0.1)	(0.106)	(0.125)	(0.16)	(0.28)	(0.43)	(0.73)
G. Peak *g* for IPSP, *v*=−0.05	4.05	13.9	20.5	34.6	72.2	>10³		
H. (Peak *v* in input compartment)	(−0.05)	(−0.05)	(−0.053)	(−0.062)	(−0.077)	<(−0.095)		

ductance is needed when synaptic input is confined to a single compartment, as compared with equal input to all compartments. Also, for a chain of equal compartments, it would be expected intuitively that the required synaptic intensity would increase with increasingly distal compartmental location, because of the electrotonic attenuation expected during passive spread from the distal compartment to the soma. To go beyond such qualitative expectation, it is best to refer to the computational results.

Rows *A* and *C* of Table 3 list the peak values of synaptic excitatory intensity (peak ε) found necessary to produce the two EPSP series (small and large) whose shapes were illustrated in Fig. 2 and summarized in Table 1; the small EPSP series had peak $v = 0.01$ in the soma compartment, while the large EPSP series had peak $v = 0.10$ in the soma compartment. In rows *A* and *C*, it can be seen for both series that the synaptic intensity (peak ε) required in compartment 1 alone was about 2.4 times that required for equal input to all compartments, and that required in compartment 2 alone was about 3.7 or 3.8 times the value for all compartments. For these three synaptic input distributions, the peak ε values of row C are between 10 and 11 times those of row A, indicating approximate linearity over this 10-fold range of EPSP amplitude. Such approximate linearity does not hold, however, for the more distal input locations. In particular, for synaptic input restricted to compartment 10, row A shows a peak ε value that was about 28 times its reference value for all compartments, while row C shows a peak ε value that was about 204 times its reference value. Put another way, the peak ε value of 234 in row C is 76 times that in row A, although it produces an EPSP which is only 10 times larger; this represents a very significant nonlinearity. For input to compartment 8, the row C value is about 19 times the row A value, and for compartment 6, the corresponding factor is about 14; both indicate significant nonlinearity. To understand the essential difference between those cases showing very significant nonlinearity and other cases showing approximate linearity, it is important to examine the amount of depolarization that takes place in the compartment which receives the synaptic input, and to bear in mind that synaptic current is proportional to the product $(1-v)\varepsilon$, as it varies with time in the input compartment.

Peak depolarization at input compartment. The time course of membrane depolarization in the input compartment (as illustrated in Fig. 3) was computed routinely in most of the synaptic potential computations. For each case in Table 3, the peak depolarization at the input compartment is tabulated as a number enclosed by parentheses. It can be seen that the values in row D are all about 10 times those in row B. However, it is instructive that in the extreme case of input to compartment 10, it was not possible for the peak v value in row D to equal 10 times that of row B, because the limiting value of v, for ε very large, is $v = 1.0$ (see METHODS). This means that the 10-fold increase of the EPSP (at the soma) was achieved in spite of the amplitude limitation at the input compartment. The very large synaptic intensity (peak $\varepsilon = 234$) produced an atypical depolarizing transient in compartment 10: its peak occurred earlier (T = 0.06 as compared with T = 0.11), it had a saturated, flat-topped shape, and its area was presumably close to 10 times that of the undistorted depolarizing transient of the small EPSP series. It is not suggested that such extreme cases need occur in nature; equally potent distal synaptic input can be achieved with smaller synaptic intensity over 2 or 3 distal compartments. The essential point is that the 10-fold increase of the EPSP at the soma corresponds, in every case, to a 10-fold increase of the depolarizing transient at the input compartment. The nonlinearities demonstrated by the upper half of Table 3 can thus be ascribed to the more than 10-fold increase of synaptic intensity required to produce the 10-fold increase of depolarization in the input compartment. This nonlinearity is greatest for dendritic input locations where the peak depolarization is greatest. In other words, peak ε must increase more than 10-fold to compensate for the decrease in driving potential $(1-v)$. This source of nonlinearity was tested quantitatively by means of an additional set of computational experiments.

Nonlinearity of EPSP amplitude increase for a 10% increase of synaptic intensity. For each of the synaptic intensity values in row *A* of Table 3, another EPSP was computed with a synaptic intensity that was 10% larger in amplitude, but had the same time course as before. The results (not shown in Table 3) demonstrate how the percentage of increase in EPSP amplitude depends upon the amount of depolarization that occurred in the input compartment. When the original peak v in the input compartment was around 0.01, the 10% increase of peak ε produced an EPSP amplitude increase of about 9.9%. Original peak v values of 0.041 and 0.063 resulted in EPSP amplitude increases of 9.64% and 9.47%. For the larger EPSP series, original peak v values of 0.405, 0.602, and 0.94, respectively, resulted in EPSP amplitude increases of 6.5, 4.6, and 1.5%, respectively. In most of these cases the percentage increase of EPSP amplitude was fairly well approximated by the expression

$$P \simeq 10(1 - 0.9y)$$

where y represents the original peak v value in the input compartment, and P represents the percentage increase of EPSP amplitude for 10% increase of synaptic intensity. As the original peak v value ranges from 0 to 1.0, the quantity inside the parentheses ranges from 1.0 to 0.1; the departure of this quantity from unity is obviously a measure of the nonlinearity for small increments of perfectly synchronous synaptic input at the same location.

This nonlinearity is similar to that derived earlier for muscle end plate potentials (7), and that derived for initial slopes and steady-state depolarizations in response to a step conductance change (12, 13). However, the end-plate potential treatment explicitly neglected reactances, and neither treatment provided for a smooth conductance transient, or for the computed peak of a transient depolarization; also neither calculation of nonlinearity provided for distant input locations. All of these difficulties are provided for in the present computations. Thus, it is useful to have determined that all of these nonlinearities are rather similar, when attention is focused on the membrane depolarization at the site of the conductance transient.

Large nonlinearities implicate dendritic conductance transients. The computed results summarized above provide the theoretical basis for a recognition of the significance of occasional large nonlinearities observed in the summation of EPSP amplitudes (1, 14). First, a significant nonlinearity is, by itself, suggestive evidence for a membrane conductance transient at the input location. Second, when the observed nonlinearity significantly exceeds that which could be accounted for in terms of the peak depolarizations at the soma, this suggests that the synaptic input occurred at dendritic locations, sufficiently distant and sufficiently circumscribed to account for the needed peak depolarization at the input location. It is not necessary that the additional synaptic input should occur at the same location as the control input; it would be sufficient for the control input to generate a depolarization which, as it spreads to the location of the additional synaptic input, is of sufficient magnitude (at the time of this additional conductance transient) to account for the nonlinearity.

Synaptic intensity with slow conductance time course. It should not be surprising that the peak synaptic intensity (peak ε) required to produce a given EPSP amplitude is reduced when the time course of the synaptic conductance is changed from the medium transient to the slow transient. This can be verified in Table 3 for the large EPSP amplitude ($v = 0.10$) at the several input locations tabulated (row E compared with row C). Since, for unit peak amplitude, the area under the slow transient is 2.3 times that under the medium transient, it is not surprising that the required peak ε for uniform input to all compartments was about half as much for the slow conductance transient as for the fast conductance transient (0.58 compared with 1.15); one can understand why the full factor of 2.3 was not obtained by noting that the slow transient has a significant tail at times after the EPSP peak is attained. For input locations near the soma, this factor is even smaller, because the EPSP peak occurs earlier. For input locations beyond compartment 5, the factor relating peak ε values exceeds 2.3, because the EPSP peaks occur later, and because the fast dendritic transients encroach farther into the nonlinear domain.

One functional implication of this result is that a small amount of temporal dispersion can enhance summation of input to a common peripheral dendritic location, while the same amount of temporal dispersion can reduce the peak summation for brief input delivered to the soma or a proximal dendritic location.

Synaptic inhibitory conductance intensity at different locations. The lower part of Table 3 shows the results of a series of computed inhibitory postsynaptic potentials (IPSP). These were computed with the slow conductance time course. It was assumed that the limiting value, $(E_j - E_r)/(E_\varepsilon - E_r) = -0.1$, and the prescribed IPSP amplitude was half of this ($v = -0.05$), corresponding to -3.5 mv if $E_\varepsilon - E_r = 70$ mv. Because this prescribed IPSP amplitude represents half the limiting amplitude, it should not be surprising that the required peak g values display very significant nonlinearity. If linearity had held perfectly, these peak g values would have been exactly 5 times the peak ε values for EPSP amplitudes of $v = .10$; however Table 3 shows ratios closer to 10, for several input locations. At compartment 6, the nonlinear saturation effect is so great that even a 100 times greater conductance peak is not sufficient. The large g values are needed to compensate for the small driving potential. An interesting functional implication of this result is that distal dendritic synaptic inhibition is not effective in producing an IPSP at the soma, although this same input could be very effective against synaptic excitation delivered to the same dendritic locations (4, 5, 12, 13).

Combinations of synaptic excitation and inhibition at different locations. It proved instructive to compute the results of combining some of the excitatory and inhibitory synaptic inputs that have already been presented separately in rows E and G of Table 3. Thus, for example, when peak $\varepsilon = 1.75$ and peak $g = 13.9$ were placed simultaneously in compartment 1, the resulting synaptic potential had a peak amplitude, $v = 0.0124$, that was significantly smaller than would have been obtained by a simple summation of the synaptic potential amplitudes, $v = +0.10$ and $v = -0.05$, obtained separately. Quite another result was obtained when peak $\varepsilon = 5.01$ and peak $g = 72.2$ were placed simultaneously in compartment 4; the resulting synaptic potential had the opposite sign; its peak amplitude, $v = -0.0146$ in compartment 1 resulted from a peak hyperpolarization, $v = -0.0224$, in compartment 4. This rather surprising result can be understood by noting that the peak g value in compartment 4 was more than 10 times the peak ε value in compartment 4, and this factor more than compensates for the 10-fold smaller inhibitory driving potential. In other words, the synaptic inhibition was more powerful than the synaptic excitation, even though the separate synaptic potential amplitudes, $v = +0.10$ and $v = -0.05$, were the same as above. This extreme example provides a further illustration of the fact that synaptic potentials observed at the soma do not provide a reliable measure of the relative potency of synaptic excitation and inhibition combined at a common dendritic location. It is more than sufficient to account for the observations (14, Fig. 7B) which we have attributed to interaction at a dendritic location.

Other computations, in which synaptic excitation and inhibition were placed in different dendritic trees of the same neuron, demonstrated that such electrotonic separation of input locations can account for the linear summation of EPSP and IPSP that is sometimes observed experimentally (14, Fig. 7A).

IV. *Effects of steady hyperpolarizing current upon EPSP shape*

There have been numerous experiments and interpretations concerned with the effects of a steady hyperpolarizing current. This current is applied inward across the soma membrane between an intracellular microelectrode and a distant extracellular electrode; after the nerve membrane has reached a steady state of hyperpolarization, an EPSP is evoked by synaptic input; the shape of this EPSP is compared with that obtained without membrane hyperpolarization. The question is: what change in EPSP shape should one expect to find for various soma-dendritic locations of synaptic input? It was pointed out in 1960 (11, p. 522–523 and 528–529) that ". . . steady state hyperpolarization of the membrane must be greatest at the soma and must decrease electrotonically with distance along the dendrites. Under such conditions (with uniformly distributed synaptic input), both the density of synaptic current and the amount of depolarization caused by the brief excitatory conductance increase must be greatest at the soma. This nonuniformity will cause a more rapid EPSP decay." At that time, however, a detailed consideration of the effects upon EPSP rising slope as compared with EPSP amplitude was not attempted. Also, at that time, the phenomenon of anomalous rectification (8) had not received much attention. Here, attention will be focused upon EPSP properties that can be predicted without complication by anomalous rectification. The focus is upon the consequences of different synaptic input locations when synaptic input is represented as a transient increase of excitatory membrane conductance.

Expected increase of EPSP slope and amplitude. For EPSP computations with such steady-state hyperpolarization, should one expect both the rising slope and the peak amplitude of the EPSP to increase by the same factor? The answer is no, in general, but yes for all cases when synaptic input is restricted to a single compartmental location. This answer has been verified by numerous examples of such EPSP computations; it is explained below in physical intuitive terms; a mathematical demonstration will be given elsewhere.

Electrotonic decrement of steady-state hyperpolarization. In an equivalent cylinder of electrotonic length, Z_m, the relative values of steady-state hyperpolarization, as a function of electrotonic distance, Z, can be expressed $\cosh(Z_m-Z)/\cosh Z_m$, on the assumption that hyperpolarizing current is applied at one end, $Z=0$, of the cylinder, and that the other end, $Z=Z_m$, is a sealed end (see ref. 9 or 10, Fig. 3). For a chain of five compartments, with $\Delta Z=0.4$ per compartment, and with $Z=0$ in compartment 1, we have $Z_m=1.6$ at the dendritic terminal in compartment 5. With this value of Z_m, consider, for example, a steady-state hyperpolarization that amounts, in compartment 1, to a 20% increase of the synaptic excitatory driving potential. For this case, the decreasing amounts of steady-state hyperpolarization in the four dendritic compartments are 14% in no. 2, 10% in no. 3, and roughly 8% in both nos. 4 and 5.

Factor of EPSP increase for single input location. When the synaptic excitatory conductance transient is restricted to a single compartment, the effect of steady-state hyperpolarization is to increase the computed EPSP amplitude by the same factor over its entire time course; thus both the rising slope and the peak amplitude are increased by precisely the same factor. This factor exactly equals the factor of increase in synaptic current, which exactly equals the factor of increase in the excitatory driving potential at the particular compartment in which the synaptic conductance transient is assumed to occur. Only when the synaptic input occurs at the soma will this factor of increase be the same as that of the excitatory driving potential at the soma; then a 20% hyperpolarization at the soma would produce a 20% increase in EPSP slope and amplitude. Such a case is illustrated by curves A_1 and A_2 in Fig. 5. In contrast, curves B_1 and B_2 result from synaptic input restricted to compartment 4 of a five-compartment chain. Here the slope and amplitude of curve B_2 are only 8% greater than those of curve B_1, and this corresponds to the 8% steady-state hyperpolarization in compartment 4 when 20% hyperpolarization is maintained at the soma compartment. In other words, the electrotonic decrement of steady-state hyperpolarization is responsible for a different increase of excitatory driving potential at each compartmental location, and it is the factor of increase in driving potential at the one-compartment receiving synaptic input that determines the factor of increase in EPSP slope and amplitude. In these cases, EPSP shape is unchanged.

EPSP shape change with compound synaptic input locations. When synaptic input is distributed to two or more compartments, the effect of steady-

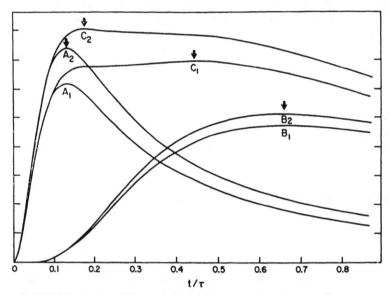

FIG. 5. Effect of steady-state membrane hyperpolarization (applied at soma), upon computed EPSP shape for (A) proximal input, (B) distal input, and (C) combined proximal and distal input. Subscript 1 designates each control EPSP computed without hyperpolarization. Subscript 2, designates the increased membrane potential transient at the soma compartment obtained with a steady-state hyperpolarization equal to 20% at the soma compartment. Computations were with a five-compartment chain, with $\Delta Z = 0.4$; the medium time course of synaptic membrane conductance was used for all cases. Case (A) corresponds to peak $\mathcal{E} = 0.10$ in compartment 1; case (B) corresponds to peak $\mathcal{E} = 0.55$ in compartment 4; case (C) corresponds to a combination of these two inputs; one unit of the ordinate scale corresponds to $\Delta v = 0.001$, for these particular peak $\mathcal{E}$ values.

state hyperpolarization upon the EPSP is more complicated. The peak amplitude is increased by a factor that is smaller than the factor of increase in the early rising slope; also, the peak occurs earlier in time, and the fall to half of peak amplitude also occurs earlier. These changes, it should be emphasized, are predicted without introducing any complications due to anomalous rectification. These changes can be understood in terms of the different amounts of increase in the synaptic excitatory driving potential at the several compartments receiving synaptic input. The input compartment nearest to the soma has the largest factor of increase in driving potential; this factor largely determines the factor of increase in the early rate of rise of the EPSP. Thus, in Fig. 5, where curves C_1 and C_2 were generated by a compound synaptic input (in compartments 1 and 4), the early slope (halfway up) is 20%

greater in C_2 than in C_1, as it is also in A_2 compared with A_1. However, the peak amplitude of C_2 is only 14% greater than that of C_1, and the time of peak is shifted from $T = .43$ to $T = .17$, providing a fairly extreme example of such a shift. Also, one can deduce that C_2 falls to one-half of its peak amplitude at an earlier time than does C_1, because the peak of C_2 is 14% greater, while the tail amplitude of C_2 is only 8% greater than that of C_1.

This one example shows why it should not be expected, in general, to have EPSP shape remain the same with and without steady-state hyperpolarization. Nevertheless, it should be added that the experimental observations (8) include cases where the rising slope is increased by as much as 20% without any significant increase of peak amplitude; in such cases, the phenomenon of anomalous rectification (8) presumably contributes as much or more to the EPSP shape change as does the compound input location effect illustrated in Fig. 3.

Different observations with hyperpolarizing current. It is possible to account for several different experimental observations that might, at first glance, appear to conflict with the theoretical predictions. For example, hyperpolarizing current can produce a large increase of EPSP amplitude with an EPSP shape of very slow time course. These slow EPSP shapes do not imply distal dendritic synaptic input; in all cases that have come to my attention, these shapes can be explained by temporal dispersion of a polysynaptic input that could be somatic or proximal dendritic.

Sometimes a 30-mv hyperpolarization produces as much as a threefold increase of EPSP amplitude. To account for this, one must bear in mind that, when both synaptic excitatory and inhibitory activity are present, the synaptic "equilibrium potential" becomes a weighted mean of the separate excitatory and inhibitory values

$$E_{eq} - E_r = \frac{(E_\epsilon - E_r)\mathcal{E} + (E_j - E_r)\mathcal{J}}{\mathcal{E} + \mathcal{J}}$$

see and compare V^* of (12) and v_s of (13). For example, if the effective driving potential, $E_{eq} - V_m$, should happen to be 15 mv, then a 30-mv hyperpolarization would increase the effective driving potential to 45 mv, and this would account for a threefold increase in synaptic potential amplitude. Whenever one cannot exclude the possibility of temporal dispersion or the possibility of mixed excitatory and inhibitory effects, one must beware of requiring the theory to account for the observations without benefit of these additional degrees of freedom.

At the other extreme, there are experiments which produce no significant increase of EPSP amplitude with steady-state hyperpolarizing current. For such cases it is relevant to ask the magnitude of the smallest increase that could have been detected, and then to ask how dendritically remote the synaptic input would have to be to account for this theoretically, without the help of anomalous rectification. Suppose, for example, that the experimental procedure would fail to detect a 4% increase, and that the hyperpolarization at the soma was 20%; this would require that the electrotonic decrement of the hyperpolarization from the soma to the synaptic input location be a factor of 5 or more. From a table of hyperbolic cosine values, one can see that $Z_m = 2.3$ would be a sufficient dendritic electrotonic length to account for this with terminal dendritic synaptic input. Alternatively, for longer dendritic electrotonic length ($Z_m \geq 4$), the synaptic input location would need only be $Z = 1.6$, to account for this much exponential decrement. In other words, an undetected increase of EPSP amplitude in such experiments need not conflict with theoretical predictions.

V. Detectability at the soma, of transient synaptic conductance at different soma-dendritic locations

The basic question to be answered here is this: given a dendritic synaptic conductance transient which generates an EPSP of respectable size at the soma, should one expect to obtain, with microelectrodes at the soma, experimental evidence that detects the synaptic conductance transient, as distinguished from a synaptic current transient? If experimental methods were perfect, the answer would certainly be yes; however, since there is significant experimental noise to contend with, the question becomes a quantitative one of estimating whether the theoretically predictable effect is large enough to detect by present experimental techniques. In fact, the theoretical results presented below suggest that the predicted effect for proximal dendritic input locations may be above the present threshold for experimental detection, while that for distal dendritic input locations may be below the present threshold for experimental detection. Future experiments may, of course, succeed in shifting the detection threshold.

Computational experiment. Although the experimental approach (15) has been to analyze transients obtained with an a-c impedance bridge technique, my own preference has been to consider a constant current applied at the soma, and to analyze the distortion of the EPSP transient that is theoretically predicted under such conditions. The results of computations for one case of transient dendritic synaptic conductance are illustrated in Fig. 6. In this case, the conductance transient was restricted to compartment 3 of a chain of five compartments (with $\Delta Z = 0.4$ per compartment). A constant current was applied to compartment 1 (the soma) at zero time; the two solid curves at left illustrate the passive response in compartment 1 to depolarizing and hyperpolarizing current. The two solid curves at right illustrate the slower and smaller passive response computed in compartment 3 for the same constant current applied at the soma. These solid curves thus represent control transients of membrane potential obtained in the absence of any synaptic conductance transient. Perfect symmetry between upper and lower curves reflects the fact that all membrane parameters are assumed to remain constant (i.e., independent of membrane potential).

Next, a synaptic conductance transient was introduced in compartment

3 (at $T = 1.0$) after the initiation of a constant current at $T = 0$. This synaptic conductance had the medium time course (defined in METHODS, and shown at lower right of Fig. 6), and the synaptic intensity was made equal to that which would produce an EPSP amplitude of $v = 0.10$ in compartment 1 in the absence of applied current. The dashed curves in Fig. 6 show the distorted membrane potential transients that were computed for compartments

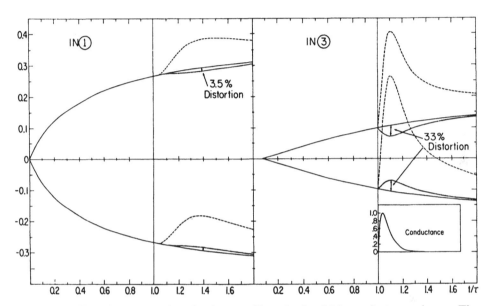

FIG. 6. Transients related to the detectability of a dendritic conductance change. The left side shows transients computed for compartment 1 in a chain of five compartments ($\Delta Z = 0.4$), while the right side shows transients computed for compartment 3. The solid curves at left and right show the voltage transients which result when a constant-current step is applied to compartment 1 at zero time; the upper solid curves result from depolarizing current; the lower solid curves result from hyperpolarizing current. The dashed curves show the change in these voltage transients computed when a brief synaptic excitatory input was put in compartment 3. The synaptic input began at $T = 1.0$, had a peak ε value of 9.52, and had the medium time course shown at lower right. The dotted curves show the deviation from the solid curves obtained in computations with the same conductance transient, but with $E_\varepsilon = E_r$. The same dotted transients were also obtained by computing one-half of the difference between the upper dashed curve and the lower dashed curve. Amplitude scale expresses dimensionless units of v.

1 and 3 for both depolarizing and hyperpolarizing applied current. When the peak amplitudes of these dashed curves are measured as departure from the solid curve control transients, a simple generalization becomes apparent. In both compartments, the upper peak (obtained with depolarizing current) has an amplitude that is 10% smaller than it would be in the absence of the applied current, while the lower peak (obtained with hyperpolarizing current) has an amplitude that is 10% larger than it would be in the absence of the applied current. This 10% change in amplitude is easily explained by the effective driving potential in compartment 3 at the time of the synaptic con-

ductance transient; at this time, the two solid curves show depolarization or hyperpolarization corresponding to $v = \pm 0.1$, implying effective synaptic excitatory driving potentials $(1-v)$, that are 10% smaller or larger than the resting value. It should be added that this 10% distortion could be doubled to 20% simply by doubling the intensity of the applied current.

Computational dissection of distortion due to conductance transient. The deviation of the dotted curves from the solid curves is a measure of the above distortion alone. This can be obtained in two different ways. The easiest way, computationally, is simply to set the excitatory emf, E_t, equal to the resting emf, E_r, in all compartments. Then, in the absence of applied polarizing current, the conductance transient would produce no voltage transient whatever, but, in the presence of applied current, the dotted curves are predicted. The effective driving potential for the deviation of the dotted curves from the solid curves is simply the $v = \pm 0.1$ polarization in compartment 3 at the time of the conductance transient.

The significance of these dotted curves is that they represent the distortion imposed upon the solid control transients by the conductance transient, but without the excitatory emf. It is this distortion that is attributable to the conductance transient alone. It is the detectability of this distortion in compartment 1 that needs to be assessed.

The alternative method of obtaining these dotted curves consists essentially of canceling the effect of E_t by taking a difference between two (dashed curve) transients. At both left and right in Fig. 6, the upper dotted curve can be obtained by taking, for every T, one-half the ordinate of the upper dashed curve minus one-half the ordinate of the lower dashed curve. Although the figure may show this imperfectly, this result was computationally precise; it is an exact mathematical consequence of assuming a linear system in which all coefficients, whether constant or time dependent, are independent of the membrane potential, and hence unchanged by both depolarizing and hyperpolarizing applied currents.

Computed distortion related to a-c bridge imbalance. The previous paragraph has been explicit about canceling the effect of E_t by taking appropriate differences between transients of opposite polarity, because this concept is rather similar to that of averaging a-c bridge imbalance over all positive and negative phases of the sinusoidal period, as in the experimental method devised by Smith et al. (15). The end result of such averaging may be regarded as roughly comparable to the dotted distortion in compartment 1 of Fig. 6. The a-c method has a number of complications which have been discussed in the APPENDIX of (15).

Computed distortion as percent distortion. As noted earlier, the magnitude of the dotted distortion in Fig. 6 could be increased by increasing the intensity of the applied current. But this would also increase the amplitude of the solid curve control transients and, presumably, also the amplitude of the experimental noise which limits the precision of experimental measurements. Thus, it seems appropriate to express the amplitude of the computed distortion as a percentage of the solid curve control amplitude. In compartment 3, this percentage is 33, but in compartment 1, where experimental observation would have to be made, the percentage distortion is only 3.5, as labeled in Fig. 6. The approximate factor of 10 relating these 2 percentages can be understood as due to a factor of nearly 3 in the electrotonic decrement of membrane polarization from compartment no. 1 to no. 3 at $T = 1.0$, and a factor of about 3.3 in the decrement of the transient peak amplitude from compartment no. 3 to no. 1. The resulting 3.5% distortion at the soma compartment probably lies close to the threshold for detection by the experimental techniques of Smith et al. (15).

Effect of different input locations. This computational experiment was repeated with different locations of the conductance transient. Each column of

Table 4. Detectability of conductance transient

A. Perturbed compartment	1	2	3	4	5	All Five
B. Synaptic intensity (peak ℰ)in perturbed cpt	1.75	4.25	9.52	19.6	44.6	1.15
C. Time of peak distortion of v in cpt 1	1.13	1.26	1.42	1.65	1.82	1.15
D. Distortion of v in cpt 1 when $E_\epsilon = E_r$	.027	.017	.010	.007	.005	.022
E. Distortion (D) expressed as percent of control response to current step alone	9.8	5.9	3.5	2.3	1.7	8.5
F. Distribution of v over five cpts, at $T = 1.0$	.266	.163	.098	.061	.044	
G. Relative values of F	1.0	.61	.37	.23	.17	

Table 4 summarizes the results of one of these experiments; column 3 is the same as that already illustrated in Fig. 6. In each case, the conductance transient had the same medium time course, and its intensity (row B of table) was made equal to that previously found necessary to produce an EPSP of amplitude, $v = 0.10$, under normal conditions. When $E_\epsilon = E_r$, the distortion in compartment 1, for each case, is expressed in dimensionless units of v, in row D of the table. To assess the detectability of each distortion, it is expressed (in row E) as a percentage of the control transient (solid curves at left in Fig. 6) at the time of peak distortion (time shown in row C). This shows that a 9.8% distortion is predicted when the conductance transient occurs in compartment 1, while only a 1.7% distortion is predicted when the conductance transient occurs in compartment 5. Also, for the case of a conductance transient distributed equally to all five compartments, the last column shows a prediction of an 8.5% distortion.

Detectability. Thus, an experimental procedure which can detect only those distortions that exceed 3.5% would be expected to detect the distortion caused by the two cases of proximal input (columns 1 and 2), and by the equal input to all five compartments; it would fail to detect the two cases of distal dendritic input (columns 4 and 5), and might barely detect the case of input to compartment 3 of the chain of five compartments. All of these cases, it should be noted, involve substantial conductance transients, each of which, under normal conditions, would produce an EPSP amplitude of $v = 0.10$ at the soma.

Electrotonic spread of membrane polarization provides key. Useful physical intuitive understanding of these results can be gained by comparing rows D and F of Table 4. Row F shows the compartmental distribution of membrane depolarization, v, (at $T = 1.0$) due to the depolarizing current step applied to compartment 1 at $T = 0$; this was the same in each experiment. When $E_t = E_r$, these values correspond to what can be regarded as the effective driving potential in each compartment, for a conductance transient applied, at $T = 1.0$, to that compartment. Inspection shows that in each of the experiments, the distortion in compartment 1 (row D) is very nearly one-tenth of this effective driving potential (row F) of the perturbed compartment; the factor of 10 reflects the fact that the EPSP amplitude had been prescribed as one-tenth the normal driving potential. Also, the relative values (row G) of the membrane depolarization at $T = 1.0$ are related to the percent distortion values (row E) by nearly a factor of 10. In other words, relative detectability at the soma depends upon the relative amount of electrotonic spread from the testing electrodes to the site of the conductance transient.

Additional generalizations. This simple generalization provides a basis for understanding several other related generalizations. *1)* If the transient conductance were initiated earlier than $T = 1.0$ for a constant current applied at $T = 0$, the electrotonic spread into the dendrites would be less, and the detectability of dendritic conductance change would be even worse than in Table 4. *2)* From these idealized considerations alone, the detectability of dendritic conductance change would be greatest when the electrotonic spread from the applied current reaches a steady state. This fact can perhaps be exploited with some neuron types; however, in the case of cat motoneurons, anomalous rectification (8) complicates such steady states. *3)* High-frequency sinusoidal applied current is useless for testing dendritic conductance change, because most of this current flows across the soma membrane capacitance (see ref. 11, p. 517 and 530). *4)* At low frequencies, such as about 100 cycles/sec, a sinusoidal steady state reaches out into the dendrites with a spatial decrement similar to that shown in rows F and G. For example, when a sinusoidal frequency of one-half cycle per τ (100 cycles/sec, if $\tau = 5$ msec) is applied to compartment 1 of a chain of five compartments, the relative steady-state sinusoidal amplitudes were found to be 1.0, 0.55, 0.30, 0.18, and 0.14, respectively (these may be compared with row G of Table 4); also, the steady-state phase lags in compartments 1 through 5 were found to be approximately 45°, 72°, 100°, 125°, and 145°, respectively. *5)* The fact that the distortion, row E, column 1, in Table 4 is very nearly 10% is no coincidence; it is a consequence of the fact that the magnitude of transient conductance in compartment 1 had already been selected to yield an EPSP amplitude equal to 10% of the normal driving potential. Thus one can guess, and it was found, that when the magnitude of the transient conductance in compartment 1 is increased (more than doubled) to that required to produce a doubled EPSP amplitude, $v = 0.20$, then the percentage distortion corresponding to row E in the first column of Table 4 becomes increased to very nearly 20%; in fact, the complete series of computational experiments for this larger prescribed EPSP amplitude results in a new set of percentage distortion values which are essentially double those in row E of Table 4. Similarly for IPSP computations, when the IPSP amplitude was prescribed as halfway from resting potential to the inhibitory equilibrium potential, the percentage distortion values were found to be essentially five times those in row E of Table 4.

Time course of transient distortion. When the conductance transient is confined to a single compartment, the time course of the distortion in compartment 1 is essentially the same as that of the corresponding EPSP. This, it should be emphasized, is significantly slower than the time course of the synaptic conductance transient, as can be seen in Fig. 6 and also in Fig. 4. The situation is more complicated when synaptic conductance transients occur in more than one compartment; it is obviously even more complicated when synaptic inhibition is present as well as synaptic excitation; in these more complicated cases, the distortion should not be expected to have the same time course as the EPSP or the EPSP-IPSP combination. For the particular case of equal conductance transients in all compartments (column 6 of Table 4) the transient distortion peaked earlier and decayed faster than the corresponding EPSP; this distortion can be understood as a weighted sum of five component distortions, with the largest weight attached to the perturbation in compartment 1, and progressively smaller weights attached to the contributions of the other compartments. These theoretical results should serve to illustrate the fact that this transient distortion, which does provide evidence for the presence of a synaptic conductance transient, does not permit a simple inference of the synaptic conductance time course.

SUMMARY

Extensive computations have been carried out with a mathematical neuron model which permits a choice of both the time course and the soma-dendritic location of synaptic input. The results provide quantitative predictions of the way in which the shape of a synaptic potential, as well as other properties of synaptic potentials, depend upon these spatial and temporal aspects of synaptic input. Quantitative details have been summarized in several tables and figures. Also, several qualitative generalizations have been developed as aids to intuitive understanding of these theoretical results. Specific applications of these theoretical results to the interpretation of experimental results from cat motoneurons are presented in a collaborative companion paper (14). The theoretical results have been presented in five parts.

Part I provides details of how the shapes of computed synaptic potentials can be characterized by means of the quantitative shape indices: time to peak, half-width, and rising slope/peak. The dependence of these shape indices upon synaptic input location, time course, and upon dendritic electrotonic length is demonstrated quantitatively and discussed in terms of electrotonic spread over the soma-dendritic membrane surface.

Part II provides a computational dissection of the several electric current transients and membrane potential transients that relate a dendritically located synaptic conductance transient to the resulting synaptic potential at the soma. These quantitative results, although not yet tested experimentally, provide insight into the distinctions that can and should be made between synaptic current, loss current due to electrotonic spread away from the input location, and the resultant, net depolarizing current. Both this net depolarizing current and the resulting membrane potential transient are distinguished at the dendritic input location and at the soma.

Part III provides details of the synaptic conductance intensities required at different locations in order to produce synaptic potentials of certain prescribed amplitudes. The nonlinearities, which tend to be greatest for distal dendritic input locations, are explained in terms of the amount of membrane depolarization occurring at the input location; significant membrane depolarization produces significant reduction in the effective driving potential. Reduced driving potential can be compensated for by increased intensity of synaptic conductance. Many examples of nonlinearity, both for various intensities of synaptic excitation and for combinations of synaptic excitation and inhibition, are illustrated and discussed.

Part IV explains the effects of steady-state hyperpolarizing current upon synaptic potentials in terms of the increase in effective driving potential at each site where a synaptic input conductance transient occurs. For single input locations, the slope and amplitude of the synaptic potential increase by the same factor, leaving the synaptic potential shape unchanged. For compound input locations, it is shown that the contribution of the proximal input location is augmented more than that of the distal dendritic input location (because of electrotonic decrement of the steady-state hyperpolarization), and a change in the shape of the synaptic potential is predicted. Comments are also made regarding anomalous rectification and other unusual observations with polarizing currents.

Part V presents quantitative results that are relevant to the detectability at the soma, of transient synaptic conductance at different dendritic locations. It is shown that relative detectability (for a given size of the control synaptic potential) depends upon the relative amount of electrotonic spread from the testing electrodes to the input location. For a suitable detection threshold, this could explain failure to detect conductance transients at distal dendritic locations under conditions which permit detection of conductance transients at proximal dendritic locations.

A theme common to all of these computations and interpretations is that results, which may appear paradoxical when examined only at the soma, can be understood quite simply when attention is directed to the synaptic input location with special attention to the effective driving potential there.

REFERENCES

1. BURKE, R. E.   Composite nature of the monosynaptic excitatory postsynaptic potential. *J Neurophysiol.* 30: 1114–1137, 1967.
2. COOMBS, J. S., ECCLES, J. C., AND FATT, P.   The inhibitory suppression of reflex discharges from motoneurons. *J. Physiol., London* 130: 396–413, 1955.
3. FATT, P. AND KATZ, B.   The effect of inhibitory nerve impulses on a crustacean muscle fibre. *J. Physiol., London* 121: 374–389, 1953.
4. FRANK, K.   Basic mechanisms of synaptic transmission in the central nervous system. *IRE Trans. Med. Electron.* 6: 85–88, 1959.
5. GRANIT, R., KELLERTH, J.-O., AND WILLIAMS, T. D.   'Adjacent' and 'remote' postsynaptic inhibition in motoneurones stimulated by muscle stretch. *J. Physiol., London* 174: 453–472, 1964.
6. HODGKIN, A. L. AND KATZ, B.   The effect of sodium ions on the electrical activity of the giant axon of the squid. *J. Physiol., London* 108: 37–77, 1949.
7. MARTIN, A. R.   A further study of the statistical composition of the end-plate potential. *J. Physiol., London* 130: 114–122, 1955.
8. NELSON, P. G. AND FRANK, K.   Anomalous rectification in cat spinal motoneurons and the effect of polarizing currents on the excitatory postsynaptic potential. *J. Neurophysiol.* 30: 1097–1113, 1967.
9. RALL, W.   *Dendritic Current Distribution and Whole Neuron Properties.* Naval Med. Research Inst., Research Rept. NM 01-05-00.01.02, 1959, p. 520–523.
10. RALL, W.   Branching dendritic trees and motoneuron membrane resistivity. *Exptl. Neurol.* 1: 491–527, 1959.
11. RALL, W.   Membrane potential transients and membrane time constant of motoneurons. *Exptl. Neurol.* 2: 503–532, 1960.
12. RALL, W.   Theory of physiological properties of dendrites. *Ann. N. Y. Acad. Sci.* 96: 1071–1092, 1962.
13. RALL, W.   Theoretical significance of dendritic trees for neuronal input-output relations. In: *Neural Theory and Modeling,* edited by R. F. Reiss. Stanford, Calif.: Stanford Univ. Press, 1964, p. 73–97.
14. RALL, W., BURKE, R. E., SMITH, T. G., NELSON, P. G., AND FRANK, K.   Dendritic location of synapses and possible mechanisms for the monosynaptic EPSP in motoneurons. *J. Neurophysiol.,* 30: 1169–1193, 1967.
15. SMITH T. G., WUERKER, R. B., AND FRANK, K.   Membrane impedance changes during synaptic transmission in cat spinal motoneurons. *J. Neurophysiol.* 30: 1072–1096, 1967.

7 EQUALIZING TIME CONSTANTS AND ELECTROTONIC LENGTH OF DENDRITES

7.1   Introduction by William R. Holmes

Rall, W. (1969). Time constants and electrotonic length of membrane cylinders and neurons. *Biophys. J.* 9:1483–1508.

Rall's paper "Time constants and electrotonic length of membrane cylinders and neurons" (1969) provides a classic example of how theory and experiment can be combined to allow insight into a major neurophysiological issue. Although the efficacy of distal synapses depended on how far they were electrotonically from the soma, the electrotonic length of various types of cells was not known. Several years earlier Wil had done some calculations based on anatomical measurements of a motoneuron and had concluded that the electrotonic length of that cell was between one and two space constants. However, these calculations were laborious. What was needed was a quick and simple procedure that could be used to estimate the electrotonic length of any cell. Such a procedure was presented in this paper.

Wil bent the rules of journal format somewhat when, immediately after the introduction, he included a three-page section titled "General Statement for Users." Perhaps he was influenced to do this by colleagues such as Bob Burke who had a "mental block activated by any differential equation" (as Bob expresses it in section 6.1). Whatever the reason, the strategy was extremely successful. This statement for users was easy to understand, and it clearly stated what had to be done to estimate electrotonic length.

With a minimum of mathematical detail, Wil showed that for cells that can be approximated as a cylinder with sealed ends, the electrotonic length, L, can be obtained from the simple formula $L = \pi[\tau_0/\tau_1 - 1]^{-1/2}$, where τ_0 and τ_1 are the first two time constants of a voltage decay transient following current input. The chief problem for the experimentalist was to get estimates for τ_0 and τ_1. Although we now have many methods to estimate time constants from transients, the most popular method in 1969 was exponential peeling because it could be done with pencil and ruler. Wil described this method in detail for the experimentalist because it was "sometimes misunderstood and done incorrectly." At the end Wil recommended estimating time constants with "a well tested computer program," although, at the time, computer programs were keypunched on cards and, assuming a computer was even available, one was lucky to get one run a day.

For most neuroscientists, the paper began and ended with this three-page section, but that was all right, because in the next two decades this simple procedure for estimating electrotonic length was followed in countless experimental studies. The term *electrotonic length* became part of the common vocabulary. Estimates of L were reported right along with resting potential and input resistance as basic properties of a neuron. In most cases reported L values were between 0.6 and 1.5, and this indicated that most synapses were close to the soma electrotonically. Thus, distal inputs could play a significant role in bringing a cell to its firing threshold.

Although investigators usually focus on the three-page statement for users, the remaining 22 pages of the paper provide a virtual treasure chest of results and insights that are still being rediscovered. To provide insight into why the electrotonic length formula worked, Wil remarked that after τ_0 the time constants of a voltage decay transient could be thought of as "equalizing" time constants governing the equalization of membrane potential over the length of the cylinder. The electrotonic length formula merely expressed a relationship between the time constants and electrotonic length obtained from the boundary conditions of the differential equation. The interpretation of the time constants as equalizing time constants became very important in future studies.

The theoretical work in this paper was not restricted to the derivation of the electrotonic length formula, and this fact is often overlooked. Wil had provided the experimentalists with a tool based on the assumption that the cell could be approximated as a cylinder with sealed ends, but he realized that, eventually, investigators would not be satisfied with this assumption. Therefore, he presented results in which he explored theoretically the effect on L estimates of various kinds of violations of the cylinder assumption. What is especially helpful is Wil's use of illustrative examples. To some, these might seem tedious, but they do provide insight, particularly for the less mathematically sophisticated reader.

Wil's theoretical treatment of a cylinder coupled to a lumped soma laid the basis for theoretical work on soma shunt models done by Durand (1984), Kawato (1984), Evans et al. (1992), and Major et al. (1993) and the formulas given in Holmes and Rall 1992a. Experimentalists found that the electrotonic length formula did not give results that were consistent with other data unless a soma with a soma shunt conductance (possibly due to electrode penetration) was included in the model. Although Wil's theoretical treatment did not explicitly mention a shunt conductance, this was implicitly included in the expression for soma conductance. Adding an isopotential patch of membrane (the soma) adds an artificial value to the L calculated with the simple formula because of its effect on τ_1. Wil gave expressions for the time constants in this case and noted that coefficients have to be determined with "special attention" (a modified orthogonality). Wil also introduced an approximate correction that one could apply to the original-formula L estimate to account for the soma conductance (equation 23).

Wil also considered theoretically the case of several dendrites coupled to a soma. Each dendrite was represented as a cylinder, but because the cylinders could have different lengths and diameters, they could not be lumped together as a single cylinder. This work laid the theoretical basis for subsequent work by Segev and Rall (1983), Evans et al. (1992), Holmes and Rall (1992a), Holmes et al. (1992), and Major et al. (1993). What was interesting here was that the interpretation of the time constants changed as one went from the single-cylinder case to the multicylinder case. The time constants after τ_0 were still equalizing time constants, but for many time constants, the equalization was along particular tip-to-tip paths in the neuron instead of from the soma to the dendritic tips. In Wil's two-cylinder example, the L estimate was equal to the sum of the L values of the two cylinders when the ρ values of the cylinders were large and approximately equal; this happened because τ_1 represented equalization between the tips of the two cylinders. In subsequent work Wil and I found that we could interpret the time constants in complex branching structures (cf. figure 7 of Holmes et al. 1992) in the same way as equalizing time constants over particular paths in the neuron. The interpretation of time constants is important because it explains how and why electrotonic length estimates can be in error when the neuron cannot be approximated as a cylinder with sealed ends.

In the last section Wil derives expressions for the time constants for current transients under voltage clamp. Two additional formulas for electrotonic length are given that use these voltage clamp time constants. What is particularly appealing about the voltage clamp time constants is that they are independent of the soma conductance and, in particular, independent of any soma shunt that might exist. Intuitively, what happens is that the voltage clamp isolates the soma from the dendrites and effectively decouples the dendrites from each other. I discovered this result with the compartmental models I was using during my postdoctoral days in Wil's lab, and I showed the result to Wil. He thought about it for a moment, his legendary intuition told him the result was correct, and he remarked that this was an insight that seemed familiar to him. I later found this result in this paper, but fortunately for me, I found it before Wil remembered it was there.

Today, it is less popular to compute L with Wil's original formula because it is now known that many cells cannot be represented as a cylinder and this causes difficulties with obtaining meaningful estimates of τ_1. What is astonishing is not that the formula is less highly regarded today but that it took two decades for the sophistication of experimental data to catch up to that of this simple theoretical expression. With more and better morphological and electrophysiological data available now, techniques for estimating electrotonic parameters of a cell have become more complex. Present methods include fitting parameters to transients (e.g., Clements and Redman 1989; Stratford et al. 1989) or finding parameter values via an inverse procedure (Holmes and Rall 1992b); see also Ali-Hassan et al. 1992. Estimating parameter values for voltage-dependent conductances has also become important as the sophistication of neuronal models has increased. Stochastic search, genetic algorithm, and simulated annealing methods are being developed to provide these estimates.

The complexity of these new techniques makes it more difficult to develop the intuitive insights that played such a large role in Wil's work. With the computer power available today, the temptation is to ignore theory and intuition until the mass of computed results reaches a point where this is no longer possible. What we can learn from this paper is that such an approach would be a mistake. Theory and intuition should be developed hand in hand with computed and experimental results to maximize insight into the issue being studied.

References

Ali-Hassan, W. A., Saidel, G. M., and Durand, D. 1992. Estimation of electrotonic parameters of neurons using an inverse Fourier transform technique. *IEEE Trans. Biomed. Engr.* 39:493–501.

Clements, J. D., and Redman, S. J. 1989. Cable properties of cat spinal motoneurones measured by combining voltage clamp, current clamp and intracellular staining. *J. Physiol. Lond.* 409;63–87.

Durand, D. 1984. The somatic shunt cable model for neurons. *Biophys. J.* 46:645–653.

Evans, J. D., Kember, G. C., and Major, G. 1992. Techniques for obtaining analytical solutions to the multicylinder somatic shunt cable model for passive neurones. *Biophys. J.* 63: 350–365.

Holmes, W. R., and Rall, W. 1992a. Electrotonic length estimates in neurons with dendritic tapering or somatic shunt. *J. Neurophysiol.* 68:1421–1437.

Holmes, W. R., and Rall, W. 1992b. Estimating the electrotonic structure of neurons with compartmental models. *J. Neurophysiol.* 68:1438–1452.

Holmes, W. R., Segev, I., and Rall, W. 1992. Interpretation of time constant and electrotonic length estimates in multi-cylinder or branched neuronal structures. *J. Neurophysiol.* 68: 1401–1420.

Kawato, M. 1984. Cable properties of a neuron model with nonuniform membrane resistivity. *J. Theor. Biol.* 111:149–169.

Major, G., Evans, J. D., and Jack, J. J. B. 1993. Solutions for transients in arbitrary branching cables. I. Voltage recording with a somatic shunt. *Biophys. J.* 65:423–449.

Rall, W. 1969. Time constants and electrotonic length of membrane cylinders and neurons. *Biophys. J.* 9:1483–1508.

Segev, I., and Rall, W. 1983. Theoretical analysis of neuron models with dendrites of unequal electrical lengths. *Soc. Neurosci. Abstr.* 9:341.

Stratford, K., Mason, A., Larkman, A., Major, G., and Jack, J. J. B. 1989. The modeling of pyramidal neurones in the visual cortex. In *The Computing Neuron*, ed. R. Durbin, C. Miall, and G. Mitchison. Workingham, U.K.: Addison-Wesley.

7.2 Time Constants and Electrotonic Length of Membrane Cylinders and Neurons (1969), *Biophys. J.* 9:1483–1508

Wilfrid Rall

(G.H1)

ABSTRACT   A theoretical basis is provided for the estimation of the electrotonic length of a membrane cylinder, or the effective electrotonic length of a whole neuron, from electrophysiological experiments. It depends upon the several time constants present in passive decay of membrane potential from an initially nonuniform distribution over the length. In addition to the well known passive membrane time constant, $\tau_m = R_m C_m$, observed in the decay of a uniform membrane potential, there exist many smaller time constants that govern rapid equalization of membrane potential over the length. These time constants are present also in the transient response to a current step applied across the membrane at one location, such as the neuron soma. Similar time constants are derived when a lumped soma is coupled to one or more cylinders representing one or more dendritic trees. Different time constants are derived when a voltage clamp is applied at one location; the effects of both leaky and short-circuited termination are also derived. All of these time constants are demonstrated as consequences of mathematical boundary value problems. These results not only provide a basis for estimating electrotonic length, $L = \ell/\lambda$, but also provide a new basis for estimating the steady-state ratio, ρ, of cylinder input conductance to soma membrane conductance.

INTRODUCTION

When membrane depolarization or hyperpolarization is distributed uniformly over the entire surface of a neuron, and the membrane potential is then allowed to decay passively to its resting value, the time course of this decay is the same at every point of the membrane and consists of a single exponential decay having a time constant known as the passive membrane time constant, $\tau_m = R_m C_m$. However, for a nonuniform distribution of membrane polarization over the neuron surface, the time course of passive decay to the resting state is not the same at all points of the membrane. In those regions where the membrane potential has been displaced farthest from the resting value, the rate of decay will be initially more rapid than elsewhere and more rapid than for the case of uniform decay; this is because there is an equalizing (passive electrotonic) spread from more polarized regions to less (or oppositely) polarized regions of the membrane surface.[1] The different decay transients expected at different membrane locations can all be expressed as different linear combinations of several specific exponential decays (Rall, 1962; also 1964).

The tendency for membrane polarization to equalize over the neuron surface during passive decay is analogous to the tendency for temperature to equalize over an unevenly heated metal surface as it cools. This analogy is helpful to physical intuition; also, the mathematical treatment of these problems is essentially the same. All of the time constants of exponential decay, namely both the passive membrane time constant and the many shorter equalizing time constants, correspond to characteristic roots (eigenvalues) of the mathematical boundary value problem.

Both the statement and solution of several boundary value problems for nerve cylinders of finite length and for a certain class of dendritic neurons were presented several years ago (Rall, 1962). That paper, however, was concerned with a problem more general than passive decay of nonuniform membrane potential; it was concerned also with the effects of nonuniform synaptic membrane conductance. Here, my purpose is to focus attention upon the equalizing time constants, and to point out their importance for an experimental estimation of effective electrotonic length in nerve cylinders and in dendritic neurons.

Application to Motoneurons

Explicit focus upon these theoretical relations is now timely because my suggestions to Drs. P. G. Nelson, H. D. Lux, and R. E. Burke have led them to seek and obtain experimental results specifically intended for such estimation of effective electrotonic length. Their experimental results (Nelson and Lux, 1969; Burke[2]) are consistent with interpreting the dendritic trees of cat motoneurons as being electrotonically equivalent to membrane cylinders of lengths in the range from about one to about two characteristic lengths. It is both interesting and gratifying that this estimated range of lengths agrees with that I obtained several years ago from entirely different calculations based upon the anatomical measurements of Aitken and Bridger (1961); although the details of these calculations have not been published, the resulting estimates have been explicitly stated (Rall, 1964, p. 83–84). Also, this same range of electrotonic lengths was found to be consistent with the range of synaptic potential shapes (monosynaptic EPSP) found in motoneurons (Burke, 1967; Rall et al. 1967, p. 1180–1181).

The fact that membrane potential transients in dendritic neurons should not be viewed as single exponential decays was recognized (Rall, 1957, 1960) in dealing with the problem of estimating the passive membrane time constant. The fact that a

---

[1] See, for example, Fig. 4 of Rall, (1960) and Figs. 6 and 7 of Rall (1962).
[2] Personal communications with R. E. Burke; this forms part of a larger study that has not yet been submitted for publication.

synaptic potential may decay in two stages was demonstrated by Fadiga and Brookhart (1960); they also noted that such two stage decay is observed at the soma when the synaptic input is delivered to the soma, but not when the input is delivered to the dendrites. Time constants for finite dendritic length were provided by (Rall, 1962; see p. 1083 and 1088). Ito and Oshima (1965) found that they could represent certain membrane potential transients as a linear combination of three exponential decays having time constants of about 25, 5, and 1 msec, respectively. With regard to shortest time constant, they discussed the possible role of dendrites, and of the endoplasmic reticulum. Their slowest time constant corresponds to some still incompletely understood slow process that underlies the over- and undershoots they studied, and possibly also the anomalous rectification studied by Nelson and Frank (1967). Whatever this underlying slow process may be, it is important to emphasize that it cannot be accounted for by the passive membrane potential theory of the present paper. Fortunately, these complications appear to be significant only in some motoneurons, and negligible in others (Nelson and Lux, 1969). Also, different neurons, such as those studied by Tsukahara, Toyama, and Kosaka (1967), appear to be free of complication by this slow process.

With regard to variety in the shapes of miniature monosynaptic EPSPs in motoneurons, the observations of Burke (1967) have been essentially confirmed in several other laboratories (Jack et al., 1967; Mendell and Henneman, 1968; Letbetter et al., 1968; and also personal communications from these groups). Essentially all of this observed variety in EPSP shape has been accounted for theoretically (except for the slow process mentioned in the previous paragraph) by means of computations (Rall, 1967; Rall et al., 1967) which imply the validity of the equalizing time constants to be explained and discussed below.

Definitions of Symbols

$V_m = V_i - V_e$ membrane potential, as intracellular minus extracellular electric potential.

$V = V_m - E_r$ deviation of membrane potential from its resting value; electrotonic potential.

r_i intracellular (core) resistance per unit length of cylinder; (ohm/cm).

r_e extracellular resistance per unit length of cylinder, if defined; otherwise set equal to zero; (ohm/cm).

r_m membrane resistance across a unit length of cylindrical membrane; (ohm cm).

c_m membrane capacity per unit length of cylindrical membrane; (farad/cm).

$\tau_m = r_m c_m$ passive membrane time constant; (sec).

$T = t/\tau_m$ time in terms of τ_m; dimensionless time variable.

$\lambda = [r_m/(r_i + r_e)]^{1/2}$ characteristic length of nerve cylinder, with r_e usually set equal to zero; (cm).

$X = x/\lambda$ distance along axis of cylinder in terms of λ; dimensionless electrotonic distance variable.

$L = \ell/\lambda$ length of cylinder in terms of λ; dimensionless electrotonic length.

$C_0, C_1, C_2, \cdots, C_n$ coefficients (independent of t) used to form a linear combination of exponential decays; (volt).

$\tau_0 = \tau_m$ passive membrane time constant; (sec).

$\tau_1, \tau_2, \cdots, \tau_n$ equalizing time constants, in parts I and II below, where n can be any positive
integer; different time constants in part III below; (sec).

α^2 separation constant, for separation of variables.

$\alpha_n{}^2$ eigenvalues of boundary value problem.

$\alpha_n = + \sqrt{\alpha_n{}^2}$ roots in form most used.

B_n constant coefficients in infinite series solutions; sometimes Fourier coefficients; (volt).

I_A current applied outward across membrane at $X = 0$; (amp).

V_A voltage (V) applied at $X = 0$; (volt).

I_S soma membrane current; (amp).

I_C current flowing into cylinder at $X = 0$; (amp).

G_S soma membrane conductance, being steady-state value of I_S/V_A; (mho).

$G_\infty = [\lambda r_i]^{-1} = \lambda/r_m = [r_i r_m]^{-1/2}$ input conductance of a cylinder of infinite length; (mho)

$G_C = G_\infty \tanh (L)$ input conductance (at $X = 0$) of a cylinder with a sealed end at $X = L$,
being steady-state value of I_C/V_A ; (mho)

$\rho = G_C/G_S = \rho_\infty \tanh (L)$ ratio of cylinder input conductance to soma membrane conductance, being steady-state value of I_C/I_S .

$\rho_\infty = G_\infty/G_S$ ratio, ρ, for limiting case when cylinder has infinite length.

$\rho_j = G_{C_j}/G_S$ ratio of cylinder input conductance (for j^{th} of several cylinders) to the membrane conductance of a common soma.

RESULTS

I. General Statement for Users

This section attempts to summarize in usable form the results judged to be of most direct importance to an experimental neurophysiologist. More detailed definitions, derivations and special cases are presented in the later sections of this paper.

The passive decay transients can be expressed as a sum of exponential decays

$$V = C_0 e^{-t/\tau_0} + C_1 e^{-t/\tau_1} + C_2 e^{-t/\tau_2} + \cdots + C_n e^{-t/\tau_n} + \cdots \qquad (1)$$

where $\tau_0 \equiv \tau_m$ represents the passive membrane time constant, and $\tau_1, \tau_2, \cdots$ $\tau_n, \cdots$ represent infinitely many equalizing time constants which are smaller than τ_0. Usually only the first one or two equalizing time constants are important to the interpretation of experimental results. The coefficients, C_n, are constants.[3]

The values of the equalizing time constants, relative to τ_0, depend upon the effective electrotonic length of the cylinder or neuron; they do not depend upon a specification of the initial non-uniform distribution of membrane potential from which the passive decay takes place. For a cylinder with both ends sealed and of electrotonic length, $L = \ell/\lambda$, the values of the equalizing time constants are given by the expression

$$\tau_n = \frac{\tau_0}{1 + (n\pi/L)^2} . \qquad (2)$$

---

[3] These coefficients are independent of t. They generally have different values at each point of observation (i.e. value of x); they are also different for different initial conditions.

This implies, of course, that

$$L = \frac{n\pi}{\sqrt{\tau_0/\tau_n - 1}}.$$
(3)

Although these equations can be used to calculate the value of L corresponding to any given value of the ratio, τ_0/τ_n, it is helpful to have a few sets of illustrative values; this is provided by Table I.

The relative values of the coefficients, $C_0,' C_1, C_2, \cdots, C_n, \cdots$ depend upon the nonuniform initial condition, upon the effective electrotonic length and, for a dendritic neuron, also upon the dendritic-to-soma conductance ratio, ρ. A completely uniform initial condition would cause all of the coefficients except C_0 to be zero. A nonuniformity that is distributed symmetrically about the mid-point of the cylinder would cause all of the odd numbered coefficients to be zero; in this case, the most important equalizing time constant would be τ_2. Usually, however, with asymmetric initial nonuniformity, the most important equalizing time constant is τ_1.

The feasibility of estimating the first one or two equalizing time constants in equation 1 from an observed decay transient depends upon three considerations: (1) C_1 and/or C_2 must not be too small relative to C_0, this is enhanced by having the initial polarization concentrated near the point of observation, and, for a dendritic neuron, also upon the dendritic-to-soma conductance ratio, ρ, not too small; (2) the effective electrotonic length must not be too long, because this would make successive time constants too close together to permit their resolution; increased length leads, in the limit, to expressions involving error functions as on p. 528 of (Rall, 1960); (3) the effective electrotonic length must not be too short, and the transient must be recorded with sufficiently high fidelity that at least one of the faster decaying components is preserved.

Although the above has all been stated for passive decay to the resting state, the same applies also to the transient approach to a nonresting steady state of passive membrane, such as when a constant current step is applied to one end of a cylinder, or to the soma of a dendritic neuron. It should be emphasized that this holds for

TABLE I
RATIO OF τ_0 TO EQUALIZING TIME CONSTANTS*

Ratio	$L = 1$	$L = \pi/2$	$L = 2$	$L = 3$	$L = 4$
τ_0/τ_1	10.9	5.0	3.5	2.1	1.6
τ_0/τ_2	40.5	17.0	10.9	5.4	4.5
τ_0/τ_3	89.8	37.0	23.2	10.9	6.6
τ_0/τ_4	159.0	65.0	40.5	18.5	10.9

* $\tau_0 = \tau_m = R_m C_m$. Ratios based on equation 16.

constant current, but not for a voltage clamp;[4] also the membrane must remain passive.

Given the favorable conditions specified above, the procedure is to "peel" the slowest exponential decay from the faster decaying portion of the transient. This procedure, long known to physicists studying multiple radioactive decays, can be carried out quite simply with the help of semilogarithmic plotting; nevertheless, it is sometimes misunderstood and done incorrectly. If we plot log V vs. t, the result (from equation 1) is a straight line only for values of t sufficiently large that faster decaying terms of equation 1 are negligibly small compared with the first (zero index) term; for such values of t, the transient has a single exponential "tail"; in other words

$$[\text{tail } V] = C_0 e^{-t/\tau_0} \tag{4 a}$$

implying that

$$\log_e [\text{tail } V] = -t/\tau_0 + \text{const.} \tag{4 b}$$

and that

$$\tau_0 = \frac{-0.4343}{\text{slope of } \log_{10} [\text{tail } V]} \tag{4 c}$$

where "slope of" means (d/dt), or slope with respect to t. In the semilog plot, we can extrapolate the straight line tail back to earlier values of the time; when these extrapolated values are subtracted from the observed values, the resulting difference is the "peeled" transient; in other words

$$[\text{peeled } V] = V - [\text{tail } V] \tag{5 a}$$

$$= V - C_0 e^{-t/\tau_0} . \tag{5 b}$$

When τ_1 and τ_2 are not too close together, and C_1 is not too small, we can find a range of values of t for which all faster decaying terms (corresponding to $n > 1$) are negligibly small compared with the term for $n = 1$; then we can write

$$[\text{peeled } V] = C_1 e^{-t/\tau_1} \tag{6 a}$$

implying that

$$\log_e [\text{peeled } V] = -t/\tau_1 + \text{const.} \tag{6 b}$$

and that

$$\tau_1 = \frac{-0.4343}{\text{slope of } \log_{10} [\text{peeled } V]} \tag{6 c}$$

for this intermediate range of t.

---

[4] See part III below for the effect of voltage clamping.

It is important to note that, over this intermediate range of t, it is not the observed V, but "peeled V," whose log has a constant slope with respect to t. When someone inadvertently fits a straight line to log V vs. t, for this intermediate range of t, the slope of that straight line is not the same as in equations 6 and will not yield a correct estimate of τ_1.

From the results above, it can be seen that

$$\tau_0/\tau_1 = \frac{\text{slope of log [peeled } V]}{\text{slope of log [tail } V]}.$$ (7)

Also, from equation 3 for a cylinder of finite length, with sealed ends, it can be seen that

$$L = \pi[\tau_0/\tau_1 - 1]^{-1/2}.$$ (8)

Thus, when they have been correctly applied to experimental data,[5] equations 7 and 8 provide an estimate of the electrotonic length of the cylinder most nearly equivalent to the whole neuron in question. Part II below also provides results for a lumped soma coupled to one or more dendritic cylinders; there it is shown to what extent the electrotonic length of the dendrites can differ from the L defined by equation 8. Results for voltage clamping are in part III.

Although it is sometimes possible to peel a sum of exponential decays in several successive steps, it is usually best to use a well tested computer program to obtain the most reliable decomposition of a linear combination of several exponential decays.

II. DERIVATION OF EQUALIZING TIME CONSTANTS

Equalization over Length or Circumference?

Because this paper is concerned with membrane cylinders (and dendritic neurons) whose lengths are much greater than their diameters, it can be shown that equalization of membrane potential over the length is of primary importance. However, it is important to note that additional time constants govern equalization of membrane potential over the circumference of the cylindrical cross section. Expressions for such circumferential equalizing time constants are derived in a companion paper (Rall, 1969). There it is estimated (for typical neuronal values) that circumferential equalization should be around a thousand times more rapid than equalization over the length of the cylinder. This provides a justification for considering only the one spatial variable, X, in the derivation that follows.

---

[5] It should be noted that such peeling can be applied also to the slope, dV/dt, because this is a differently weighted sum of the same exponential decays. This is useful in situations where the level but not the direction of the baseline is uncertain. Also, peeling this sum of exponentials is aided by the greater weight of the equalizing terms relative to the uniform decay term.

Statement of Boundary Value Problem, for Cylinder with Sealed Ends

The partial differential equation for passive membrane potential distributions in a nerve cylinder is well established; it can be expressed

$$\frac{\partial^2 V}{\partial X^2} = V + \frac{\partial V}{\partial T} \tag{9}$$

for all values of X and T. For a cylinder of finite electrotonic length, L, we restrict consideration of this differential equation to the range $0 \leq X \leq L$. We assume a "sealed end" (Rall, 1959, p. 497) at both ends of this cylinder; this corresponds to the mathematical boundary conditions

$$\frac{\partial V}{\partial X} = 0, \quad \text{at } X = 0, \quad \text{for } T > 0, \tag{10}$$

and

$$\frac{\partial V}{\partial X} = 0, \quad \text{at } X = L, \quad \text{for } T > 0. \tag{11}$$

The initial condition can be expressed

$$V(X, 0) = F(X), \quad \text{for } 0 \leq X \leq L. \tag{12}$$

Taken together, equations 9–12 define a boundary value problem which has a unique mathematical solution obtainable by classical methods (Churchill, 1941; Carslaw and Jaeger, 1959; and Weinberger, 1965).

Equalizing Time Constants, for Cylinder with Sealed Ends

Because of present interest in these time constants, we wish to pay particular attention to the way in which they are determined by the differential equation and the boundary conditions. First, we note that a solution of the partial differential equation 9 can be expressed

$$V(X, T) = (A \sin \alpha X + B \cos \alpha X)e^{-(1+\alpha^2)T} \tag{13}$$

This solution, obtained by the classical method of separation of variables,[6] represents $V(X, T)$ as the product of two functions, one of which is a function of X only, the other being a function of T only; the constant, α^2, is known as the separation constant. The fact that this is a solution can be verified by differentiation and substitution in equation 9; it should be noted that equation 9 is satisfied for any arbitrary combination of values for the constants A, B and α.

---

[6] See, for example, Chapter IV in Weinberger (1965), or pages 25–27 in Churchill (1941).

In order to apply the boundary conditions (equations 10 and 11), we must consider the partial derivative with respect to X,

$$\frac{\partial V}{\partial X} = (\alpha A \cos \alpha X - \alpha B \sin \alpha X)e^{-(1+\alpha^2)T}.$$

At $X = 0$, $\sin \alpha X = 0$ and $\cos \alpha X = 1$; therefore the boundary condition (equation 10) at $X = 0$ requires that $\alpha A = 0$, and this, in fact, requires that we set $A = 0$; (A could differ from zero only in the special case when $\alpha = 0$; then $\sin \alpha X = 0$, and again $A \sin \alpha X$ vanishes in equation 13). With $A = 0$, the other boundary condition (equation 11) at $X = L$ then requires that

$$\alpha B \sin \alpha L = 0. \tag{14}$$

This condition is satisfied when $\alpha = 0$, and also by every value of α for which αL is equal to some integral multiple of π, because then $\sin \alpha L = 0$. Thus, the infinitely many roots of equation 14 can be expressed

$$\alpha_n = n\pi/L \tag{15}$$

where n is any positive integer,[7] or zero. It may be noted that the numbers, α_n^2, correspond to the "eigenvalues" or the "characteristic numbers" of classical boundary value problems.

For $n = 0$, $\alpha = 0$, and it follows that the time dependent part of equation 13 becomes simply

$$e^{-T} \equiv e^{-t/\tau_m} \equiv e^{-t/\tau_0}$$

which represents exponential decay with the passive membrane time constant, $\tau_m = r_m c_m$, which we here identify also as τ_0.

When n is any positive integer, the corresponding α_n of equation 15 implies that the exponent in equation 13 has the value

$$-[1 + (n\pi/L)^2]t/\tau_0 \equiv -t/\tau_n$$

from which it follows that

$$\tau_0/\tau_n = 1 + (n\pi/L)^2. \tag{16}$$

This result defines the equalizing time constants, τ_n, for n equal to any positive integer. This provides the basis for equations 2 and 3 and the illustrative values of Table I, in part I above.

---

[7] For all of these values of n, the functions (equation 13) are linearly independent of each other; negative integer values of n also satisfy equations 14 and 15, but their use in equation 13 would not provide any additional independent eigenfunctions.

Comment on Solution as a Sum of Exponentials

The preceding section has shown that the two boundary conditions (equations 10 and 11) constrain two of the arbitrary constants in equation 13, which defines a class of solutions of the partial differential equation 9. The resulting class of solutions can be expressed

$$V(X, T) = B \cos (\alpha_n X) e^{-(1+\alpha_n^2)T}$$

where B is still an arbitrary constant, and each solution corresponds to a particular value of α_n, as defined by equation 15.

Because equation 9 is linear, any linear combination of these distinct solutions is also a solution. The class of all such linear combinations can be expressed as the following infinite series

$$V(X, T) = \sum_{n=0}^{\infty} B_n \cos (n\pi X/L) e^{-[1+(n\pi/L)^2]T} \tag{17}$$

where the B_n are still arbitrary constants. Only when we impose the constraint provided by the initial condition (equation 12) of the complete boundary value problem, do the coefficients, B_n, become constrained to particular values. These particular values can be defined as the Fourier coefficients,

$$B_0 = (1/L) \int_0^L F(X) \, dX$$

and, for $n > 0$,

$$B_n = (2/L) \int_0^L F(X) \cos (n\pi X/L) \, dX.$$

Then equation 17 expresses a unique solution of the boundary value problem originally defined by equations 9–12; see Churchill (1941), or Weinberger (1965). Explicit solutions for particular choices of $F(X)$ will be presented in a separate paper.

This solution obviously represents a sum of exponentials like equation 1 in part I, above. Any particular point of observation corresponds to a particular value of X; then the coefficients of equation 1 are related to those of equation 17 by the expression

$$C_n = B_n \cos (n\pi X/L).$$

Coupling of Single Cylinder to Lumped Soma

The point, $X = 0$, is taken as the point where a lumped soma membrane is coupled with the origin of the membrane cylinder (Rall, 1959). This cylinder may be thought of as a single cylinder of finite length, with a sealed end at $X = L$; it may also be thought of as an "equivalent cylinder" representing an entire dendritic tree, or even several dendritic trees which have the same electronic length (Rall, 1962, 1964).

The boundary condition at $X = 0$ is more complicated than before. The current flowing outward across the lumped soma membrane can be expressed

$$I_s = G_s(V + \partial V/\partial T)$$

where G_s represents soma membrane conductance. The current flowing into the cylinder at $X = 0$ can be expressed

$$I_c = (1/r_i)[-\partial V/\partial x]_{x=0}$$
$$= (1/\lambda r_i)[-\partial V/\partial X]_{X=0}.$$

If there is a current, I_A, applied outward across the membrane at $X = 0$, continuity requires that

$$I_A = I_S + I_C.$$

Hence, the boundary condition at $X = 0$ can be expressed

$$[\partial V/\partial X]_{X=0} = \lambda r_i[-I_A + G_S(V + \partial V/\partial T)]. \tag{18}$$

The symbol, ρ, has previously (Rall, 1959) been used to represent the ratio of cylinder input conductance to soma membrane conductance; this ratio equals the ratio of the steady-state values of I_c and I_s, above; thus

$$\rho = \frac{(1/\lambda r_i)V_0 \tanh L}{G_S V_0}$$
$$= \frac{\tanh L}{\lambda r_i G_s}$$

where V_0 is the steady-state value at $X = 0$ and

$$V = V_0 \cosh [L - X]/\cosh L$$

is the steady-state solution in the cylinder.

Using the above expression for ρ, and setting $I_A = 0$ in equation 18, we obtain the expression

$$\rho \partial V/\partial X = (V + \partial V/\partial T) \tanh L, \quad \text{at } X = 0 \tag{19}$$

as the boundary condition expressing cylinder-to-soma coupling during passive membrane potential decay.

The mathematical boundary value problem to be solved differs from that defined by equations 9–12 only in that the previous boundary condition (equation 10) at $X = 0$ is now replaced by equation 19 above. This difference, however, results in a changed set of equalizing time constants and in a solution that involves a generalized Fourier expansion in which special attention is required to obtain correct values of the coefficients.[8]

Equalizing Time Constants for Cylinder with Soma

Because the differential equation is the same as before, we again use a solution of the same general form as equation 13, above, except that we replace the argument, αX, by the argument, $\alpha(L - X)$, to take advantage of the fact that the simpler boundary condition is at $X = L$. Thus, we consider the solution

$$V(X, T) = [A \sin \alpha(L - X) + B \cos \alpha(L - X)]e^{-(1+\alpha^2)T}. \quad (20)$$

The boundary condition (equation 11) at $X = L$ requires that $A = 0$, and the boundary condition (equation 19) at $X = 0$ then requires that

$$\rho\alpha B \sin \alpha L = (-\alpha^2 B \cos \alpha L) \tanh L.$$

This requirement is satisfied by $\alpha = 0$, and by values of α which are roots of the transcendental equation

$$\alpha L \cot \alpha L = -\rho L/\tanh L = -C \quad (21)$$

where C is a positive constant; the roots of this equation have been tabulated.[9] The equalizing time constants can be expressed

$$\tau_n = \frac{\tau_0}{1 + (\alpha_n)^2} \quad (22)$$

where each α_n is a root of equation 21. The consequences of equations 21 and 22 are summarized in Fig. 1, which shows the dependence of τ_0/τ_1 upon L for several different values of ρ. It is apparent that any given value of τ_0/τ_1 corresponds to many possible combinations of values for ρ and L. For example, a value of 6 for the ration, τ_0/τ_1, corresponds approximately to $L = 1.1$ for $\rho = 2$, or to $L = 1.25$ for $\rho = 5$, or $L = 1.4$ for $\rho = \infty$; of course, ρ need not be an integer, and many other combinations are possible.

Some intuitive grasp of the possible values of the roots, α_n, can be obtained by considering briefly the limiting cases for ρ very large and ρ very small.

The limiting case, $\rho = \infty$, corresponds to *complete dendritic dominance* (Rall,

---

[8] This has been done for several cases, but the results have not yet been submitted for publication.
[9] See Table II of Appendix IV in Carslaw and Jaeger (1959); note that their α corresponds to αL here.

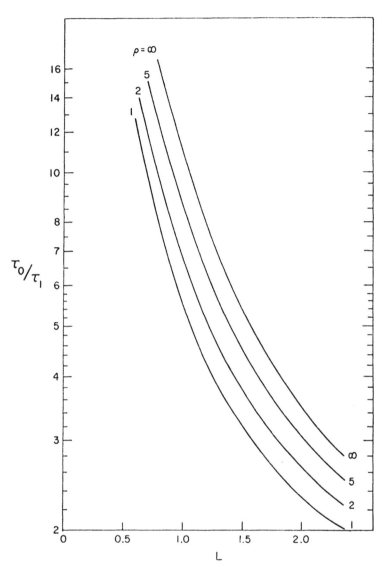

FIGURE 1   Dependence of the time constant ratio, τ_0/τ_1, upon the value of L, for several values of ρ. Calculations based upon equations 21 and 22.

1959) or to a *vanishing soma admittance* at $X = 0$; it is equivalent to the zero slope boundary condition at $X = 0$, and implies that

$$\alpha_n = n\pi/L \qquad (\text{for } \rho = \infty)$$

where n may be zero or any positive integer; (cf. earlier equations 14–16).

   The other limiting case, $\rho = 0$, corresponds to *vanishing dendritic admittance*, or to an *infinite soma admittance* at $X = 0$; it is equivalent to a voltage clamp at $X = 0$, and implies that

$$\alpha_n = (2n - 1)\pi/2L, \quad \text{(for } \rho = 0)$$

where n may be any positive integer; (cf. equations 27 and 29, below).

Illustrative Example   For any finite value of ρL, $\alpha_0 = 0$, and $\pi/2 < \alpha_1 L < \pi$. For example, if $L = 1.5$ and $\rho = 4.82$, then $\rho L/\tanh L = 8.0$, and the first nonzero root of the transcendental equation 21 is $\alpha_1 L = 2.80$, or, since $L = 1.5$, $\alpha_1 = 1.87$; it follows that $\tau_0/\tau_1 = 4.5$ for this particular case. This time constant ratio for the cylinder-coupled-to-soma may be compared with two related cases of a cylinder alone, with sealed ends at both $X = 0$ and $X = L$, where equation 16 applies. First consider the cylinder alone with $L = 1.5$; then $\tau_0/\tau_1 = 5.4$ is implied. However, this cylinder alone has an electrotonic length that is less than that of the previous combination of soma with cylinder. Therefore, we consider a longer cylinder, lengthened by the factor, $(\rho + 1)/\rho$, to allow for the soma membrane surface as an extension of the cylinder instead of as a lump; for this length

$$\tau_0/\tau_1 = 1 + \left[\frac{\pi}{L(\rho + 1)/\rho} \right]^2$$

which equals 4.0 in the case of this particular example. It may be noted that the correct τ_0/τ_1 value of 4.5, found above for the soma coupled to the cylinder, lies between the two values 5.4 and 4.0, found for the two different lengths of a cylinder alone just considered.

From the foregoing, it can be seen that when the inverse problem of estimating L from a τ_0/τ_1 value is considered, simple use of equation 8 yields an L value for that cylinder which best approximates the whole neuron or cylinder being studied. If we know at least an approximate value of ρ and wish to estimate the L value for the equivalent *dendritic* cylinder, the value provided by equation 8 would be too large by a factor, f, where $1 < f < (\rho + 1)/\rho$. A reasonable approximation is provided by either $f \simeq (1 + 0.5/\rho)$, or $f \simeq \sqrt{1 + 1/\rho}$. Thus, we can write the approximate expression

$$L \simeq \pi \left[\frac{\rho/(\rho + 1)}{\tau_0/\tau_1 - 1} \right]^{1/2} \tag{23}$$

for an estimate of L (of the equivalent dendritic cylinder) when the values of ρ and τ_0/τ_1 are known. This expression gives results in agreement with Fig. 1.

Several Dendrites Coupled to Single Soma

When the several dendritic trees of a neuron correspond to equivalent cylinders of significantly different electrotonic length, it is not correct to represent them all together as one cylinder. Here we show that it is possible to obtain correct equalizing time constants even for such more complicated problems. The previous analysis shows that the current flowing into one cylinder could be expressed

$$I_C = \frac{\rho G_s}{\tanh L} \left[-\frac{\partial V}{\partial X} \right]_{X=0}.$$

Now, if we have several cylinders, k in number, and the jth cylinder has a lenght, L_j, and a cylinder input conductance to soma membrane conductance ratio, ρ_j, the total dendritic input current can be expressed

$$I_D = G_s \sum_{j=1}^{k} \frac{\rho_j}{\tanh L_j} \left[-\frac{\partial V_j}{\partial X_j} \right]_{X=0}. \tag{24}$$

In each cylinder, there is a solution of the form (equation 20), with $A = 0$ and with α_n required to satisfy the following generalization of equation 21

$$\alpha = -\sum_{j=1}^{k} \frac{\rho_j \tan \alpha L_j}{\tanh L_j}. \tag{25}$$

Consider, for example, $k = 2$, $L_1 = 1$, with $\rho_1/\tanh L_1 = 3$ and $L_2 = 2$, with $\rho_2/\tanh L_2 = 5$; then the transcendental equation is

$$\alpha = -3 \tan \alpha - 5 \tan 2\alpha.$$

Obviously, $\alpha = 0$ is a root. Seeking, by trial and error, a root between 0 and $\pi/2$, we find $\alpha_1 \simeq 1.10$, because then $\tan \alpha \simeq 1.96$ and $\tan 2\alpha \simeq -1.37$, which values nearly satisfy the above equation. Between $\pi/2$ and π, we find $\alpha_2 \simeq 1.97$, because then $\tan \alpha \simeq -2.37$ and $\tan 2\alpha \simeq 1.03$, which values also nearly satisfy the above equation. Notice, for α_1 and α_2, $\tan \alpha$ and $\tan 2\alpha$ have opposite signs. However, near π, we find the root, $\alpha_3 \simeq 2.92$, because then $\tan \alpha \simeq -0.22$ and $\tan 2\alpha \simeq -0.47$, which values have the same sign and nearly satisfy the above equation. For $n > 3$, it can be shown that $\alpha_n \simeq n\pi/3$, which is rather interesting because this is the same as equation 15, where the denominator here represents $L_1 + L_2$, the sum of the lengths of the two cylinders. In fact, this simple rule provides first approximations to the smaller roots as well. On reflection, it is obvious that this simple result would hold best when both ρ are large and approximately equal; then the whole neuron can be approximated as an equivalent cylinder of length, $L_1 + L_2$, with the soma located not at $X = 0$ but at a point L_1 from one end.

Although the roots of equation 25 can also be found for any particular case of three or more cylinders coupled to a single soma, little purpose would be served by another illustrative example. It will be clear to anyone who has carefully considered the example above, that the addition of a third cylinder of a different length must increase the number of roots between 0 and π, because of the greater number of possibilities of positive and negative contributions to the summation in equation 25.

III. VOLTAGE CLAMP AND RELATED PROBLEMS

Drastic Effect of Voltage Clamp

When the membrane potential is held to a constant value at one end of the cylinder, or at the point $(X = 0)$ of soma-to-cylinder coupling, the boundary value problem becomes very significantly changed: the time constants are changed and should not be called "equalizing" time constants; furthermore these new time constants are independent of ρ; in fact, after the initial instantaneous charging of the soma to its clamped value, the soma membrane draws a constant current from the voltage clamp, while the transient component of the clamping current flows entirely into the cylinder (cf. Rall, 1960, p. 514–515 and 529–530 for the case of a cylinder of infinite length).

Before demonstrating it mathematically, it can be understood physiologically, that simple passive decay and simple equalizing decay cannot take place when there is a voltage clamp placed across the cell membrane at any point. The voltage clamp has much in common with a short circuit; whereas passive membrane decay requires that the membrane have its normal membrane conductance (also capacitance and EMF) everywhere. A short circuit, or a voltage clamp, must make the decay to a steady state be more rapid than a simple passive decay. Nevertheless, these faster time constants may also be useful for estimation of L by means of equation 33 below.

Time Constants for Voltage Clamp at $X = 0$

The boundary value problem differs from that stated earlier with equations 9–12 in that the previous condition (equation 10) at $X = 0$ is replaced by

$$V(0, T) = V_0 . \tag{26}$$

It is simplest to show the effect of voltage clamping upon the time constants by considering first the particular case of $V_0 = 0$. Thus, the boundary condition

$$V(0, T) = 0 \tag{27}$$

requires that the coefficient, B, in the solution (equation 13) be set equal to zero. Then the zero slope boundary condition (equation 11) at $X = L$ requires that

$$\alpha A \cos \alpha L = 0. \tag{28}$$

Although this equation is satisfied by $\alpha = 0$, this root is trivial because it makes $\sin \alpha X = 0$ for all X. However, equation 28 is satisfied by $\alpha L = \pi/2$, and by every value of α for which αL is equal to $\pi/2$ plus $(n - 1)\pi$, because then $\cos \alpha L = 0$. Thus, the infinitely many roots of equation 28 can be expressed

$$\alpha_n = (2n - 1)\pi/2L \tag{29}$$

where n may be any positive integer. In this case, the infinite series solution to the boundary value problem can be expressed

$$V(X, T) = \sum_{n=1}^{\infty} A_n \sin (\alpha_n X) e^{-(1+\alpha_n^2)T} \qquad (30)$$

where the α_n are defined by equation 29 and the A_n are the Fourier coefficients defined by

$$A_n = \frac{2}{L} \int_0^L F(X) \sin (\alpha_n X) \, dX. \qquad (31)$$

Here, the time constants implied by equations 29 and 30 are quite different from those considered earlier; here

$$\tau_n = \frac{\tau_m}{1 + (2n - 1)^2 (\pi/2L)^2} \qquad (32)$$

where n may be any positive integer. We note again that $\alpha_0 = 0$, which would have given a $\tau_0 = \tau_m$, has been excluded because such an α_0 would make $\sin (\alpha_0 X)$ in equation 30 vanish for all X. Thus, even the largest time constant, τ_1, is smaller than τ_m. For example, if $L = \pi/2$, $\tau_1 = 0.5 \tau_m$ and $\tau_2 = 0.1 \tau_m$; see also Table II.

These time constants are obviously different from the equalizing time constants discussed in parts I and II above. Nevertheless, if both τ_1 and τ_2 can be measured reliably, the following expression, obtained from equation 32 above, permits an estimate of L,

$$L = (\pi/2)(9\tau_2 - \tau_1)^{1/2}(\tau_1 - \tau_2)^{-1/2}. \qquad (33)$$

When the clamped value, V_0, is different from zero, the time constants are the same, but solution becomes

$$V(X, T) = V_0 \frac{\cosh (L - X)}{\cosh L} + \sum_{n=1}^{\infty} A_n \sin (\alpha_n X) e^{-(1+\alpha_n^2)T}$$

TABLE II

RATIO OF τ_m TO TIME CONSTANTS* UNDER VOLTAGE CLAMP‡

Ratio	$L = 1$	$L = \pi/2$	$L = 2$	$L = 3$	$L = 4$
τ_m/τ_1	3.5	2.0	1.6	1.27	1.15
τ_m/τ_2	23.2	10.0	6.5	3.5	2.4
τ_m/τ_3	62.6	26.0	16.4	7.9	4.9
τ_m/τ_4	121.9	50.0	31.2	14.4	8.5

* Ratios based on equation 32. Note that these time constants need not be referred to τ_m; they can be referred to each other, as in equation 33.
‡ Voltage clamp applied at one end.

where the A_n are obtained from equation 31 provided that $F(X)$ is replaced by the difference, $F(X) - V_0 \cosh (L - X)/\cosh L$, in equation 31.

At $X = 0$, this transient simply gives $V = V_0$, as it should. However, referring back to equation 18, we can express the voltage clamping current, minus the constant current to the soma, as proportional to $[-\partial V/\partial X]$ at $X = 0$, as follows,

$$[I_A - I_s] \propto \left[V_0 \tanh L - \sum_{n=1}^{\infty} \alpha_n A_n e^{-(1+\alpha_n{}^2)T} \right] \tag{34}$$

where the A_n are the same as those of the preceding paragraph, and the α_n and the resulting time constants are the same as equations 29, 32, and 33 above.

Special Case of Voltage Clamps at $X = 0$ and $X = L$.

This special case merits brief mention because the time constants turn out to be the same as the equalizing time constants found earlier for the cylinder with both ends sealed, except that here there is no $\tau_0 = \tau_m$. The boundary conditions can be expressed,

$$V(0, T) = V_0, \quad \text{and} \quad V(L, T) = V_L$$

where V_0 and V_L are both constants. The steady-state solution can be expressed

$$V(X, \infty) = [V_0 \sinh (L - X) + V_L \sinh X]/\sinh L. \tag{35}$$

Now, if we consider the function

$$U(X, T) = V(X, T) - V(X, \infty) \tag{36}$$

we obtain a boundary value problem in which the partial differential equation for $U(X, T)$ has the same form as equation 9, and the boundary conditions become simplified to

$$U(0, T) = 0 = U(L, T).$$

When a general solution of the form (equation 13) is subjected to the boundary condition at $X = 0$, we find that $B = 0$, and then the boundary condition at $X = L$ requires that

$$A \sin \alpha L = 0$$

which has the roots

$$\alpha_n = n\pi/L. \tag{37}$$

The solution for $U(X, T)$ can thus be expressed

$$U(X, T) = \sum_{n=1}^{\infty} A_n \sin{(n\pi X/L)}e^{-[1+(n\pi/L)^2]T}. \tag{38}$$

Although the α_n are the same as in equation 17, equation 38 differs significantly both by being a sine series instead of a cosine series, and by summing from $n = 1$ instead of $n = 0$.

This solution would be of practical value in those axons, dendrites or muscle fibers where it may be possible to voltage clamp at two points and observe the time course of the transient at a location between the two clamped points. This would have the merit of being completely undisturbed by any activity outside the region between the two voltage clamps.

Killed-End at $X = L$

The killed-end boundary condition corresponds to a short circuit between interior and exterior media; this means that $V_m = 0$, at $X = L$, and since $V = V_m - E_r$, we have the boundary condition,

$$V(L, T) = - E_r = V_L$$

which is equivalent to a voltage clamp at $X = L$.

If the boundary condition at $X = 0$ is a voltage clamp, the problem becomes the same as that of the preceding section. However, if the boundary condition at $X = 0$ is a zero slope, then the problem becomes the same as that of equations 26–33 with the ends reversed.[10] These results would be relevant to experiments in which one would apply a voltage clamp to a neuron soma, and measure time constants both before and after severing or killing the dendritic terminals.

For a current clamp at $X = 0$ with cylinder-to-soma coupling, it would be necessary to use a modification of the analysis previously used (equations 18–22). First, we define $G(X)$ as the steady state (equation 35) for $I_A = 0$ and $V = V_L = -E_r$ at $X = L$. Then, for the function

$$W(X, T) = V(X, T) - G(X)$$

we have the boundary conditions

$$W(X, T) = 0 \quad \text{at} \quad X = L$$

---

[10] Very recently, I learned that Lux (1967), treated the problem of constant current at $X = 0$, with a differently defined short circuit at $X = L$. By using Laplace transform methods, he obtained time constants that agree with those obtained here (equation 32). These same time constants have also been obtained by Jack and Redman (personal communication) using still another method.

and

$$\gamma \partial W / \partial X = (W + \partial W / \partial T) \coth L, \quad \text{at} \quad X = 0.$$

This second boundary condition differs from previous equation 19 because

$$\gamma = \frac{(1/\lambda r_i) W_0 \coth L}{G_S W_0}$$

is a steady-state (conductance) ratio with respect to W, whereas the true ρ would be

$$\rho = \frac{(1/\lambda r_i)(W_0 \coth L - [dG/dX]_0)}{G_S (W_0 + G_0)}$$

where the zero subscript designates values at the point, $X = 0$. When these boundary conditions are applied (cf. equations 20 and 21 above) we set $B = 0$ and find that

$$-\gamma \alpha A \cos \alpha L = (-\alpha^2 A \sin \alpha L) \coth L$$

which can be rewritten as the transcendental equation

$$\alpha L \tan \alpha L = \gamma L \tanh L \qquad (39)$$

where $\gamma L \tanh L$ is a positive constant. The roots of this equation have been tabulated by Carslaw and Jaeger (1959, Appendix IV, Table I). The solution for $W(X, T)$ is thus of the form (equation 30), where here each α_n is a root of equation 39.

Case of Leaky End at $X = L$

Instead of a short circuit by an infinite conductance at $X = L$, consider a leaky end having a finite conductance, G_L, between interior and exterior media at $X = L$. At this end, the leakage current must equal the core current

$$G_L V_m = (1/\lambda r_i)[-\partial V_m / \partial X], \quad \text{at} \quad X = L.$$

This can be expressed more simply as the boundary condition

$$\partial V_m / \partial X = -h V_m, \quad \text{at} \quad X = L \qquad (40)$$

where $h = G_L \lambda r_i$. Let the other boundary condition be

$$\partial V_m / \partial X = 0, \quad \text{at} \quad X = 0. \qquad (41)$$

Then the solution takes the form

$$V_m(X, T) = \sum_{n=1}^{\infty} B_n \cos (\alpha_n X) e^{-(1+\alpha_n^2)T} \qquad (42)$$

where the roots, α_n, must satisfy the transcendental equation

$$\alpha L \tan \alpha L = hL \qquad (43)$$

where hL is a positive constant. The roots of this equation have been tabulated by Carslaw and Jaeger (1959, Appendix IV, Table I).

If instead of the boundary condition (equation 41), the value of V_m were clamped to zero at $X = 0$, but still satisfied equation 40 at $X = L$, then the solution takes the form (equation 30) where the roots, α_n, must satisfy the transcendental equation

$$\alpha L \cot \alpha L = -hL. \qquad (44)$$

These roots have also been tabulated by Carslaw and Jaeger (1959, Appendix IV, Table II).

Effect of Series Resistance with Voltage Clamp

In actual experimental situations, it may be difficult to prevent the presence of a series resistance between the clamped voltage, V_A, and the voltage at $X = 0$. This means that the soma-dendritic system is not truly voltage clamped at $X = 0$. Instead, the apparatus provides an applied current,

$$I_A = G_*(V_A - V), \qquad \text{at} \quad X = 0$$

where G_* is the reciprocal of the series resistance,[11] V_A is the applied constant voltage, and V is the transient voltage at $X = 0$. Then, previous equation 18 can be used to obtain the boundary condition

$$\partial V/\partial X = \lambda r_i [G_*(V - V_A) + G_S(V + \partial V/\partial T)], \qquad \text{at} \quad X = 0$$

for G_* finite. If we take the other boundary condition as $\partial V/\partial X = 0$ at $X = L$, and if we consider the function

$$U(X, T) = V(X, T) - V(X, \infty)$$

then, the boundary value problem for U has the boundary condition

$$\rho \partial U/\partial X = kU + (U + \partial U/\partial T) \tanh L, \qquad \text{at} \quad X = 0$$

where $k = (G_*/G_S) \tanh L$ is a positive constant of finite magnitude; this result may be compared with equations 19 and 40. The other boundary condition is $\partial U/\partial X = 0$

---

[11] In this section G_* is finite, and V at $X = 0$ differs from V_A when there is current, I_A, flowing In the limit, as $G_* \to \infty$, $V \to V_A$, and perfect voltage clamping is restored; then the boundary condition of the present section is replaced by one like equation 26, and the transcendental equation 45 is replaced by equation 28, which implies the roots given by equation 29.

at $X = L$. Then, using a solution of the form (equation 20), the boundary conditions require that

$$\rho \alpha B \sin \alpha L = kB \cos \alpha L - \alpha^2 B \cos \alpha L \tanh L$$

which is not satisfied by $\alpha = 0$. In this case, the α_n are roots of the transcendental equation

$$\alpha L \tan \alpha L = [G_*/G_s - \alpha^2](L/\rho) \tanh L \qquad (45)$$

which differs from all previous examples. It may be noted that for large G_*/G_s the right hand side is approximately independent of α for small α_n ; then equation 45 can be treated almost like equation 39; as G_*/G_s becomes very large the voltage clamp condition is approached.[12] At the other limit, as $G_* \rightarrow 0$, equation 45 reduces to equation 21. Intermediate cases must be treated individually.

Illustrative Example Suppose that the whole neuron steady state conductance is 6×10^{-7} mho, and that $\rho = 5$; then the soma membrane conductance, $G_s = 10^{-7}$ mho. Suppose also that $L = 1.5$ and $G_* = 2 \times 10^{-5}$ mho. Then the equation for the α becomes

$$\alpha L \tan \alpha L = (200 - \alpha^2)(0.272).$$

Because G_*/G_s is large, we know that $\alpha_1 L$ is close to $\pi/2$; then $\sin \alpha_1 L \simeq 1.0$ and $\cos \alpha_1 L \simeq \pi/2 - \alpha_1 L$. Thus, we have

$$\alpha_1 L \simeq (\pi/2)C/(C + 1)$$

where

$$C = [G_*/G_s - (\pi/2L)^2](L/\rho) \tanh L.$$

In the above example, $C \simeq 54$, giving $\alpha_1 L \simeq 1.54$, $\alpha_1 \simeq 1.03$, and a value of about 2.06 for τ_m/τ_1 .

Experimental values obtained in voltage clamping experiments on cat motoneurons can be found in papers by Frank, Fuortes and Nelson (1959), Araki and Terzuolo (1962), and Nelson and Frank (1963).

DISCUSSION AND CONCLUSIONS

This paper presents solutions to a number of mathematical boundary value problems which characterize transient distributions of membrane potential in passive membrane cylinders and in neurons whose dendritic trees can be represented as equiva-

---

[12] See footnote 11.

lent cylinders.[13] These solutions can all be expressed as the sum of a steady state component plus several transient components which decay to zero; together these transient components represent a linear combination of exponential decays. This linear combination is actually an infinite series, whose coefficients (in the simpler cases) are Fourier coefficients determined by the initial condition of the boundary value problem; more complicated cases involve coefficients of generalized Fourier expansions; these will be presented explicitly in a separate publication.

Solutions have been obtained for a variety of boundary conditions. All of the cases in parts I and II of the Results have in common that the membrane is nowhere short-circuited in any way; the ends of the cylinders are either sealed or coupled to a soma; constant current electrodes are also permitted. However, voltage clamping electrodes, and killed-end or leaky-end boundary conditions are excluded from parts I and II, and are dealt with separately in part III.

The essential difference between these two classes of solutions is that uniform passive decay with the passive membrane time constant, τ_m, can occur and usually does occur[14] under the conditions of parts I and II; it cannot occur under the conditions of part III. Also, the time constants, τ_1, τ_2, τ_3, ... etc. in parts I and II have meaning as equalizing time constants; the time constants in part III are usually quite different,[15] and should be thought of not as equalizing, but as governing the transient approach to the steady state associated with the given voltage clamp or leak.[16]

Special attention has been given to explaining how the equalizing time constants arise from the boundary conditions, and how the effective electrotonic length can be estimated from time constant ratios, especially the ratio, τ_0/τ_1, of the passive membrane time constant, $\tau_0 = \tau_m$, to the first equalizing time constant, τ_1; see equations 8 and 23 in parts I and II above. In contrast, for voltage clamp conditions, the effective electrotonic length can be estimated from a different relation; see equation 33 in part III above.

For those cases which include the coupling of a cylinder to a lumped soma membrane, the ratio, ρ, of cylinder input conductance to soma membrane conductance,

[13] The class of dendritic trees that can be represented as equivalent cylinders has been defined (Rall, 1962) and discussed (Rall, 1964); this class has the property, $dA/dx \propto dZ/dx$, which means that the rate of increase of dendritic surface area, with respect to x, remains proportional to the rate of increase of electrotonic distance, with respect to x. A larger class of dendritic trees has the more general property, $dA/dZ \propto e^{KZ}$, where K is a constant that may be positive or negative (Rall, 1962). Mathematical solutions have been obtained for this larger class, and will be presented in a separate publication in collaboration with Steven Goldstein.

[14] It does not occur when the initial condition does not contain a uniformly distributed component; then $C_0 = 0$, in equation 1.

[15] Compare Table II with Table I. However, for voltage clamping at both ends, see equation 37.

[16] Although it is true that $[V(X, T) - V(X, \infty)]$ decays to zero everywhere in all of these cases, uniform decay is possible only in parts I and II, where the boundary conditions at $X = 0$ and $X = L$ are either $\partial V/\partial X = 0$ or coupling to an intact soma. Uniform decay is not possible in part III, because a point of short-circuit or of voltage clamp imposes nonzero $\partial V/\partial X$ at that point.

effects the value of L (for the cylinder) estimated from a given τ_0/τ_1 value; this is displayed in Fig. 1 above. By using $\rho = \infty$ (which is equivalent to cylinder without soma) we obtain the value of L for that cylinder which best approximates the whole neuron. However, to estimate the value of L for the cylinder which best approximates a dendritic tree as distinct from the soma, it is necessary to have an estimate of ρ, when working with the equalizing time constants and Fig. 1.

In contrast to the above, it is significant that the different time constants obtained with voltage clamping at the soma do not depend upon ρ at all, for ideal clamping, and the effect of ρ is very small even when there is a moderate amount of series resistance in the system; see illustrative example following equation 45 in part III above. This means that the value of L for the cylinder can be estimated without knowing ρ; this can be done either with τ_1 and τ_2 in equation 33, or by using τ_1 from voltage clamp together with τ_m obtained either with current clamp or unclamped passive decay, and using equation 32 with $n = 1$.

It is noteworthy that using both current clamping and voltage clamping at the soma could thus provide a new method of estimating ρ. Obtain τ_m from current clamp; also obtain τ_1 and, if possible, τ_2 with voltage clamp; these provide an estimate of L for the cylinder (from equations 32 and 33). Now using this L and the equalizing time constants obtained with current clamping, one can estimate ρ from Fig. 1, or from equations 21 and 22.

There are two other electrophysiological methods of estimating ρ. One is based upon sinusoidal stimulation applied to the soma (Rall, 1960; Nelson and Lux, 1969). Because the original theory was based upon the assumption of a cylinder of infinite length, it should be remarked that finite length has less effect upon the steady-state AC input admittance of the cylinder than upon the steady-state DC input conductance of the cylinder.[17] The other method is based upon equations 6 and 12 of (Rall, 1960) for the slope, dV/dt, of the response to an applied current step. This method was used by Lux and Pollen (1966). It also is based upon the assumption of a cylinder of infinite length; however, the early part of the transient should be little changed by finite length. The amount of error can be evaluated by adding to the transient, $V(0, T)$, the transient, $V(2L, T)$. This is because a matched current step applied at $X = 2L$ would result, by symmetry, in making $\partial V/\partial X = 0$ at the point, $X = L$, halfway between the two current sources; this $\partial V/\partial X = 0$ at $X = L$ is equivalent to the sealed-end boundary condition used in the present paper. For longer times, it becomes necessary to consider more terms, corresponding to $X = 4L$, $X = 6L$, etc.;[18] however, these additional terms are not needed for the early portion of the slope.

---

[17] An explicit solution for sinusoidal steady states in cylinders of finite length (with sealed ends) has been worked out and will be published separately; see also Lux (1967) for a case of finite length with a different terminal boundary condition.

[18] These additional terms are more complicated. They have been derived and computed by Jack and Redman (personal communication), as part of an extensive program of theory, computations and ex-

In conclusion, it can be seen that it is now appropriate to explore various procedures for estimating the most consistent set of the parameters, ρ, L, R_m and $\tau_m = R_m C_m$ which determine the electrical properties of a passive neuron, for particular neurons and neuron types. Such exploration has now begun.[19] At present, it is too early to say which of the several possible combinations of theory and experiment will provide the best simultaneous estimate of the values of these parameters; this will be determined largely by the limitations of experimental precision.

Notes Added in Response to Referee Comments.   I thank one referee for drawing my attention to the recent work of Koike, Okada, Oshima, and Takahashi (*Exp. Brain Res.* 1968. **5:**173–188 and 189–201. Following Ito and Oshima (1965), the authors have applied a "triple exponential analysis" to pyramidal tract cells of cat's cerebral cortex.

One referee expressed reservations about assuming the same passive dendritic membrane properties for the soma and the dendrites. This is a simplifying assumption that has been discussed earlier (Rall, 1959, p. 494 and 523–524; Rall, 1960, p. 514–515, 519, and 529). Fortunately, careful experiments with voltage clamping at the soma, compared with current clamping at the soma, can provide a test of this simplifying assumption for each neuron type.

One referee questioned the assumption that the membrane itself should have only one passive membrane time constant; he asks why I did not include another membrane time constant corresponding to the tubular system of muscle fibers; see Ito and Oshima (1965). My approach has been to investigate how much can be accounted for by a consideration of finite dendritic length without the addition of more complicated membrane models. If electron microscopy should reveal similar tubular systems in certain neuron membranes, this question would merit further study in those neurons. In the case of cat motoneurons, the EPSP shape analysis (Rall et al., 1967) supports the notion that the faster time constant depends upon finite length, and that the weight of its contribution to the observed transient depends upon the nonuniformity (over dendritic length) of the membrane depolarization.

I am grateful to Dr. J. Z. Hearon and to Drs. P. G. Nelson and R. E. Burke for helpful comments on an earlier draft of this manuscript.

---

periments that they and their collaborators have carried out. They have used Laplace transform methods to obtain the terms of their mathematical series; these terms are expressed in terms of parabolic cylinder functions (or, alternatively, in terms of error functions). This mathematical series is quite different from the sums of exponential decays presented here. It is interesting that these different mathematical approaches are not contradictory; they are complementary.

Jack and Redman have recently read a draft of this paper, and I have recently read drafts of two of their unpublished manuscripts. Although we have not yet had the opportunity to make detailed quantitative comparisons, we do find our results to be in substantial agreement. Also, we know that the sums of exponentials converge most poorly for small values of t, while the sums of terms involving error functions converge most poorly for large values of t.

[19] For example, Nelson and Lux (1969), and Burke (earlier footnote 2); also, Jack and Redman (earlier footnote 18) have devised a particular set of procedures for estimating values of these parameters. Furthermore, the parameter, K (see earlier footnote 13), as well as the long time constant of Ito and Oshima (1965) need to be taken into account for some neurons.

REFERENCES

AITKEN, J. and J. BRIDGER. 1961. *J. Anat.* **95**:38.

ARAKI, T. and C. A. TERZUOLO. 1962. *J. Neurophysiol.* **25**:772.

BURKE, R. E. 1967. *J. Neurophysiol.* **30**:1114.

CARSLAW, H. S. and J. C. JAEGER. 1959. Conduction of Heat in Solids. Oxford Press, London. 510.

CHURCHILL, R. V. 1941. Fourier Series and Boundary Value Problems. McGraw-Hill, New York. 206.

CLARK, J. and R. PLONSEY. 1966. *Biophys. J.* **6**:95.

FADIGA, E. and J. M. BROOKHART. 1960. *Amer. J. Physiol.* **198**:693.

FRANK, K., M. G. F. FUORTES, and P. G. NELSON. 1959. *Science.* **130**:38.

ITO, M. and T. OSHIMA. 1965. *J. Physiol. (London).* **180**:607.

JACK, J. J. B., S. MILLER, and R. PORTER. 1967. *J. Physiol. (London).* **191**:112.

LETBETTER, W. D., W. D. WILLIS, JR., and W. M. THOMPSON. 1968. *Fed. Proc.* **27**:749.

LUX, H. D. 1967. *Pflügers Archiv.* **297**:238.

MENDELL, L. and E. HENNEMAN. 1968. *Fed. Proc.* **27**:452.

NELSON, P. G. and K. FRANK. 1963. *Actual. Neurophysiol.* **15**:15.

NELSON, P. G. and K. FRANK. 1967. *J. Neurophysiol.* **30**:1097.

NELSON, P. G. and H. D. LUX. 1969. *Biophys. J.* In Press.

RALL, W. 1957. *Science.* **126**:454.

RALL, W. 1959. *Exp. Neurol.* **1**:491.

RALL, W. 1960. *Exp. Neurol.* **2**:503.

RALL, W. 1962. *Ann. N. Y. Acad. Sci.* **96**:1071.

RALL, W. 1964. *In* Neural Theory and Modeling. R. F. Reiss, editor. Stanford University Press, Stanford, Calif. p. 73–97.

RALL, W. 1967. *J. Neurophysiol.* **30**:1138.

RALL, W. 1969. *Biophys. J.* **9**:1509.

RALL, W., R. E. BURKE, T. G. SMITH, P. G. NELSON, and K. FRANK. 1967. *J. Neurophysiol.* **30**:1169.

TSUKAHARA, N., K. TOYAMA, and K. KOSAKA. 1967. *Exp. Brain Res.* **4**:18.

WEINBERGER, H. F. 1965. Partial differential equations. Blaisdell, Waltham, Mass. 446.

8 ANALYSIS OF RESPONSE TO SINGLE INPUTS IN A COMPLEX DENDRITIC TREE

8.1 Introduction by Charles Wilson with Supplemental Comments by John Rinzel

Rall, W., and Rinzel, J. (1973). Branch input resistance and steady attenuation for input to one branch of a dendritic neuron model. *Biophys. J.* 13:648–688.

Rinzel, J., and Rall, W. (1974). Transient response in a dendritic neuron model for current injected at one branch. *Biophys. J.* 14:759–790.

Although it may not have been immediately obvious to everyone in 1959 and 1960 that synapses located out on the distal portions of the dendritic tree were important in neuronal function, it certainly was in 1973. By that time the issue of whether or not dendrites were important was considered settled, at least by students and other open-minded people (I was a student then). The emphasis of the discussion had shifted to making concrete predictions based on a knowledge of synaptic distributions on dendrites. The early 1970s was a period of great progress in neuroanatomy, riding on several revolutionary technical advances and spearheaded by the application of the electron microscope. The landmark book *The Fine Structure of the Nervous System* by Peters, Palay, and Webster, first published in 1970 (current edition, 1991), was having an impact that cannot easily be appreciated today. Investigators studying neurons in every part of the brain were discovering highly structured synaptic arrangements revealing the remarkable specificity of synaptic connections. The Golgi method (100 years old in 1973) was enjoying a renaissance; students were reading the work of Cajal and Lorente de Nó as enthusiastically as that of more contemporary authors. The spatial organization of inputs on a neuron was clearly shown to be one of the defining characteristics of a cell type and seemed certain to determine a large part of the functional properties of cells and circuits in the brain. Neuroanatomists looking for support for this notion were elated to find that there was an emerging theory of neuronal function based specifically on this concept. During the same period, many neurophysiologists abandoned the central nervous system of mammals, looking for more secure recording conditions, better characterized neuronal circuitry, and geometric simplicity in the somata of giant neurons of invertebrates. Because it is so difficult to record from more than one part of a neuron at a time, the announcement that the neuron is not isopotential is not always taken as good news by the neurophysiologist.

There's no question that these are difficult papers for the neuroscientist to read. They were written for the small audience of mathematical neuroscientists and published in the *Biophysical Journal*, an excellent journal but certainly not read by everyone at the time. Unlike the widely read experimental work, these papers could not be read in one sitting but required (for most of us at least) many hours of careful study. Still, because of the multidisciplinary mood in neuroscience at the time, and the enormous interest of the topic to so many neuroscientists, these papers were widely discussed, and many brave attempts were made to understand them by scientists and students who would not normally have read mathematical work. Folklore about the implications of dendrites and synaptic integration in dendritic neurons was more plentiful than understanding of what Rall and others had actually accomplished up to that time, however, and this remained so for some time. Despite the obvious successes of theoretical work before 1973, there was really no general mathematical theory of synaptic integration in dendritic neurons prior to the Rall and Rinzel (1973) paper. The equivalent cylinder model, which had come to represent electrotonic theory in the minds of most people, was a spatially lumped model, not a model of distributed synaptic interactions. It was ideally suited for the analysis of the available neurophysiological data, in which the vicinity of the soma and the signals recorded there required exact representation but accuracy in the details of distal dendritic events was less important. The compartmental model, while computationally able to handle any problem, offered little in the way of insight. Its utility for simulating spatially complex situations had been demonstrated (Rall 1964), but it did not offer an analytical solution, whose special cases and asymptotic behavior could be enumerated and used to create a mental picture of the entire range of behavior of the system. An analytical solution, suitable for developing such a thorough understanding for the steady state, was provided by the Rall and Rinzel paper, and the later Rinzel and Rall article (1974) completed the analysis for time-varying signals.

What was attempted in these papers was not a model of the motoneuron or any other actual cell. The solution was for an idealized, simplified neuron. It included input to (the very end of) a single branch of a dendritic tree of a neuron consisting of several equivalent dendritic trees. The neuron had no soma other than that formed by the junction of the dendritic trees. There was no axon, and no action potentials. It was clear that this was not intended to be a realistic model of any particular neuron, and perhaps some very practical readers discounted the papers on this basis. The value of this model was actually as an abstraction applicable to all neurons. Anyone who has tried to make a model of a biological system knows that the art is not in deciding what details should be included in the model but in deciding what details should be excluded. In these papers, the things excluded were those which distinguished one neuron from another. The model was based on a set of carefully chosen symmetries that simultaneously (almost miraculously) abstracted the neuron and simplified the mathematics. Of course the most important (and widely discussed) simplification was the assumption of electrotonic continuity at dendritic branch points (the famous 3/2 power rule). Discussions of which, if any, real neurons obey this constraint have continued unchecked since it was introduced in earlier papers. There are only two possible approaches to the issue. One is to select a particular geometry to use as a template for an abstracted neuron, and the other is to obtain a solution that explicitly includes the geometry of the cell, and so will serve for all neuron shapes. Rall and Rinzel took the first approach. Since the publication of their papers, several approaches for the solution for passive neurons of arbitrary geometry have been offered, and they continue to be presented (Butz and Cowan 1974; Holmes 1986; Horowitz 1981; Koch and Poggio 1985; Cao and Abbott 1993; Majors et al. 1993). These important contributions, inspired by the work of Rall and Rinzel, continue to enrich neuron theory. But, to obtain the solution for an arbitrary geometry, these authors have been forced to abandon the search for a closed solution and have pursued recursive methods whose utility is comparable to that of the compartmental model.

The closed solution, with its potential for generating understanding and insight (not simply the correct answer) is still available only for one branching pattern, the one chosen by Rall and Rinzel. Time has proved the wisdom of their approach. The fundamental principles that have emerged from theoretical studies of such abstracted dendrites apply rather well to neurons of all geometry. The selection of one simple abstract neuron whose solution can be understood revealed the principles that govern synaptic interactions in linear neurons. To this day, if one wishes to analyze the implications of dendritic branching on synaptic inputs, rather than the effects of any particular branching pattern, the assumptions of the Rall and Rinzel paper should be adopted. For analysis of any specific neuron, a comparison should probably be made with results obtained using the generic branching pattern. Otherwise, one is not sure if the result of interest is due to the specific characteristics of the neuron type or is expected for any branching neuron. Thus, although not a numerically accurate model of any cell, this model gave, for the first time, the general form for the input impedance and for the propagation of synaptic potentials for all dendritic neurons.

The most obvious accomplishments of the analysis should be enumerated. These papers offer the first and best description of branch attenuation, which continues to be an important issue in studies of synaptic interaction. They also point out the surprisingly large effect of branching on the propagation of synaptic potentials. One still often hears the argument that because the total electrotonic length between an input and a recording site is small, the attenuation of the signal recorded should likewise be small. The fallacy in this argument is that it is based on the equivalent cylinder model. While very useful for some purposes, the equivalent cylinder model was not Rall's model of synaptic potential propagation in a branched neuron. In these papers, the crucial effect of impedance loading at branch points is very clearly and beautifully explained. A related result, the fact that voltage attenuation within branching dendrites depends greatly upon the direction of signal propagation, proved critical for theoretical studies of the functional effects of dendritic spines and was very clearly presented in these papers. The finding that the time course of the somatic response to transient current injection in the dendrites is independent of how the current is distributed among the various branches, but depends only upon distance from the soma, proved important for neurophysiological studies of EPSP shapes. In the second paper, the relationship between transient and steady-state solutions was clarified in a section on the time integral of voltage and the distribution of charge dissipation in the dendrites. The approach was to use a single characteristic of the transient response at any location on the dendrites and solve for it in a manner similar to the steady-state solution for voltage. This is an excellent source of insight into the behavior of the model that cannot be duplicated in strictly numerical simulations of neurons. A similar approach, used recently by Agmon-Snir and Segev (1993) for analysis of the time course of synaptic potentials propagating throughout a neuron, was undoubtably inspired by the Rinzel and Rall treatment. For those of us pursuing computer simulations to deal with the complexity of nonideal, nonlinear neurons, these relationships serve as an essential template for the interpretation of our results.

These papers also explored the fundamental relationship between input resistance, local synaptic potential, and synaptic effectiveness. Although it may seem obvious now, the high input resistance of distal dendritic sites was not well appreciated at the time and had been dealt with only briefly in theoretical work (e.g., MacGregor 1968). The dramatic potential for saturation of synaptic current due to giant local synaptic potentials (which do not seem giant when seen from the soma) was not well appreciated until clearly explained in the Rall and Rinzel papers. The importance of the duration of synaptic conductances, both in the local saturation effects and in propagation within the dendrites, was also explained there for the first time. The possibility that synaptic current might be limited by factors dependent upon the shape of the postsynaptic neuron, of course, laid the groundwork for all subsequent work on changes in cell shape as mediators of synaptic plasticity. This issue later acquired great importance for students of dendritic spines, and it is obvious that Rall and Rinzel saw the application of their approach to the dendritic spine problem at the time these papers were written. Of course, they also successfully applied the approach explicitly to the issue of dendritic spines.

Most important, the papers laid out the symmetry rules that became the basis for our intuitive understanding of signal propagation in branching dendritic trees. This intuition is still valuable, and those wishing to develop it within themselves can do no better than to consult these two papers. Because much of what is explained there continues to be discussed, rediscovered, and misunderstood today, these papers continue to be on the list of required reading for those who would understand synaptic interactions or interpret synaptic potentials in dendritic neurons.

References

Agmon-Snir, H., and Segev, I. (1993) Signal delay and input synchronization in passive dendritic structures. *J. Neurophys.* 70:2066–2085.

Butz, E. G., and Cowan, J. D. (1974) Transient potentials in dendritic systems of arbitrary geometry. *Biophys. J.* 14:661–689.

Cao, B. J., and Abbott, L. F. (1993) A new computational method for cable theory problems. *Biophys. J.* 64:303–313.

Holmes, W. R. (1986) A continuous cable method for determining the transient potential in passive dendritic trees of known geometry. *Biol. Cyber.* 55:115–124.

Horowitz, B. (1981) An analytical method for investigating transient potentials in neurons with branching dendritic trees. *Biophys. J.* 36:155–192.

Koch, C., and Poggio, T. (1985) A simple algorithm for solving the cable equation in dendritic trees of arbitrary geometry. *J. Neurosci. Meth.* 12:303–315.

MacGregor, R. J. (1968) A model for responses to activation by axodendritic synapses. *Biophys. J.* 8:305–318.

Major, G., Evans, J. D., and Jack, J. J. B. (1993) Solutions for transients in arbitrarily branching cables: I. Voltage recording. *Biophys J.* 65:423–449.

Peters, A., Palay, S. L., and Webster, H. deF. (1991) *The Fine Structure of the Nervous System. Neurons and Their Supporting Cells.* New York: Oxford Univ. Press.

Rall, W. (1964) Theoretical significance of dendritic trees for neuronal input-output relations. In *Neural Theory and Modeling*, ed. R. Reiss. Stanford: Stanford Univ. Press.

Rall, W., and Rinzel, J. (1973) Branch input resistance and steady attenuation for input to one branch of a dendritic neuron model. *Biophys. J.* 13:648–688.

Rinzel, J., and Rall, W. (1974) Transient response in a dendritic neuron model for current injected at one branch. *Biophys. J.* 14:759–790.

Supplemental Comments by John Rinzel

In 1968, I came to the NIH with no post-high-school biology background (I had a B.S. in engineering and an M.S. in applied mathematics) to serve in the U.S. Public Health Service. My alert supervisor in the computer division directed me to some of Wil's papers and then introduced us. Coming from outside the field, I had little appreciation of Wil's scientific stature. I did not realize that he was heading a revolution in neurophysiology and drastically affecting the way many neuroscientists thought about dendritic function. His pleasant, soft-spoken, gentle presentation did not fit any stereotype I had of a revolutionary. He did not direct a large working group; in fact, he usually worked with one, sometimes two, young scientists. Fortunately, Wil took me on as a collaborator. We were going to consider questions related to dendritic spines, and I was to carry out the computations (at which I was well experienced for physics problems). It soon became clear that this man was superextraordinary. His time and availability seemed limitless, and his patience with my ignorance of biophysics, impressive. He was fostering me, and I was learning so many new things.

For our initial computations, I was conservative, concerned about numerical accuracy, and I used a rather fine spatial discretization for solving the cable equation with a single spine in an explicitly branched dendritic architecture. This became a costly task on the NIH computers, in spite of my numerical and programming tricks. This constraint was a factor in our search for an alternative strategy, an analytical one. In addition, Wil knew, of course, that the input resistance at the spine site was an important quantity for us to determine. Earlier (Rall 1959), he had developed a recursive formula for dendritic input resistance, but the solution was not in closed form. Formulating a solvable, idealized model problem became the next challenge, at which point I saw Wil's creative mastery begin to strike.

As a young mathematical scientist, I was excited to see Wil put mathematical physics to work on a biological problem. His keen physical intuition played a key role. First, he used the principle of superposition to simultaneously formulate and solve this problem, physically. Then we expressed the solution mathematically, computed some examples, and, again with Wil leading, we developed the physiological implications of our theoretical results. All of the essential results for these two papers, as well as those from our modeling of passive dendritic spines, were obtained before I returned to graduate school in 1970. (The writing came significantly later, due partly to Wil's worsening vision problems and partly to his high standards and dedicated effort to communicate theoretical results clearly.)

Without question, Wil's mentoring was inspirational and career determining for me. We bonded, beyond the level of scientific colleagues, and his outlook on life has been a guide for 25 years.

Supplemental Reference

Rall, W. (1959) Branching dendritic trees and motoneuron membrane resistivity. *Expt. Neurol.* 1:491–527.

8.2 Branch Input Resistance and Steady Attenuation for Input to One Branch of a Dendritic Neuron Model (1973), *Biophys. J.* 13:648–688

Wilfrid Rall and John Rinzel

ABSTRACT Mathematical solutions and numerical illustrations are presented for the steady-state distribution of membrane potential in an extensively branched neuron model, when steady electric current is injected into only one dendritic branch. Explicit expressions are obtained for input resistance at the branch input site and for voltage attenuation from the input site to the soma; expressions for AC steady-state input impedance and attenuation are also presented. The theoretical model assumes passive membrane properties and the equivalent cylinder constraint on branch diameters. Numerical examples illustrate how branch input resistance and steady attenuation depend upon the following: the number of dendritic trees, the orders of dendritic branching, the electrotonic length of the dendritic trees, the location of the dendritic input site, and the input resistance at the soma. The application to cat spinal motoneurons, and to other neuron types, is discussed. The effect of a large dendritic input resistance upon the amount of local membrane depolarization at the synaptic site, and upon the amount of depolarization reaching the soma, is illustrated and discussed; simple proportionality with input resistance does not hold, in general. Also, branch input resistance is shown to exceed the input resistance at the soma by an amount that is always less than the sum of core resistances along the path from the input site to the soma.

INTRODUCTION

It seems now generally accepted that the many synapses distributed over the dendritic surface of a neuron can make significant contributions to the integrative behavior exhibited by this neuron as it responds to various spatiotemporal patterns of afferent input. In some theoretical studies it has been useful to lump the effects of neighboring synapses and to lump regional groupings of the dendritic branches belonging to a neuron (e.g., Rall, 1962, 1964, 1967). Nevertheless, it is clear that any particular one of these synapses is located upon one particular dendritic branch; also, when a synapse is made with a dendritic spine, that spine is attached to a particular dendritic branch. This gives rise to questions about the input resistance that would be "seen" or confronted by a particular synapse on a particular dendritic branch. Questions arise also about the amplitude of membrane depolarization generated at the synaptic site, and about the attenuation of amplitude as this membrane depolarization spreads (electrotonically) from the synaptic site to other locations, both in the same dendritic tree, at the neuron soma, and in other dendritic trees of the same neuron. Such questions have been noted and discussed, for example, by Katz and Miledi (1963, p. 419), Arshavskii et al. (1965), Rall (1967; 1970, p. 184), and Kuno (1971).

This is the first of several closely related papers which provide mathematical solutions and contribute biophysical intuition toward the understanding of effects of synaptic input to one branch of an extensively branched neuron model. This first paper is restricted to the steady-state problem. For a steady current applied across the membrane at one site in one branch of the neuron model, the complete steady-state solution for the distribution of electrotonic potential throughout all branches and trees of the neuron model is obtained. This steady-state solution provides expressions for branch input resistance and for steady-state attenuation of electrotonic potential from the branch input site to the neuron soma; numerical examples are tabulated, illustrated, and discussed.

The second paper[1] treats the corresponding transient problem, for the injection of a brief current at the branch input site. Our solution of this more difficult problem depends upon the conceptual approach (mathematical superposition of simpler boundary value problems) that is introduced, illustrated, and discussed in the first paper. In addition to providing a mathematical derivation of the required transient response functions, the second paper also illustrates and discusses specific computed examples.

Subsequent papers of this series will deal with the additional theoretical complications involved in treating synaptic input to a dendritic spine. The effect of a synaptic excitatory conductance at the spine head is coupled to the dendritic branch by means of the spine stem current. Our solution of this problem depends partly upon the transient response functions derived in the second paper of this series. Also, the steady-state interpretations of synaptic input to a dendritic spine make use of the steady-state results in the first paper of this series. A consideration of these theoretical results in relation to recent neuroanatomical studies of dendritic spines has led to a recognition of possible functional implications of spine stem resistance; a paper presenting and discussing these implications is in preparation.

---

[1] Rall, W., and J. Rinzel. Manuscript in preparation.

Brief communications of various portions of this research have already been presented on several occasions.[2]

ASSUMPTIONS OF NEURON MODEL

Symmetry and Idealized Branching

Much of our biophysical intuition and many of our mathematical results have been facilitated by several assumptions of symmetry in our idealized neuron models. If we had been interested only in the steady-state problem, we could have dispensed with these symmetry assumptions completely: we could have solved the problem by the same stepwise procedure (which permits arbitrary branch lengths and diameters) that was outlined earlier (Rall, 1959) for the case of steady current injection at a neuron soma. The symmetry assumptions are of greatest value in obtaining the transient solutions;[1] they permit us to apply the mathematical principle of superposition to construct the solution of a complicated boundary value problem as a combination of several simpler boundary value problems. Because it simplifies our exposition of the particular superpositions we have used, we have chosen to introduce the method in this steady-state paper. Also, we simplify our presentation by beginning with more severe symmetry assumptions than superposition actually requires; the effects of relaxing the severity of these assumptions are examined later in the Appendix.

Most of our results are expressed for an idealized neuron model composed of several equivalent dendritic trees (N in number) in which there are several orders (M) of symmetric dendritic branching. A diagram of one particular example (Fig. 1 A) shows six equal dendritic trees in which there are two orders of symmetric dendritic branching. It should be pointed out immediately that the angles between the trees and between the branches are of no importance. These angles do not enter into any of the mathematics.[3] It is the lengths and diameters of the trunks and branches that are important. Fig. 1 A is intended merely to bring out the equivalences between corresponding lengths and diameters. The soma of this neuron model is represented by the common origin of the six dendritic trees.

In addition to the symmetry assumptions already noted, we have restricted our treatment to dendritic trees whose branch diameters satisfy the constraint for trans-

---

[1] The use of symmetry and superposition to obtain these solutions was included in a presentation for the American Association for the Advancement of Science Symposium on Some Mathematical Questions in Biology, Boston, December, 1969. The mathematical and numerical treatment of coupling the dendritic spine to a branch of the model was presented at the Society for Industrial and Applied Mathematics National Meeting, Denver, June, 1970. Functional implications for dendritic spines were presented at the 25th International Congress of Physiological Sciences, Munich, July, 1971, and at the first annual meeting of the Society for Neuroscience, Washington, D. C., October, 1971.

[3] This follows from the assumption of extracellular isopotentiality; see Other Simplifying Assumptions section below.

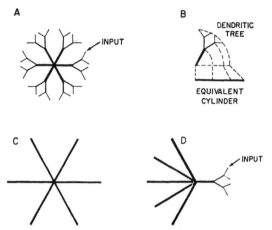

FIGURE 1   Diagrams illustrating features of the idealized neuron model. A represents the neuron model composed of six identical dendritic trees. B indicates the relation of a dendritic tree to its equivalent cylinder. C represents the same model as A, with each dendritic tree replaced by an equivalent cylinder. D represents the same model as A and C, with dendritic branching shown explicitly only for the tree which receives input current injected into the terminal of one branch; the five other trees of the model are represented by their equivalent cylinders, here shown gathered together. In diagrams A, C, and D, the point of common origin of the trees or equivalent cylinders is regarded as the neuron soma; see text.

formations between a tree and an equivalent cylinder (Fig. 1 B; also Rall, 1962, 1964). Except in the Appendix, we have assumed symmetric bifurcations that yield daughter branches of equal diameter. Together, these assumptions imply that at every branch point, each daughter branch diameter is about 63% of its parent branch diameter; strictly, the requirement is that the 3/2 power of each daughter diameter be exactly half as great as the 3/2 power of its parent diameter. With such branching, an entire dendritic tree can be shown to be mathematically equivalent to a cylinder (Rall, 1962); increments Δx of actual dendritic length are expressed as increments of electrotonic length, $\Delta X = \Delta x/\lambda$, where λ is the characteristic length of each cylinder as defined below. This equivalence applies to spatiotemporal spread from the trunk into the dendritic branches; it applies also to spread from the dendrites to the trunk, when the input is delivered equally to all terminal branches of that dendritic tree.

The equivalent cylinder concept can be used to reduce the idealized (branched) neuron model of Fig. 1 A to simpler versions (Figs. 1 C and D) for appropriate conditions. Thus, for example, if current is injected equally to all terminal branches of just one of the six dendritic trees of Fig. 1 A, this tree can be treated as an equivalent cylinder which receives input at its distal end. The origin of this cylinder can be coupled to the origins of five other equivalent cylinders, as in Fig. 1 C. These other cylinders have the same dimensions as the input cylinder but differ in receiving no input at their distal ends; they receive equal shares of the current that reaches them at their common origin (soma) from the input cylinder. The six cylinders in Fig. 1 C represent the same neuron model as that in Fig. 1 A; the existence of the branches makes no difference under the stated condition of input delivered equally to all terminal branches of the one tree. However, when the input current is injected to only one branch terminal of one dendritic tree, it is necessary to include the branching details of that tree but not the branching of the other trees, as shown in Fig. 1 D. The five equivalent cylinders which do not receive input have been oriented more together in this figure to emphasize their equivalence with each other in sharing equally the current that flows to the origin (soma) from the input tree; the angles between the cylinders have no other significance, as noted earlier.[3] This last case (Fig. 1 D) is an illustrative example of the problem we solve below.

Other Simplifying Assumptions

Here we briefly note several other simplifying assumptions of dendritic neuron models (cf., Rall, 1959, 1962). All dendritic trunks and branches are treated as cylinders of uniform passive nerve membrane. Extracellular resistivity is neglected, implying extracellular isopotentiality. This, together with the usual core conductor assumptions, permits each cylinder to be treated as a one-dimensional cable of finite length (see Rall [1969 b] for discussion and references). At all branch points, membrane potential is assumed to be continuous, and core current is conserved. Dendritic terminals are assumed to be "sealed" or "insulated," implying zero leakage current across the terminal membrane; except for a terminal where current is injected, this implies a zero slope ($dV/dX = 0$) boundary condition, just inside (not across) the terminal membrane.

The assumption of extracellular isopotentiality brings with it several useful simplifications. It means that spatial orientation of the dendritic trees and branches can have no effect upon the distribution of membrane potential over the dendritic surfaces; only electrotonic distances and boundary conditions are important. It also provides simpler expressions for the characteristic length λ and for the various input resistances. It should be noted that this assumption represents a good approximation for some experimental situations, but not for others. For a single dendritic neuron placed in a volume conductor (which is assumed not to be subjected to an externally applied electric field) the current flow generated by activity of that neuron results in gradients of extracellular potential that are negligible relative to the much larger gradients of intracellular potential along the intracellular core resistance and across the relatively large membrane resistance (for estimates, see Rall, 1959, 1969 b). When extracellular space is severely restricted, however, either by glial sheaths or by simultaneous activity in a large population of closely packed cells, extracellular potential gradients can become comparable with or even greater than the intracellular potential gradients; see, for example, synchronous activity of granule cells in olfactory bulb (Rall and Shepherd, 1968, pp. 887–890, 901–904).

Under such conditions, one must avoid assuming extracellular isopotentiality and assume an appropriate extracellular resistance per unit length for each cylinder; also, the effects of tree and branch orientation would then need to be considered.

Because it might be objected that we should not treat the soma as merely the point of common origin of the dendritic trees, we comment. The superposition methods of this paper and its transient sequel would lose much of their simplicity if a lumped soma were explicitly included at the origin of the neuron model. This can be verified by examining the effect of a lumped soma upon previously published theoretical transient results (Rall, 1969 a, pp. 1492–1496; see also Rall, 1960, as well as Jack and Redman, 1971). Our present assumption of a point soma can be qualified with the thought that a finite soma surface area could be designated, if needed, as being composed of several initial length increments, one from each dendritic trunk. Finally, we note also that the neuron model of the present paper does not include an axon- or a spike-generating locus; our focus of attention is upon the contribution of passive membrane electrotonus to the integrative properties of the extensively branched neuron model.

SYMBOLS

For Membrane Cylinders

$V_m = V_i - V_e$	Membrane potential, as intracellular minus extracellular electric potential; (volts).
$V = V_m - E_r$	Electrotonic potential, as deviation of membrane potential from its resting value E_r; (volts).
R_i	Resistivity of intracellular medium; (ohms centimeters).
R_m	Resistance across a unit area of membrane; (ohms square centimeters).
d	Diameter of membrane cylinder; (centimeters).
$r_i = 4R_i/(\pi d^2)$	Core resistance per unit length; (ohms centimeters^{-1}).
$\lambda = [(R_m/R_i)(d/4)]^{1/2}$	Characteristic length of membrane cylinder, when extracellular resistance is neglected; (centimeters).
x	Actual distance along a cylinder axis; (centimeters).
$\Delta X = \Delta x/\lambda$	Increment of electrotonic distance; (dimensionless).
$X = \int_0^x (1/\lambda)\, dy$	Electrotonic distance from origin; in a tree, λ changes at each branch point; (dimensionless).
$R_\infty = \lambda r_i = (2/\pi)(R_m R_i)^{1/2}(d)^{-3/2}$	Input resistance at origin of membrane cylinder of semi-infinite length; (ohms).

For Membrane Cylinders of Finite Length

L	Electrotonic distance from origin ($X = 0$) to the end of cylinder ($X = L$).
$R_{CL,\,ins}$	Input resistance at end ($X = L$) for a *cylinder insulated* ($dV/dX = 0$) at the origin; Eq. 7.
$R_{CL,\,clp}$	Input resistance at end ($X = L$) for a *cylinder clamped* ($V = 0$) at the origin; Eq. 9.

For Idealized Neuron Model

N	Number of equivalent dendritic trees (or their equivalent cylinders) that are coupled at $X = 0$.
L	Electrotonic length of each of those trees or equivalent cylinders.
M	Number of orders of symmetric branching, specifically in the dendritic tree which receives the input.
X_1	Electrotonic distance from the origin to the first point of branching.
X_k	Electrotonic distance from the origin to the kth-order branch points.
R_{T_∞}	Value of R_∞ for the *trunk* cylinder of one dendritic tree.
R_N	Whole *neuron* input resistance at the point $(X = 0)$ of common origin of the N trees or equivalent cylinders; Eq. 11.
R_{NCL}	Input resistance at the end $(X = L)$ of one equivalent *cylinder* of the neuron model, for current applied as in Fig. 2 F; Eq. 14.
R_{BL}	Input resistance at the end $(X = L)$ of one terminal *branch* of the neuron model, for current applied as in Figs. 1 A and D; Eq. 22.
V_{BL}	Steady value of V at input *branch* terminal.
V_0	Steady value of V at the *origin* of the neuron model.
$AF_{BL/0} = V_{BL}/V_0$	Attenuation factor from input branch terminal to soma; Eq. 26.

For the Discussion

V_{in}	Steady value of V at some synaptic site.
R_{in}	Input resistance at this synaptic site.
g_ϵ	Synaptic excitatory conductance at this synaptic site.
$V_\epsilon = E_\epsilon - E_r$	Synaptic excitatory equilibrium potential, being the difference between the excitatory emf and the resting emf.
$(V_\epsilon - V_{in})$	Effective steady driving potential for synaptic current.
V_{in}/V_ϵ	Normalized steady synaptic depolarization; Eq. 32.
$\Delta X = L/(M + 1)$	For equal electrotonic increments.

THEORY

For the usual assumptions of one-dimensional cable theory, steady-state distributions of membrane potential along the length of a passive membrane cylinder must satisfy the ordinary differential equation

$$d^2V/dX^2 - V = 0, \tag{1}$$

where X and V are explicitly defined in the list of Symbols. Because we wish to exploit even and odd symmetry about the origin, we express the general solution of Eq. 1 in terms of hyperbolic functions,[4] as follows,

$$V = A \sinh X + B \cosh X, \tag{2}$$

---

[4] The hyperbolic sine and cosine are defined and tabulated in standard mathematical tables. Because $\sinh(-X) = -\sinh(X)$, this function has odd symmetry about the origin. Because $\cosh(-X) = \cosh(X)$, this function has even symmetry about the origin.

where A and B are arbitrary constants to be determined by the boundary conditions.

When a steady current I is injected at the terminal $(X = L)$ of a cylinder of finite length, the terminal boundary condition can be expressed

$$dV/dX = IR_\infty, \qquad \text{at } X = L, \tag{3}$$

where R_∞ represents the input resistance for a semi-infinite length of such a cylinder. It may be noted that both the diameter and the materials of the cylinder are included in the definition of R_∞ ; see the list of Symbols. To understand this boundary condition, it is helpful to note that the intracellular (core) current (flowing parallel to the cylinder axis and taken as positive when in the direction of increasing x) can be given several alternative[5] expressions

$$(-dV_i/dx)/r_i = (-dV_i/dX)/(\lambda r_i) = (-dV/dX)/R_\infty .$$

When the injected current is positive, the resulting core current is negative, because it must flow from $X = L$ toward the origin. Furthermore, we assume that none of the injected current can leak out through the sealed terminal of the cylinder; therefore, the core current must equal exactly $-I$ at $X = L$, and Eq. 3 must hold. It should be added that for a cylinder which extends from the origin to a terminal at $X = -L$, the sign becomes reversed, because a positive current injected at this terminal would result in a positive core current flowing from $X = -L$ toward the origin. Thus, the boundary condition for current injection at $X = -L$ differs from Eq. 3 by a minus sign.

Even Symmetry for 2L; or Length L Insulated at the Origin

For a cylinder of length $2L$ diagram A in Fig. 2 illustrates the case of even symmetry, where the same steady current $I/2$ is injected at both ends $(X = \pm L)$ of the cylinder. This symmetry requires[4] that $A = 0$ in Eq. 2; the value of B can be determined from the boundary condition at either end. Because the core current at $X = L$ must equal minus $I/2$ in this example, we see (from Eq. 3, above) that the boundary condition here can be expressed

$$dV/dX = (I/2)R_\infty, \qquad \text{at } X = L. \tag{4}$$

Together with $A = 0$ in Eq. 2, this boundary condition implies that $B = (I/2)R_\infty/$

---

[5] The first expression simply represents Ohm's Law. The second uses the substitution, $dx = \lambda dX$, which follows from the definition of X. The third expression depends upon two substitutions: $\lambda r_i = R_\infty$, by definition, and $dV_i/dX = dV/dX$, because $V = V_i - V_e - E_r$, and both V_e and E_r are assumed to be constants (independent of X).

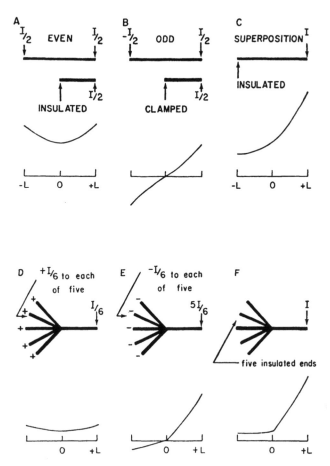

FIGURE 2 Diagrams illustrating superposition of component boundary value problems characterized by even and odd symmetry; see text. A, B, and C refer to a cylinder of length 2L. A shows even symmetry for equal source currents at both ends; the graph of V with distance shows zero slope at origin ($X = 0$), corresponding also to insulated boundary condition at origin. B shows odd symmetry for a source current at $X = L$ with a matching sink current at $X = -L$; the graph shows $V = 0$ at origin, corresponding also to voltage-clamped boundary condition at origin. C shows the superposition of A and B; the graph shows zero slope at $X = -L$, corresponding to insulated boundary condition at $X = -L$. D, E, and F refer to a neuron model composed of six equal cylinders of length L like Fig. 1 C; one cylinder extends to the right, to distinguish it from the other five, shown gathered to the left of the common origin. D shows even symmetry for equal source currents $I/6$ applied to the distal ends of all six cylinders; the graph shows zero slope at the origin. E shows the result of five source-sink current pairs, where one cylinder receives all five source currents, while each of the other five cylinders receives one of the ($-I/6$) sink currents; the graph shows discontinuous slope at origin, where the one cylinder has a slope which is five times as steep as that in each of the five other cylinders. F shows the superposition of D and E, where the resultant current is all applied to one cylinder; the graph shows that the five other cylinders satisfy a zero slope (insulated) boundary condition at their distal ends; graph also shows a fivefold discontinuity of slope at the origin, in agreement with E.

sinh L, and that the solution for this case of even symmetry can be expressed

$$V(X) = (I/2)R_\infty \cosh X/\sinh L, \qquad (5)$$

for the entire range, $-L \leq X \leq L$. It should be noted that the case of even symmetry necessarily implies the condition

$$dV/dX = 0, \qquad \text{at } X = 0, \qquad (6)$$

which corresponds also to an insulated or sealed boundary at $X = 0$, as noted in Fig. 2 A.

The input resistance at $X = L$, for this case of a cylinder insulated at the origin, is the ratio of the steady input voltage, $V(X)$ at $X = L$, to the steady input current $I/2$. It follows from Eq. 5 that this input resistance can be expressed

$$R_{CL,\text{ ins}} = R_\infty \coth L. \qquad (7)$$

For example, if $L = 1.0$, this input resistance is 1.313 times R_∞. For values of L greater than 2.65, this resistance differs from R_∞ by less than 1%.

Odd Symmetry for 2L; or Length L Clamped at the Origin

For a cylinder of length $2L$ diagram B in Fig. 2 illustrates the case of odd symmetry, where a steady source current $I/2$ is injected at $X = L$, and a matching steady sink current $-I/2$ is applied at $X = -L$. This odd symmetry requires that $B = 0$ in Eq. 2; the value of A can be determined from the boundary condition at either end. The boundary condition at $X = L$ can be expressed in the same form as Eq. 4, but here, with $B = 0$ in Eq. 2, this boundary condition implies that $A = (I/2)R_\infty/\cosh L$, and that the solution for this case of odd symmetry can be expressed

$$V(X) = (I/2)R_\infty \sinh X/\cosh L, \qquad (8)$$

for the entire range, $-L \leq X \leq L$. It should be noted that the case of odd symmetry necessarily satisfies the condition $V = 0$ at $X = 0$ which is equivalent to a voltage-clamped boundary condition at $X = 0$, as noted in Fig. 2 B.

Setting $X = L$ in Eq. 8, we see that the input resistance at $X = L$ can be expressed, for this case of a cylinder clamped ($V = 0$) at the origin, as

$$R_{CL,\text{ clp}} = R_\infty \tanh L. \qquad (9)$$

For example, if $L = 1.0$, this input resistance is 0.762 times R_∞. For values of L greater than 2.65, this resistance differs from R_∞ by less than 1%.

Whole Neuron Input Resistance at Origin (Soma) of Neuron Model

Consider a neuron model composed of N equal dendritic trees coupled to a common origin (Fig. 1 A). Each tree has a trunk whose diameter and materials can be characterized by $R_{T\infty}$, the input resistance at the origin of a trunk cylinder extended to semi-infinite length. Each dendritic tree is assumed to have a finite electrotonic length L and, in those situations (such as current injection at the origin) where it is not necessary to distinguish between separate dendritic branches, each dendritic tree can be represented as an equivalent cylinder (Figs. 1 B and C) of electrotonic length L. We assume all dendritic terminals to have sealed (insulated) ends; this implies a zero slope ($dV/dX = 0$) boundary condition at $X = L$. If the current, I is injected at the common origin of N such cylinders, I/N flows into each cylinder, and the steady potential distribution can be expressed, for each cylinder, as

$$V(X) = (I/N)R_{T\infty} \cosh (L - X)/\sinh L, \qquad (10)$$

which satisfies the boundary conditions at $X = 0$ and at $X = L$. The whole neuron input resistance R_N at the origin of this model is the ratio of the steady input voltage $V(X)$ at $X = 0$ to the steady input current I. It follows from Eq. 10 that this input resistance can be expressed

$$R_N = (R_{T\infty} \coth L)/N. \qquad (11)$$

For example, consider $L = 1.0$ and $N = 6$; then R_N is 0.219 times $R_{T\infty}$. For values of L greater than 2.65, R_N differs from $R_{T\infty}/N$ by less than 1%.

Effect of Restricting Input Current to One Cylinder of Neuron Model

Suppose that a steady current I/N is injected at the end of each cylinder, as illustrated in Fig. 2 D for the case of $N = 6$. Then there is even symmetry with respect to the origin, and Eqs. 4–7 apply, with I/N replacing $I/2$, and $R_{T\infty}$ replacing R_∞. Next, instead of this even symmetry, suppose that a steady source current I/N is injected at the end of only one cylinder, while a steady sink current $-I/N$ is applied to the end of one other cylinder. For the special case of $N = 2$, this is exactly the same as Fig. 2 B and Eqs. 8 and 9. For N greater than 2, it should be noted that the additional cylinders would not be disturbed by the single source-sink pair just described.[6] Thus, as shown in Fig. 2 E, we can superimpose $(N - 2)$ additional source-sink pairs, with the result that one cylinder receives a combined source current $(N - 1)I/N$ at its end $X = L$ while each of the $(N - 1)$ other cylinders receive separate sink currents each of which equals $-I/N$; note that this

---

[6] The several cylinders are connected only at the origin, and the source-sink pair satisfies two conditions: $V = 0$ at the origin, and the current reaching the origin from the source is exactly matched by the current flowing from the origin toward the sink.

superposition of source-sink pairs preserves the voltage-clamped condition ($V = 0$) at the origin (Fig. 2 E).

Now we can superimpose the N sources of Fig. 2 D with the $(N - 1)$ source-sink pairs of Fig. 2 E to obtain the combined result of Fig. 2 F, where one cylinder receives a combined current injection I at $X = L$, while the complete cancellation of the source and sink currents at the ends of the $(N - 1)$ other cylinders implies that their ends receive zero resultant input current and thus correspond to insulated ends.

As is indicated in Fig. 2 F, it is convenient to let the input cylinder be represented by positive values of X, and to let the $(N - 1)$ other cylinders be represented by negative values of X. Thus, the superimposed solution can be represented mathematically (using Eqs. 5 and 8 with $I/2$ replaced by I/N, and R_∞ replaced by $R_{T\infty}$) by the following two expressions: for the input cylinder (i.e., for $0 \leq X \leq L$),

$$V(X) = (I/N)R_{T\infty} \, [\cosh X/\sinh L + (N - 1) \sinh X/\cosh L], \qquad (12)$$

while, for each of the $(N - 1)$ other cylinders (i.e., for $-L \leq X \leq 0$),

$$V(X) = (I/N)R_{T\infty} \, [\cosh X/\sinh L + \sinh X/\cosh L]. \qquad (13)$$

It may be noted that this steady-state solution does satisfy continuity of V and conservation of core current at the origin; it also satisfies the current input boundary condition ($dV/dX = IR_{T\infty}$) at $X = L$ of the input branch, as well as the zero slope boundary condition at each terminal ($X = -L$) of the $N - 1$ other cylinders of the neuron model.

Setting $X = L$ in Eq. 12 and dividing by the steady input current I we see that the input resistance at $X = L$ of the input cylinder can be expressed, for this case of current injection at the end of one cylinder of the neuron model, as

$$R_{NCL} = R_{T\infty}[\coth L + (N - 1) \tanh L]/N. \qquad (14)$$

It can be seen that for $N = 1$, this equation reduces to Eq. 11, as it should. Also, for large L, where both the hyperbolic tangent and hyperbolic cotangent differ negligibly from unity, this resistance differs negligibly from $R_{T\infty}$, as would be expected from the physical intuitive consideration that the boundary condition at the origin should have negligible effect upon the terminal input resistance when L is large enough. Additional insight into this result can be obtained by referring this result to the insulated and "clamped" (even and odd) results of Eqs. 7 and 9; then the present result can be expressed

$$R_{NCL} = [1/N]R_{CL, \, ins} + [(N - 1)/N]R_{CL, \, clp}, \qquad (15)$$

where we have identified $R_{T\infty}$ (of Eq. 14) with R_∞ (of Eqs. 7 and 9).

A physical interpretation of this result is that a fraction $1/N$ of the input current is completely dissipated in the input cylinder (as though there were insulation at the origin; see Figs. 2 A and D), while the remaining fraction $(N - 1)/N$ of the input current dissipates partly in the input cylinder and partly in the other cylinders (as though the origin were clamped to $V = 0$; see Fig. 2 E).

In view of earlier Eq. 11 for the whole neuron input resistance R_N at the origin, we can use Eq. 14 to express the ratio

$$R_{NCL}/R_N = 1 + (N - 1)(\tanh L)^2. \tag{16}$$

For example, if $L = 1.0$ and $N = 6$, the input resistance R_{NCL} defined by Eqs. 14–16 is 3.9 times R_N, or 0.86 times $R_{T\infty}$. For large values of L, the input resistance ratio of Eq. 16 is nearly N.

It is also interesting to note that the special case $N = 2$ which reduces Fig. 2 F to Fig. 2 C, also reduces Eq. 14 to the simpler expression

$$R_{2CL} = R_{T\infty}(\coth L + \tanh L)/2$$

$$= R_{T\infty} \coth (2L), \tag{17}$$

where the second form follows from a standard identity. This agrees, as it should, with Eq. 7 for a doubling (from L to $2L$) of the distance from the insulated end to the input end of a cylinder; compare Fig. 2 C with the right half of Fig. 2 A.

Effect of Restricting Input Current to One Dendritic Branch Terminal

We consider first the case where there is only one order of symmetric dendritic branching. Diagrams A, B, and C in Fig. 3 illustrate the superposition method for this case. If both branch terminals of one tree receive the same steady input current $I/2$ (as in Fig. 3 A) the distribution of steady membrane potential must be exactly the same in both branches. Given that the branch diameter satisfies the constraint for transformation of this tree to an equivalent cylinder, this case is equivalent to the injection of I at $X = L$ in the equivalent cylinder. In other words, the case of Fig. 3 A is equivalent to that of Fig. 2 F, and the steady-state solution is the same as that given by eqs. 12 and 13.

Now we consider the particular kind of odd symmetry illustrated by Fig. 3 B, where a steady source current $I/2$ is injected at one branch terminal, while a matching steady sink current $-I/2$ is applied at the other branch terminal. Let $X = X_1$, define the (first-order) branch point. The odd symmetry between the two branches implies that $V = 0$ at $X = X_1$, and that all of the current flowing to $X = X_1$ from the source branch must exactly equal all of the current flowing from $X = X_1$ into the sink branch. This source-sink pair supplies no current or voltage to the trunk or the other trees, which is why they are dotted in Fig. 3 B. The distribution of steady

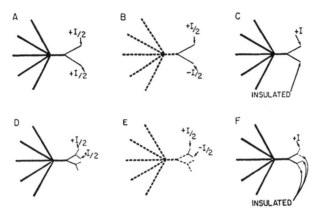

FIGURE 3 Extension of superposition method to dendritic branching in one tree; see text. Diagrams A, B, and C, represent the simplest case of only one order of branching, with a pair of equal branches. A shows even branch symmetry, with equal source currents to both branch terminals. B shows odd branch symmetry, with a source current applied to one branch terminal and a matching sink current applied to the other; no current flows in the dotted regions. C shows the superposition of A and B, where the resultant current is all applied to one first-order branch terminal. Diagrams D, E, and F represent the extension to second-order branching. D shows even branch symmetry only for the pair of secondary branches belonging to one primary branch, with equal sources currents to both of these secondary branch terminals. E shows odd branch symmetry, for a source-sink current pair applied to one pair of secondary branch terminals. F shows the superposition of D and E, where the resultant current is all applied to a single secondary branch terminal.

potential in the source branch, due to this source-sink pair alone, can be expressed

$$V(X) = (I/2)(2R_{T\infty}) \sinh (X - X_1)/\cosh (L - X_1), \qquad (18)$$

for the range, $X_1 \leq X \leq L$; the sister (sink) branch has corresponding negative values. This odd symmetry may be compared with that of Fig. 2 B and Eq. 8. Here, we note that $(I/2)$ is the amount of the source current, and that $(2R_{T\infty})$ is the R_∞ value for each branch cylinder; this R_∞ value follows from the equivalent cylinder constraint which requires that symmetric branches each have a $d^{3/2}$ value equal to half the trunk value.

Steady-State Solution for One Order of Branching

By superimposing the odd branch symmetry of Fig. 3 B with the even branch symmetry of Fig. 3 A, we obtain the case of input to a single branch of first order, Fig. 3 C. Within this input branch, the resultant solution is given by the sum of Eqs. 12 and 18 (i.e., the righthand sides) for the range $X_1 \leq X \leq L$. For the sister branch, the solution is given by Eq. 12 minus Eq. 18. For the trunk ($0 \leq X \leq X_1$), Eq. 12 alone is still the solution; also, for the $(N - 1)$ other trees, Eq. 13 is still the solution assuming ($-L \leq X \leq 0$) as before.

This result has the interesting implication that the solution in the trunk and in the other trees is completely unaffected by whether the input current I is injected entirely into one branch terminal or divided equally between the two branch terminals, and this is easily generalized to include any apportionment of this input current between these two branch terminals.

Extension to Higher Orders of Branching

Diagrams D, E, and F of Fig. 3 illustrate the additional superposition required when we add a second order of symmetric branching. When the same steady input current $I/2$ is delivered to the terminals of the two secondary branches belonging to the same parent primary branch (Fig. 3 D), the distribution of steady membrane potential is the same in both of these secondary branches and is equivalent to that of Fig. 3 C, just solved above.

Now we consider the case of odd symmetry between this pair of secondary branches (Fig. 3 E), with a steady source current $I/2$ injected at the terminal of one secondary branch, while a matching steady sink current $-I/2$ is applied at the terminal of its sister branch. Let $X = X_2$ be the electrotonic distance, from origin to second-order branch point. In analogy with the previously considered odd symmetry between a pair of primary branches (Fig. 3 B), this case of odd symmetry between a pair of secondary branches has $V = 0$ at $X = X_2$, and supplies no current or voltage to any of the regions shown dotted in Fig. 3 E. The distribution of steady potential in the source branch, due to this source-sink pair alone, will be expressed in the more general form that applies to a branch pair of kth order, where the particular case $k = 2$ corresponds to the secondary branches of Fig. 3 E; this general form is

$$V(X) = (I/2)(2^k R_{T\infty}) \sinh (X - X_k)/\cosh (L - X_k), \qquad (19)$$

for the range, $X_k \leq X \leq L$; the sister (sink) branch has corresponding negative values. We note that $(I/2)$ is the amount of the source current (of the source-sink pair), and that $(2^k R_{T\infty})$ is the R_∞ value for a kth-order branch, on the assumption of symmetric branching in a tree satisfying the equivalent cylinder constraint. It may be noted that Eq. 19 agrees, when $k = 1$, with Eq. 18, as it should.

The case of input restricted to the terminal of a single secondary branch (Fig. 3 F) is obtained by superimposing the odd (secondary branch) symmetry of Fig. 3 E with the even (secondary branch) symmetry of Fig. 3 D, where we have already noted that the latter is equivalent to the case of Fig. 3 C, for one order of branching. This method can now be generalized by using Eq. 19 in successive superpositions, as the order k is stepped from 1 to M in unit steps.

Steady-State Solution for Branch Terminal Input with M Orders of Branching

When there are M orders of symmetric branching in the input tree, the method of successive superpositions (using Eqs. 12 and 19) leads to the following general expression for the distribution of potential in this neuron model when the steady current I is injected only at the terminal of one branch,

$$V(X) = IR_{T\infty}\left\{\frac{\cosh X}{N \sinh L} + \frac{A \sinh X}{N \cosh L} + \sum_{k=1}^{M} 2^{(k-1)} \frac{B_k \sinh (X - X_k)}{\cosh (L - X_k)}\right\}, \quad (20)$$

where A and B_k are simple constants whose values are specified according to location, as follows:

in the input tree $A = N - 1$;
   in the input branch $B_k = 1$, for all k from 1 to M;
   in the sister branch   same, except $B_M = -1$;
   in the parent branch   same, except $B_M = 0$;
   in first cousin branches   same, except $B_M = 0$, and $B_{M-1} = -1$;
   in grandparent branch   same, except $B_M = 0$, and $B_{M-1} = 0$;

    . . .

   in the input trunk $B_k = 0$, for all k; (cf. Eq. 12);
  in the other trees $\begin{cases} A = 1, \text{ assuming, }^{7} X < 0, \text{ and} \\ B_k = 0, \text{ for all } k; \text{ (cf. Eq. 13).} \end{cases}$

A specific example of such solutions is presented and illustrated in the Results section below.

By differentiating Eq. 20 with respect to X and setting $X = L$, we can verify that the boundary condition at the input-receiving branch terminal is correctly satisfied; thus

$$(\mathrm{d}V/\mathrm{d}X)_{X=L} = IR_{T\infty}\left\{(1/N) + (N - 1)/N + \sum_{k=1}^{M} 2^{(k-1)}\right\}$$

$$= 2^{M} IR_{T\infty}, \quad (21)$$

which is I times the R_∞ value of a Mth-order branch cylinder, as it should be, according to Eq. 3. For the sister branch, the corresponding expression for its terminal boundary condition reduces to zero because the last term of the summation has a minus sign. A zero slope boundary condition is similarly satisfied at the ends of all terminal branches (except the input branch) of this neuron model. The other boundary conditions, continuity of V and conservation of core current at every branch point, have been satisfied also by the method of superposition used; each odd function that was superimposed at a branch point contributed zero to the value of V at that point, and contributed a source-sink pair of currents whose net contribution was also zero at that point.

Input Resistance for Current Injected to a Single Branch Terminal

We can now give the general expression for the input resistance R_{BL} for current injected at the terminal ($X = L$) of one dendritic branch of a neuron model com-

---

[7] This sign convention agrees with Figs. 2 D, E, F and with Eq. 13. Alternatively, if the other trees are represented by positive values of X, as in Fig. 4 and in expression 27 below, then $A = -1$.

posed of N equal dendritic trees, with M orders of symmetric dendritic branching (which satisfy the equivalent cylinder constraint). By setting $X = L$ in Eq. 20 (for the input branch) and dividing by the steady input current I we obtain the input resistance

$$R_{BL} = R_{T\infty} \left\{ \frac{\coth L}{N} + \frac{(N-1)\tanh L}{N} + \sum_{k=1}^{M} 2^{(k-1)} \tanh (L - X_k) \right\}. \quad (22)$$

For the special case of no dendritic branching, $M = 0$ and the summation expression in Eq. 22 contributes nothing; this equation then reduces to Eq. 14. Also, the special case of a long input branch makes all of the hyperbolic tangent and hyperbolic cotangent values close to unity; then (as seen with Eq. 21) the expression for R_{BL} reduces essentially to $2^M R_{T\infty}$, which is the R_∞ value of an Mth-order branch cylinder, as would be expected from physical intuitive considerations.

In this expression, the size and the materials of the neuron model are incorporated in $R_{T\infty}$, which is the limiting value of the input resistance of a dendritic trunk cylinder, when extended to semi-infinite length. In experimental situations, however, it is the value of the whole neuron input resistance R_N at the soma that is the most useful reference value. Also, referring to Eq. 11 for R_N, we see that it is not difficult to express the ratio of these two input resistances, R_{BL} and R_N, as follows:

$$R_{BL}/R_N = 1 + (N-1)(\tanh L)^2 + N \tanh (L) \sum_{k=1}^{M} 2^{(k-1)} \tanh (L - X_k). \quad (23)$$

This is the expression that was used to compute the table of illustrative values given in the Results section below; a more general expression is derived in the Appendix.

Steady-State Attenuation Factor from Branch Terminal to Soma

Attenuation factors are usually defined as the ratio of an amplitude or intensity at the input location to the smaller (attenuated) value found at a point of observation or output. So defined, the attenuation factor is a number greater than one; also, increased attenuation results in an increased attenuation factor. For the present problem of steady-state voltage attenuation, the voltage at the terminal of the input branch of the neuron model can be obtained most simply as

$$V_{BL} = IR_{BL}. \quad (24)$$

The corresponding voltage at the origin (soma) can be obtained by setting $X = 0$ in Eq. 12, 13, or 20; this gives

$$V_0 = IR_{T\infty}/(N \sinh L)$$

$$= IR_N/\cosh L, \quad (25)$$

where the second expression makes use of Eq. 11 for R_N.

Now, by taking the ratio of V_{BL} to V_O, we can write the following expression for the attenuation factor, from input branch terminal to the soma,

$$AF_{BL/O} = (R_{BL}/R_N) \cosh L, \qquad (26)$$

where the ratio of input resistances inside the parentheses is precisely that defined by Eq. 23, above. This tells us that the attenuation factor is closely related to, but not identical with, the ratio of the input resistances at the input branch terminal and at the soma; the attenuation factor is always larger, because $\cosh (L)$ is greater than unity for all L values greater than zero. Illustrative values are given in the Results section, below; a more general expression is derived in the Appendix.

Note on Generalization of Theory

The Appendix provides more general results for branch input resistance and for attenuation factor. The input current can be applied at any point of any branch. Daughter branches need not be equal, but their diameters still must satisfy the more general equivalent cylinder constraint. Also, the dendritic trees need not be of equal trunk diameter, and the results are even further generalized to provide for trees that need not have the same electrotonic length. The final section of the Appendix provides results for AC steady-state impedance and attenuation.

ILLUSTRATIVE RESULTS

Example of Potential Distribution throughout Neuron Model

The method of solution described above has been used to compute the particular example illustrated in Fig. 4. This is a case of six dendritic trees with three orders of branching, i.e., $N = 6$ and $M = 3$. Here each tree has an electrotonic length $L = 1$ which is divided into four equal electrotonic increments, $\Delta X = 0.25$, for each trunk and each order of branching. The steepest gradient of membrane potential occurs in the input branch (BI); most of the input current reaches the parent branch point (P). Very little of this current flows out into the sister branch (BS); most of it flows through the parent branch where the gradient with respect to X is roughly half as steep as that in the input branch, because the R_∞ value of the parent branch cylinder is half that of the input branch cylinder. At the grandparent branch point (GP), relatively little current flows into the first cousin branches (BC-1), and most of the current flows through the grandparent branch, where the gradient with respect to X has been roughly halved again. In contrast to the steep gradients in the input branch and the parent and grandparent branches, the dashed curve in Fig. 4 shows the smaller gradient obtained if the same total amount of input currently were divided equally between the eight terminal branches of one dendritic tree. This dashed curve is continuous with the curve for this tree trunk; in fact, the solution in this trunk would be the same for any apportionment of the

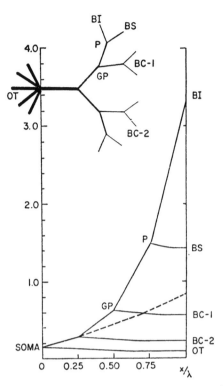

FIGURE 4   Branching diagram (upper left) and graph (below) showing steady-state values of V as a function of X in all branches and trees of the neuron model, for steady current injected into the terminal of one branch. BI and BS designate the input branch and its sister branch; P and GP designate their parent and grandparent branch points; BC-1 and BC-2 designate first and second cousin branches, with respect to the input branch; OT designates the other trees of the neuron model. The model parameters are $N = 6, L = 1, M = 3$, with equal electrotonic length increments $\Delta X = 0.25$ assumed for all branches. Ordinates of graph express $V/IR_{T\infty}$ values, as defined by Eqs. 12, 13, and 20; see also expressions 27–31 and commentary in text.

same total input current between these eight branch terminals. Also, the solution from the soma into the five other trees (OT) is the same for any such apportionment of the same input.

The values of membrane potential shown in Fig. 4 are given as the dimensionless ratio of $V(X)$ to $IR_{T\infty}$. For the other trees (OT), these values were obtained from the expression

$$0.142 \cosh X - 0.108 \sinh X, \tag{27}$$

which follows from Eq. 13; (the minus sign is used here together with positive values of X for these cylinders). For the trunk of the input tree and for the dashed curve in Fig. 4, the values were obtained from the expression

$$0.142 \cosh X + 0.54 \sinh X, \tag{28}$$

which follows from Eq. 12. For the grandparent branch, which extends from $X = 0.25$ to $X = 0.5$, one must add to the value of expression 28, the value of

$$\sinh (X - 0.25)/\cosh (0.75), \qquad (29)$$

based on Eq. 18. However, for the other half of this tree, extending from $X = 0.25$ to the four terminals of the second cousin branches (BC-2), the value of expression 29 was subtracted from that of expression 28.

For the parent branch, extending from $X = 0.5$ to $X = 0.75$, one must add to the value of expressions 28 plus 29 also the value of

$$2 \sinh (X - 0.5)/\cosh (0.5), \qquad (30)$$

based on Eq. 19 with $k = 2$. For the input branch, extending from $X = 0.75$ to $X = 1.0$, one must add to the value of expressions 28 plus 29 and 30 also the expression

$$4 \sinh (X - 0.75)/\cosh (0.25), \qquad (31)$$

based on Eq. 19 with $k = 3$. For the sister branch (BS), the value of expression 31 was subtracted from that of expressions 28 plus 29 and 30. In that portion of the tree which extends from the grandparent branch point (GP) to both terminals of the first cousin branches (BC-1), the value of expression 30 was subtracted from that of expressions 28 plus 29.

Examples of Input Resistance Ratio and Attenuation Factor

In Fig. 4, the value plotted for $V/IR_{T\infty}$ at the input terminal is about 3.4, while that at the origin (soma) is 0.142; the ratio of these two numbers gives a value of 23.9 for the attenuation factor from input terminal to soma. Alternatively, one can use Eq. 23 to obtain a value of 15.5 for the input resistance ratio R_{BL}/R_N, and then use Eq. 26 to obtain a value of 23.9 for the attenuation factor. Many additional examples have been calculated and listed in Table I.

All of the values in Table I depend upon specifying the values of N, L, and M for a symmetrically branched neuron model, with the additional simplifying assumption that the successive branch points X_k are equally spaced, with increments in X given by $\Delta X = L/(M + 1)$. The value inside each parenthesis in Table I gives the input resistance ratio R_{BL}/R_N, defined by Eq. 23. The value immediately below each parenthesis gives the corresponding attenuation factor, defined by Eq. 26. Several useful rough generalizations about the effects of changing the value of N, L, or M separately can be made from inspection of the values in Table I.

Effect of increasing L, with N and M constant. Consider the effect of doubling the value of L from 1.0 to 2.0; this means doubling all trunk and branch lengths, when expressed in units of X. Comparison of the first two columns of

TABLE I

INPUT RESISTANCE RATIO (R_{BL}/R_N) AND STEADY-STATE
ATTENUATION FACTOR $AF_{BL/0}$

M	$N = 6$		$L = 1.5$	
	$L = 1.0$	$L = 2.0$	$N = 6$	$N = 10$
2	(9.5)	(17.4)	(14.3)	(23.6)
	14.7	65.5	33.6	55.4
3	(15.5)	(30.4)	(24.2)	(40.2)
	23.9	114	56.8	94.4
4	(26.0)	(53.6)	(41.7)	(69.4)
	40.1	202	98.0	163
5	(44.6)	(95.4)	(73.1)	(122)
	68.8	359	172	286
6	(78.0)	(172)	(130)	(216)
	120	647	305	508
7	(138)	(311)	(233)	(388)
	213	1170	548	912
8	(248)	(569)	(422)	(704)
	352	2140	992	1650

Table I shows that the input resistance ratio is roughly doubled, and that the attenuation factor increases roughly fivefold. With the larger M values, these factors of increase are somewhat larger.

Effect of increasing N, with L and M constant. We examine the effect of increasing N from 6 to 10, when $L = 1.5$ and M is constant, by comparing the last two columns of Table I. Both the input resistance ratio and the attenuation factor increase by a factor that is very close to 10/6. We can understand this most easily by considering, for example, that the dendritic trees are not changed in size (i.e., $R_{T\infty}$ is held constant). Then R_{BL} is little changed, because the distribution of input current in the input tree is almost unchanged; it is only slightly affected by the boundary condition (at the origin) with the other trees. However, the value of R_N is very significantly changed; the parallel input resistance of 10 trees must be reduced to exactly 6/10 of that for 6 trees of the same size. For such conditions, the increase in the input resistance ratio and in the attenuation factor can be attributed almost entirely to the 6/10 factor in R_N.

Effect of increasing M, with N and L constant. The previous example of $N = 6$, $L = 1$, and $M = 3$ implied trunk and branch increments of $\Delta X = 0.25$ (see Fig. 4). If we preserve these values of N and L, and increase M by four orders of branching to $M = 7$, this results in $\Delta X = 0.125$, with eight increments. The values in Table I show an approximately ninefold increase, from 15.5 to 138 for the input resistance ratio, and from 23.9 to 213 for the attenuation factor. Throughout Table I, an increase of M by four orders, while N and L are held constant, results in around a 9- or 10-fold increase. In other words, the factor of increase per unit increase in M is given roughly by the square root of three, for the values in Table I. We gain some additional insight by noting that changes in M can have no effect upon the value of R_N when N, L, and $R_{T\infty}$ are held constant (see Eq. 11). Under such conditions, the increase in the input resistance ratio and in the attenuation factor, with increase in M, can be attributed entirely to the increase of R_{BL}, which can be attributed, in turn, to the smaller diameters of the higher order branches.

Nonreciprocity of Branch Attenuation

Comparison of the attenuation along the input branch and its sister branch (in Fig. 4) is instructive because neurophysiologists sometimes argue, erroneously, that the attenuation along a dendritic branch should be the same, whether it takes place in the centripetal or the centrifugal direction. This fallacy presumably results from noting that the core resistance is the same in both directions, while forgetting the importance of the boundary conditions. In Fig. 4, the attenuation from the parent branch point (P) to the terminal of the sister branch (BS) is rather small because of the insulated (zero slope) boundary condition at the terminal; in contrast, the attenuation from the terminal of the input branch (BI) to the parent branch point (P) is much larger because the boundary condition at P permits a large amount of current to flow from the input branch into the thicker parent branch. Here, the input branch and its sister branch have exactly the same core resistance; the difference results entirely from the boundary conditions. Similarly, in Fig. 2 the graphs show how attenuation from $X = L$ to the origin depends upon the boundary condition at the origin. An earlier publication (see Eq. 3 and Fig. 3, pp. 496–498, Rall, 1959) provides both a mathematical expression and a graphical illustration for such dependence of attenuation upon boundary conditions.

DISCUSSION

Application of Theoretical Results to Motoneurons

Motoneurons of cat spinal cord are large neurons whose input resistance values (R_N usually between 0.5 and 2.5 MΩ) are lower than for most other neurons in the mammalian central nervous system. The notion that the equivalent cylinder constraint might apply to motoneurons, at least as a rough approximation, was suggested some time ago (Rall, 1959) on the basis of preliminary evidence. Recently, Lux et al. (1970) checked 50 dendritic bifurcations in 7 carefully studied motoneurons and reported that the ratio of the summed $d^{3/2}$ of the daughter branches to the parent $d^{3/2}$ ranged from 0.8 to 1.2, with a mean of 1.02 ± 0.12 (SD). Also, Barrett and Crill (1971) found that (except for a sharp initial taper of the dendritic trunks) the summed $d^{3/2}$ value decreases only rather gradually with distance. These results, together with unpublished calculations based upon the data of Aitken and

Bridger (1961), imply that motoneuron dendritic trees may reasonably be approximated by equivalent cylinders, and furthermore, that the electrotonic length L for soma plus dendritic tree ranges between 1 and 2, with a mean value around 1.5 (see also Rall, 1964, 1969 a, 1970; Nelson and Lux, 1970; Burke and ten Bruggencate, 1971; Jack et al., 1970, 1971; Lux et al., 1970; Barrett and Crill, 1971). The study of Lux et al. (1970) is unusual in providing the first examples of estimation of L values by two independent methods on the same neuron; one method (Rall, 1959) depends upon anatomical measurements of branch lengths and diameters, together with the R_N measurement; the other method (Rall, 1969 a) is entirely electrophysiological, depending upon the theoretical relation between L and the time-constant ratio obtained by peeling the sum of exponential decays. Barrett and Crill (1971, plus personal communication) have recently also determined L by both methods on the same neuron.

Dendritic trees of different size occur on a single motoneuron. Also, the larger motoneurons tend to have both more numerous and larger dendritic trees than do the smaller motoneurons; see Kernell (1966), and also Gelfan et al. (1970). Such differences in tree size need not imply differences in electrotonic length L because the larger trunk diameters imply larger λ values. Thus, we have supposed that the separate L values of the separate dendritic trees belonging to a particular motoneuron could be nearly the same, in spite of differences in tree size. This supposition obtains support from the observation by Burke and ten Bruggencate (1971) that there is no significant correlation between whole motoneuron size (as indicated by R_N) and the L value estimated for the whole motoneuron; in other words, the observed range of L values was found to be the same for small motoneurons as for larger motoneurons. Because the large motoneurons possess more large dendritic trees, this result implies that the large dendritic trees do not have significantly larger L values. The measurements reported by Lux et al. (1970) and by Barrett and Crill (1971) also support this conclusion.

The early measurements of Coombs et al. (1955) and of Frank and Fuortes (1956) provided a range of cat motoneuron input resistance values of from 0.5 to 2.5 MΩ; this range was discussed in relation to dendritic anatomy by Rall (1959) and by Kernell (1966) and Burke (1967 a). Although these last two authors found a few larger R_N values, around 6–8 MΩ, most cat motoneuron input resistance values still lie in the original fivefold range. R_N values of 0.5 MΩ correspond to the largest motoneurons having the highest axonal conduction velocity and belong to fast twitch, phasic-type motor units; R_N values of 2–3 MΩ correspond to significantly smaller motoneurons having lower axonal conduction velocity and usually belonging to slow twitch, tonic-type motor units (Burke, 1967 a; cf., Wuerker et al., 1965; Kernell, 1966).

For this fivefold range in R_N, the terminal branch input resistance R_{BL} in a tree having about six or seven orders of branching, would be estimated in the range from roughly 40 to 350 MΩ for $L = 1.0$, and from roughly 65 to 750 MΩ for $L = 1.5$–2.0, using Table I. For a dendritic tree with only three orders of branching, a range of smaller values, roughly 7.5–75 MΩ for $L = 1.0$–2.0 would be estimated for R_{BL}; however, so few orders of branching would be expected only in a small dendritic tree with small trunk diameter. For input to a midbranch ($X = L/2$) reference to the corresponding sections of the Appendix and Discussion suggest an input resistance roughly in the range from 1.5 to 20 MΩ, depending upon branch order.

Because we have specified branch order, but not branch diameter, in the examples above, it is useful to consider what branch diameters are implied by different orders of symmetric branching. For example, a tree with a trunk diameter of 5 μm and 7 orders of symmetric branching would imply a terminal branch diameter of 0.2 μm; a tree with a large trunk diameter of 20 μm would imply a 7th-order branch diameter of 0.8 μm, or a 10th-order branch diameter of 0.2 μm. These particular examples were chosen because 0.2 μm corresponds to the smallest terminal branch diameters observed by histologists (Golgi material and light microscopy by Dr. Aitken, personal communication; electron microscopy by Doctors Reese and White, personal communication).

With regard to steady-state voltage attenuation from a branch input site to a motoneuron soma, it is important to note the evidence that the dendritic membrane of cat motoneurons is normally passive. This is provided by the observation that whenever the combination of two excitatory postsynaptic potentials (EPSP) departs significantly from linearity, that departure has been a small deficit (Burke, 1967 *b*, pp. 1116–1120; Rall et al., 1967, pp. 1184–1185; see also Kuno and Miyahara, 1969). It is well known that such small deficits can be accounted for theoretically with the usual assumption that synaptic excitation consists of a conductance change in the postsynaptic membrane, where neither this synaptic conductance nor the adjacent passive membrane has voltage-dependent (regenerative) properties (Martin, 1955; Rall, 1967, p. 1157; Rall et al., 1967, p. 1183; Kuno, 1971; see also Eq. 32 below). On the other hand, if a small nonlinearity were caused by active membrane properties (local response), one would expect an excess (not a small deficit) of membrane depolarization; such small excess has not been reported for normal motoneurons. However, the abnormal "partial responses" of chromatolyzed motoneurons have been attributed to active properties of abnormal dendritic membrane, as contrasted with normally passive properties (Eccles et al., 1958; Kuno and Llinas, 1970). Thus, assuming normal membrane properties, our earlier example of a trunk diameter of 5 μm and a seventh-order terminal branch of 0.2 μm (with $N = 6$ and $L = 1.5$ in Table I) implies $R_{BL}/R_N = 233$ and a steady-state attenuation factor of 548. If this branch terminal were depolarized by 55 mV, the steady effect at the soma from this one steady input would be 0.1 mV.

Application to Other Neuron Types

Pioneering quantitative treatment of dendritic branching in cerebral cortex was provided by Bok (1936, 1959) and by Sholl (1953, 1956). The variety of dendritic patterns in different neuron types has been emphasized and illustrated by Ramon-Moliner (1962, 1968) and by the Scheibels (1970). Improved quantitative methods were described and illustrated by Mannen (1966). The contributions of many other anatomists are reviewed in the papers cited above.

In order to apply the present theoretical results to any particular neuron type, one would like to have at least approximate answers to several questions. Does the dendritic branching approximately satisfy the equivalent cylinder constraint? Has an approximate range of R_N values been determined experimentally? Do the several dendritic trees seem to have similar electrotonic lengths, and, if so, has the range of such L values been estimated from experiment? Are estimates of N, M, and terminal branch diameter available? When the answers to these questions are affirmative, branch input resistance values can be estimated by means of the present theoretical results. If the branching does not satisfy the equivalent cylinder constraint, one must use the general method (Rall, 1959) for arbitrary branch lengths and diameters. For neurons where the evidence suggests active (nonlinear, regenerative) dendritic membrane properties, the attenuation factor expressions of the present paper do not apply.

Input resistance values have been measured for only a few types of neurons other than motoneurons; nearly all of these values have been larger, indicating that the neurons are smaller, and this accounts for the increased difficulty in obtaining reliable measurements with intracellular microelectrodes. Spencer and Kandel (1961) reported an average estimate of 13 MΩ for hippocampal neurons. Takahashi (1965) reported R_N values from 1.5 to 15 MΩ for pyramidal tract neurons, reporting a mean of 5.9 MΩ for 26 fast conducting cells and 10.1 MΩ for 10 slow conducting cells (see also Koike et al., 1968). Lux and Pollen (1966) obtained a range from 4.5 to 10 MΩ for identified Betz cells, and a wider range of 4.4–15.2 MΩ for nonidentified cortical cells (see also Creutzfeldt et al., 1964; Jacobson and Pollen, 1968). It seems reasonable to attribute R_N values around 4.5 MΩ to the larger pyramidal cells, and R_N values around 10–15 MΩ could be attributed to smaller pyramidal cells. Still larger R_N values would be expected for the smaller neurons of stellate and other cell types.

Calculations involving electrotonic distance in the apical dendrite of a pyramidal cell have been reported by Jacobson and Pollen (1968); see also Humphrey (1968) where emphasis was more upon extracellular potentials. Although the apical dendrite is usually much longer than the basilar dendrites, it is important to point out that this does not necessarily imply a larger L value, because the apical diameter is also larger. Furthermore, the well-known taper of apical dendritic diameter does not necessarily mean significant departure from the equivalent cylinder constraint, because the apical dendrite gives off side branches as it reduces its diameter. Jacobson and Pollen (1968) published a brief summary of their measurements and calculations based on a large sample of pyramidal cells. They mention seeing between 3 and 12 side branches of betwen 1 and 2 μm diameter along the major stretch of the apical shaft; they also reported apical dendritic diameter at 50 μm intervals along a 250 μm length, both for the five largest pyramidal cells and for 80 small- and medium-sized pyramidal cells. It is interesting that the following examples, which are in general agreement with Jacobson and Pollen's data, also satisfy the equivalent cylinder constraint on $d^{3/2}$: a 2.2 μm apical diameter with a 1.0 μm side branch emerging from a 2.6 μm parent diameter; a 3.1 μm apical diameter with a 1.5 μm side branch emerging from a 3.8 μm parent diameter; a 4.6 μm apical diameter with a 2.0 μm side branch emerging from a 5.4 μm parent diameter. Because of the unequal branching, dendritic input resistances would be calculated by means of the general results in the Appendix. Also, with regard to electrotonic length estimation, we can use Jacobson and Pollen's apical diameters for the five largest pyramidal cells, plus their rough estimate of a 250 μm long secondary branch tapering from 2.5 to 2.0 μm diameter, and a 250 μm tertiary branch tapering from 2.0 to 1.5 μm. For the larger membrane resistivity (R_m = 4,500 Ω cm²) we get ΔX values of about 0.3, 0.4, and 0.5 for these primary, secondary, and tertiary segments, giving a sum of about 1.2 for the apical value of L minus the still higher order branches; for the smaller R_m value of 1,500 Ω cm², the ΔX values are about 0.5, 0.7, and 0.8, giving a larger sum of about 2.0 for the apical value of L minus the still higher order branches. Unfortunately, we do not have the corresponding information on the basilar dendrites of these same cells. For several ranges of values, however, Jacobson and Pollen (1968) themselves obtained estimates of steady-state electrotonic attenuation over the apical dendritic length. Their results imply attenuation factors of about 3 or 4 from the major branch point (V_1) to soma, about 18 from the next branch point (V_2) to soma, and about 33–50 from the next branch point (V_3) to soma.

Local Synaptic Depolarization Not Proportional to Input Resistance

Because it is quite commonly believed that the amplitude of synaptic depolarization at the synaptic site should be expected to be directly proportional to the input resistance at that site, it seems important to draw attention to several reasons why such a strict proportionality should not be expected to hold, in general. It may be noted, however, that such proportionality can be a useful approximation for some situations; see, for example, Katz and Thesleff (1957), Katz and Miledi (1963), and Katz (1966); see also Kuno (1971), and MacGregor (1968).

First, it should be noted that brief synaptic input results in a transient EPSP, and even if the synaptic current generated at two different input sites were the same, the EPSP amplitude would depend not simply upon the input resistance at each site, but upon the different transient response function at each site. Furthermore, if there is significant depolarization of different amounts at the two synaptic sites, equal synaptic conductance transients would not produce equal synaptic current transients (Rall, 1967). Thus, in general, when comparing two synaptic sites, the synaptic currents would be unequal, the transient response functions would not be related by any simple ratio, and the resulting peak depolarizations should not be expected to exhibit the input resistance ratio. The steady-state aspect of this problem is treated explicitly below; the transient details are included in the companion paper.[1] In any case, it is clear that when the effect of synaptic input to a fine dendritic branch having high input resistance is compared with that of equal synaptic input to a thicker branch having lower input resistance, the local depolarization (at the synaptic site) is larger at the site with the larger input resistance. This has led some (at least in conversation) to infer, erroneously, that such a larger local effect would produce a larger EPSP at the soma. The error here consists of forgetting that the attenuation from the synaptic site to the soma would be increased by a factor that is usually greater than the factor of input resistance increase (see Eq. 26); also, as noted already, the local depolarization at the synaptic site would be increased by a factor that is likely to be smaller than the factor of input resistance increase. The following example illustrates these two effects for a steady state; the overall discrepancy would be even greater for transients.

For a steady synaptic excitatory conductance g_ϵ we can express the steady synaptic current as

$$(V_\epsilon - V_{in})g_\epsilon = V_{in}/R_{in}.$$

Where $V_\epsilon = E_\epsilon - E_r$ is the excitatory equilibrium potential, relative to the resting potential, and V_{in} is the resulting steady depolarization at the input site whose input resistance is R_{in}. Rearrangement of this expression provides the following useful expression for a single input,

$$(V_{in}/V_\epsilon) = (R_{in}g_\epsilon)/(1 + R_{in}g_\epsilon), \tag{32}$$

where it can be seen that steady V_{in} is proportional to $(R_{in}g_\epsilon)$ only when the value of $(R_{in}g_\epsilon)$ is much smaller than unity. Suppose, for example, that $g_\epsilon = 10^{-8}$ mho, and suppose, at the soma, $R_{in} = R_N = 10^6$ Ω; then Eq. 32 gives 0.01/1.01 for (V_{in}/V_ϵ). Next, suppose we place the same steady-state synaptic conductance at a branch terminal, where, for example, $R_{in} = R_{BL} = 10^8$ Ω, or 100 times the previous input resistance; then Eq. 32 gives $(V_{in}/V_\epsilon) = 1/2$, which is 50 rather than 100 times the previous steady depolarization. To carry this example further, consider the attenuation from the branch terminal to the soma, and compare this attenuated amplitude with that found previously for input at the soma. In this example, $R_{BL}/R_N = 100$, and if we also assume $L = 1.5$, Eq. 26 implies an attenuation factor of 235; then the steady value of 1/2 for (V_{in}/V_ϵ) at the input branch terminal implies a value of $(V/V_\epsilon) = 0.00212$ at the soma, or about one-fifth the value obtained when the same synaptic conductance was applied directly to the soma. To recapitulate this example, when the synaptic excitatory conductance was shifted from the soma to a branch terminal whose input resistance was 100 times as great as that at the soma, the steady depolarization at the synaptic site was increased 50 times, not 100 times; also, the steady attenuation factor of 235 from the input branch terminal to the soma resulted in a soma depolarization that was about one-fifth the reference value obtained with synaptic input at the soma.

Nonlinear Summation of Adjacent Dendritic Synaptic Inputs

It has already been pointed out elsewhere (Rall, 1967, pp. 1155–1156, 1167–1168; Rall et al., 1967, pp. 1183–1184) that the larger depolarization at a dendritic synaptic site can be responsible for significant nonlinearity of synaptic summation. This nonlinearity results because the depolarization due to one synapse reduces the synaptic driving potential $(V_\epsilon - V_{in})$ at the adjacent synapse;[8] the larger the local depolarization, the greater the nonlinear effect. In fact, we have argued that when an observed nonlinearity significantly exceeds the amount which could be accounted for by the depolarization at the soma, it is reasonable to suppose that the synaptic input sites must have been dendritic and sufficiently near each other for the depolarization produced by one to sufficiently reduce the effective synaptic driving potential of the other. Essentially the same concept has been used by Kuno and Miyahara (1969) to account for nonlinearities they observed. Also, MacGregor (1968) has recently stressed nonlinear effects in dendritic regions.

How Branch Input Resistance Differs from Core Resistance

It is of interest to examine the simple notion that branch input resistance might be estimated as the series resistance composed of R_N plus successive core resistance along the direct line from the input branch terminal to the soma. Such a resistance estimate can be shown mathematically (see below) to exceed the correct value of R_{BL}; a large discrepancy results with large electrotonic branch lengths, while smaller discrepancies result with small L and short electrotonic branch lengths. The physical intuitive explanation is that simple core resistance neglects the spread of current into the sister and cousin branches, and it also neglects the leakage of current across the dendritic membrane surface; in other words, it neglects the branching and cable properties of the dendrites. However, when a branch is short, little current leaks across its membrane, and consequently, the gradient of potential along its core is nearly constant; this can be seen in Fig. 4, where the slopes along the main line are nearly constant, and the slopes in the sister and cousin branches are rather small because they must be zero at their terminals. In this particular case, the series resistance estimate is 3.97 times $R_{T\infty}$, which is about 17% larger than the correct value of R_{BL}. A larger discrepancy results when we double L from 1.0 to 2.0, keeping $N = 6$ and $M = 3$. Then the series resistance estimate is 7.67 times $R_{T\infty}$, which is about 46% larger than the correct value of R_{BL}.

---

[8] In particular, if n equal synapses are active in very close proximity, we can replace g_ϵ by the product ng_ϵ in Eq. 32 to obtain the resultant local depolarizing effect.

To explain these results, we note first that for a length, $\Delta X = \Delta x / \lambda$, of a cylinder characterized by $R_\infty = \lambda r_i$, the core resistance can be expressed $r_i \Delta x = R_\infty(\Delta x / \lambda) = R_\infty \Delta X$. Thus, the core resistance of a kth order branch segment, extending from $X = X_k$ to $X = X_{k+1}$ of the neuron model, can be expressed as

$$2^k R_{T\infty}(X_{k+1} - X_k).$$

The proposition we wish to prove can be expressed

$$R_{BL} < R_N + R_{T\infty}\left\{X_1 + \sum_{k=1}^{M} 2^k(X_{k+1} - X_k)\right\}, \tag{33}$$

where the right side of this inequality represents the series resistance estimate composed of R_N plus successive core resistance segments along the direct route from the input branch terminal to the origin (soma).

In order to prove this inequality, we refer to Eq. 22 for R_{BL} and note a useful property of the hyperbolic tangent: although tanh (x) approximately equals x when x is small, it is always less than x; in fact, the first two terms of the series expansion (for values of x less than unity) give that tanh $(x) = x - x^3/3$. Thus, we can examine each term of the summation in Eq. 22 and express a corresponding inequality. We do this here for $k = M$, $k = M - 1, \ldots$, $k = 1$, and for the term in tanh (L):

$$2^{(M-1)} \tanh (L - X_M) < (L - X_M)2^{(M-1)}, \tag{34}$$

$$2^{(M-2)} \tanh (L - X_{M-1}) < (L - X_M)2^{(M-2)} + (X_M - X_{M-1})2^{(M-2)}, \tag{35}$$

$$\cdots \qquad\qquad \cdots \qquad\qquad \cdots$$

$$2^0 \tanh (L - X_1) < (L - X_M) + (X_M - X_{M-1})$$
$$+ \ldots + (X_2 - X_1), \tag{36}$$

$$[(N - 1)/N] \tanh (L) < (L - X_M) + (X_M - X_{M-1})$$
$$+ \ldots + (X_2 - X_1) + X_1. \tag{37}$$

It should be noted that the sum of the column composed of the first expression to the right of each inequality sign simplifies to $2^M(L - X_M)$; this times $R_{T\infty}$ is equal to the core resistance of the input branch. Furthermore, the sum of all the right-hand terms of inequalities 34–37 yields the expression inside the brackets of previous inequality 33, and this times $R_{T\infty}$ is equal to the series core resistance along the direct route from the input branch terminal to the origin. Thus, referring again to Eq. 22, we can see that if we multiply the left and right sides of inequalities 34–37 by $R_{T\infty}$ and then add R_N (Eq. 11) to both the sum of the left sides and the sum of the right sides of the above inequalities, the result is precisely the inequality 33 which we set out to prove.

This proof not only demonstrates that R_{BL} is always less than this series resistance estimate, it also provides a detailed breakdown into component inequalities which can be examined to see how much each contributes. This, as well as several other points, can be illustrated by reference to Table II.

Components of Input Resistance and of Core Resistance. In Table II, the first row corresponds to inequality 34 and five subsequent rows correspond to inequalities 35–37, for the particular case of $N = 6$, $L = 1.5$, and $M = 5$, with equal increments, $\Delta X = 0.25$, for all branches. Columns A and B display the component terms of $R_{BL}/R_{T\infty}$, as defined by Eq. 22. It can be seen that the highest order term (3.92) makes the largest contribution to the numerical result; also, it differs least from its corresponding term in column C, because the hyperbolic tangent has the smallest argument. The fact that the two highest order terms are nearly equal in column B, and exactly equal in column C, results from two simplifying assumptions: the assumption of equal electrotonic length for the input branch and its parent branch, and the assumption of equal daughter diameters that satisfy the equivalent cylinder constraint. Subsequent terms in column B become progressively smaller, as the power of 2 becomes smaller in column A. The smallest term, 0.184, in column B corresponds to $R_N/R_{T\infty}$; it must be included to obtain the correct total for $R_{BL}/R_{T\infty}$, as defined by Eq. 22. When this total, 13.46, is divided by the value of $R_N/R_{T\infty}$, we obtain a value of 73.1 for R_{BL}/R_N, in agreement with the value given earlier in Table I, for $L = 1.5$, $N = 6$, and $M = 5$.

The core resistance of a kth-order branch is $2^k R_{T\infty}\Delta X$, for equal electrotonic length increments ΔX; see explanation in the sentences preceding inequality 33. For the present example, the value of the core resistance divided by $R_{T\infty}$ is 8.0 for

TABLE II

COMPONENTS OF INPUT RESISTANCE AND CORE RESISTANCE

(Using inequalities 34–37 for $N = 6$, $L = 1.5$, $\Delta X = 0.25$)

A		B		C		D	E	F			
$2^4 \tanh (0.25)$	$=$	3.92	$<$	4.0	$=$	4.					
$2^3 \tanh (0.50)$	$=$	3.70	$<$	4.0	$=$	2. $+$	2.				
$2^3 \tanh (0.75)$	$=$	2.54	$<$	3.0	$=$	1. $+$	1. $+$	1.			
$2^1 \tanh (1.0)$	$=$	1.52	$<$	2.0	$=$	½ $+$	½ $+$	½ $+$	½		
$2^0 \tanh (1.25)$	$=$	0.85	$<$	1.25	$=$	¼ $+$	¼ $+$	¼ $+$	¼ $+$	¼	
$(5/6) \tanh (1.5)$	$=$	0.75	$<$	1.50	$=$	¼ $+$	¼ $+$	¼ $+$	¼ $+$	¼ $+$	¼
		13.28	$<$	15.75	$=$	8. $+$	4. $+$	2. $+$	1. $+$	½ $+$	¼
		$+$		$+$							
$(1/6) \coth (1.5)$	$=$	0.184	$=$	0.184	$=$	$R_N/R_{T\infty}$					
$R_{BL}/R_{T\infty}$	$=$	13.46	$<$	15.93	$=$	$(R_N + R_{\text{CORE}})/R_{T\infty}$					

the input branch, 4.0 for its parent branch, and 2.0 for its grandparent branch. These values are to be found in Table II as the following column sums: sum of column D for the input branch, sum of column E for the parent branch, and sum of column F for the grandparent branch. Furthermore, the sum of all terms of the right-hand side of inequalities 34–37 provides the value 15.75 for the series core resistance divided by $R_{T\infty}$ along the direct route from the input terminal to the origin. By adding $R_N/R_{T\infty} = 0.184$ to this value, we obtain 15.93 for the right-hand side of inequality 33 divided by $R_{T\infty}$. This result exceeds the branch input resistance value, $R_{BL}/R_{T\infty} = 13.46$, by more than 18%. Even larger discrepancies result with larger values for L.

Effect of a Middendritic Input Location

Up to this point of the paper, we have considered only the input site at a dendritic terminal. What is the effect of shifting the input site to a middendritic location? One can guess, immediately, that the input resistance should be smaller than at the terminal for two reasons: the input branch diameter is larger, and the input current splits immediately into centripetal and centrifugal components. The exact mathematical consequences are derived in the Appendix; comparison of Eq. A 8 with Eq. 22 shows several changes. If the input site is at $X = X_i$ on a branch of order $k = k_i$, Eq. A 8 has X_i in place of L in the arguments of the numerators, and the summation runs only to $k = k_i$ instead of $k = M$; also, there is a factor, $\cosh (L - X_i)$ present. Suppose, for example, that $X_i = 0.5$ is used with $N = 6$, $L = 1.0$, and $M = 3$, or $M = 7$. This input site is exactly middendritic in terms of electrotonic distance. For $M = 3$, Eq. A 8 gives

$$R_{BX}/R_{T\infty} = (1.13)(0.16 + 0.28 + 0.20) = 0.72,$$

which is about 21% of the value (3.40) obtained for a terminal input site. For $M = 7$, Eq. A 8 gives $(1.13)(0.16 + 0.28 + 0.27 + 0.39 + 0.42)$ or 1.72 for $R_{BX}/R_{T\infty}$, which is only about 6% of the value (30.3) obtained for a terminal input site.

Effect of Unequal Branching

All of the results, so far, have been based upon the assumption of symmetric bifurcations along the input portion of the input tree; this makes the R_∞ value of the terminal branch cylinder equal to exactly $2^M R_{T\infty}$. However, it is important to note that these results have not depended upon symmetric branching in the other portions of the input tree, or in the other trees of the neuron model; this other branching can be profuse or sparse in terms of the number of orders M, and it can be asymmetric, provided that the equivalent cylinder constraint is satisfied, and that all terminals correspond to the same electrotonic distance $X = L$ from the origin. This generality holds because the equivalent cylinder for the (noninput) sister branch is all that enters into each superposition along the input branch lineage.

What, however, is the effect of asymmetric bifurcations along the input branch lineage? The solution to this problem is derived in the Appendix. Briefly, the R_∞ value of the input branch becomes generalized from $2^\mu R_{T\infty}$ to the product, $\gamma_1 \gamma_2 \ldots \gamma_M R_{T\infty}$, where each of these γ_k is the ratio of the R_∞ of the input carrying daughter cylinder at the kth branch point, to the R_∞ of its parent cylinder. For symmetric branching, each γ_k would equal 2; when the input carrying daughter cylinder is thinner than its sister branch, γ_k is greater than 2. In the expression for R_{BL}, the factor, $2^{(k-1)}$ in the summation expression becomes replaced by a product, $\gamma_1 \gamma_2 \ldots (\gamma_k - 1)$; compare Eq. A 9 with earlier Eq 20. Clearly, if all of the γ_k are greater than 2, both R_{BL} and the R_∞ value of the terminal branch cylinder would be greater than for the case of symmetric bifurcations; also, the attenuation factor would be greater. On the other hand, for randomized asymmetries where γ_k values less than 2 are as probable as values greater than 2, these effects will tend to cancel. Any specific example can be computed in detail.

Effect of Unequal Trees

Although the body of this paper presents a model composed of equal dendritic trees, the superposition method can be generalized to treat unequal trees. It is simplest to consider different trunk diameters while preserving a common electrotonic length L for all trees. However, Eqs. A 9–A 12 of the Appendix show how unequal L values can also be provided for. These expressions involve the ratio γ which equals the ratio of the combined input conductance of all dendritic trees (from their common origin) to the input conductance of the input tree alone. Each tree must still have branch diameters that satisfy the equivalent cylinder constraint, but the N equivalent cylinders can now have different lengths and diameters. If these lengths and diameters are all made equal, the ratio γ reduces to N.

SUMMARY

(a) Mathematical solutions and numerical illustrations are presented for the steady-state distribution of membrane potential in an extensively branched neuron model, when steady electric current is injected into only one dendritic branch. The model assumes that the dendritic membrane is passive and that the dendritic trees satisfy the equivalent cylinder constraint on branch diameters. Although the initial derivation assumes equal dendritic trees and symmetric dendritic branching, these simplifying assumptions are dispensed with in the Appendix. Also, the initial derivation limits the site of current injection to the end of a terminal branch, while the generalization in the Appendix permits the input site to be located anywhere on any branch or trunk of a dendritic tree.

(b) These solutions provide us with explicit expressions for input resistance at a branch input site, and for the attenuation factor for voltage attenuation from the input site to the soma. It is useful to express the branch input resistance relative to the whole neuron resistance R_N measured at the soma (origin) of the model. The attenuation factor is related to, but always greater than, this input resistance ratio.

(c) Table I illustrates many numerical examples of this input resistance ratio and the attenuation factor, for the case of symmetric branching, with equal electrotonic increments per branch, and with input injected at a branch terminal; the input resistance ratios range from about 10 to 700, while the attenuation factors range from about 15 to 2,000, for the ranges of N, L, and M assumed for this table. Increasing the number of orders of branching M, while keeping the number of trees N and their electrotonic length L constant, increases both the input resistance ratio and the attenuation factor approximately threefold for a two unit increase in M. Increasing N, while L and M are held constant, increases both the input resistance ratio and the attenuation factor in nearly direct proportionality with the increase in N. Doubling L from 1.0 to 2.0, with N and M held constant, approximately doubles the input resistance ratio, and increases the attenuation factor about fivefold.

(d) The application to cat spinal motoneurons is discussed with attention to recent experimental evidence showing that these neurons satisfy the various assumptions of the model to at least a reasonable approximation. Terminal branch input resistance values are estimated to lie in the range from roughly 40 to 750 MΩ; for middendritic input sites the range would be smaller, roughly 1.5–20 MΩ, or more for high orders of middendritic branching.

(e) Although applicability of the theory to other neurons is handicapped by insufficient information, the requirements are discussed and the case of pyramidal tract neurons is reviewed.

(f) The theoretical solution in the dendritic trunk (and at the soma) is the same whether injected current is applied entirely to one branch or is divided between several branches of the same tree, provided that the injection sites are all at the same electrotonic distance from the soma. This does not hold for input as a synaptic membrane conductance.

(g) Membrane depolarization at the site of a steady synaptic conductance input is not, in general, directly proportional to the input resistance. While a high input resistance does yield a larger local depolarization, this depolarization itself causes a deficit in synaptic current, because it decreases the effective synaptic driving potential. Also, because of increased electrotonic attenuation, the large depolarization at a dendritic synaptic site yields less soma depolarization than if the same synaptic conductance input were delivered directly to the soma.

(h) It is shown that branch input resistance exceeds the input resistance at the soma by an amount that is always less than the series sum of core resistances along the path from the input site to the soma.

(i) Several significant generalizations of the theoretical results are provided in the Appendix: the dendritic trees can be unequal in trunk diameter and in electrotonic length; daughter branch diameters can be unequal but must satisfy the equivalent cylinder constraint; the site of current injection can be anywhere on a branch of any order.

(j) Expressions are also derived for input impedances and attenuation for AC steady states.

APPENDIX

MORE GENERAL THEORETICAL RESULTS

Additional Symbols Used in Appendix

X_i	Electrotonic distance from the origin to the point of current *injection*, not restricted to $X = L$.
V_i	Value of V at the point of current *injection*.
$R_{C, \text{ins}}(X_i, L, R_\infty)$	Input resistance at the point $(X = X_i)$ in a *cylinder insulated* $(dV/dX = 0)$ at the origin as well as at $X = L$; Eq. A1.
$R_{C, \text{clp}}(X_i, L, R_\infty)$	Input resistance at the point $(X = X_i)$ in a *cylinder clamped* $(V = 0)$ at the origin, but insulated at $X = L$; Eq. A 2.
$R_{NC}(X_i, L, N, R_{T\infty})$	Input resistance at the point $(X = X_i)$ of one equivalent *cylinder* of the *neuron* model; or parallel input resistance of all branches (at $X = X_i$) belonging to one dendritic tree of the neuron model; Eq. A 5.
k_i	Branching order of the one branch which receives input at $X = X_i$.
R_{BX}	Input resistance at the point $(X = X_i)$ on one dendritic *branch* of order (k_i); function of $(X_i, k_i, L, N, R_{T\infty})$ with symmetric branching; Eq. A 8.
R_B	More general *branch* input resistance at the point $(X = X_i)$ for nonsymmetric branching and unequal trees (branching must still satisfy equivalent cylinder constraint); see Eq. A 11.
γ	Ratio of combined input conductance of all dendritic trees (at their common origin) to the input conductance of the input tree; Eq. A 10; reduces to N for equal trees.
γ_1	Ratio of the $d^{3/2}$ value for the trunk of the input tree to the $d^{3/2}$ value for the first-order branch which leads to the input site.
γ_k	Ratio at kth-order branch point of the parent $d^{3/2}$ value to the $d^{3/2}$ value of the input carrying daughter branch.
p_k	Product which reduces to $2^{(k-1)}$ for symmetric branching; see Eqs. A 9–A 12.
$AF_{BX/0}$	General attenuation factor from $X = X_i$ to soma; Eq. A 12.
$\omega = 2\pi f$	Angular frequency for a sinusoidal steady state.
$j = (-1)^{1/2}$	For complex variable notation.
$q = (1 + j\omega\tau)^{1/2} = (Y_m/G_m)^{1/2}$	Complex function of frequency; function of membrane admittance to conductance ratio.
$r = (1 + \omega^2\tau^2)^{1/2} = a^2 + b^2$	Modulus of q^2.
$a = [(r + 1)/2]^{1/2}$	Real part of q.
$b = [(r - 1)/2]^{1/2}$	Imaginary part of q.

$\alpha = 2aL;\ \alpha_k = 2a(L - X_k).$

$\beta = 2bL;\ \beta_k = 2b(L - X_k).$

$Z_{CL,\,\text{ins}}$ Input impedance at the end $(X = L)$ for a *cylinder insulated* $(dV/dX = 0)$ at the origin; Eq. A 15.

$Z_{CL,\,\text{clp}}$ Input impedance at the end $(X = L)$ for a *cylinder clamped* $(V = 0)$ at the origin; Eq. A 16.

Z_N Whole *neuron* input impedance at the point $(X = 0)$ of common origin of N equal dendritic trees or equivalent cylinders; Eq. A 17.

Z_{BL} *Branch* input impedance at the end $(X = L)$ of one terminal branch of the neuron model.

Effect of Input Site Not Restricted to X = L

When the point of current injection is located at the electrotonic distance, $X = X_i < L$, from the origin, the injected current divides into a centrifugal and a centripetal component. For a single cylinder of length $2L$ even symmetry (compare earlier Fig. 2 A and Eqs. 4–7) would require a source current of $I/2$ at $X = -X_i$ as well as $X = +X_i$. This even symmetry implies $dV/dX = 0$ at $X = 0$, and insulated ends also imply that $dV/dX = 0$ at $X = \pm L$. For positive values of X, we need to match solutions for the two regions that join at $X = X_i$. We can write

$$V(X) = V_i \cosh X/\cosh X_i, \quad \text{for } 0 \leq X \leq X_i,$$

and

$$V(X) = V_i \cosh (L - X)/\cosh (L - X_i), \quad \text{for } X_i \leq X \pm L.$$

which provide continuity of $V(X)$ at $X = X_i$, and which also satisfy $dV/dX = 0$ at $X = 0$ and $X = L$. In other words, these three boundary conditions have been used to determine three of four arbitrary constants; the remaining constant V_i must be determined from the requirement that $I/2$ equal the amount of core current flowing away from $X = X_i$. This can be expressed

$$I/2 = (V_i/R_\infty)[\tanh X_i + \tanh (L - X_i)]$$

$$= (V_i/R_\infty) \sinh L/[\cosh X_i \cosh (L - X_i)].$$

From this it follows that the input resistance, $V_i/(I/2)$, can be expressed

$$R_{c,\,\text{ins}}(X_i, L, R_\infty) = R_\infty \cosh (L - X_i) \cosh X_i/\sinh L, \qquad (\text{A 1})$$

for a cylinder of length L insulated at both $X = 0$ and $X = L$, with steady input current injected at $X = X_i$. This input resistance clearly depends upon three parameters, L, R_∞, and X_i. When $X_i = L$, this reduces to Eq. 7; it can be seen that $X_i = 0$ also gives the same result.

For the corresponding case of odd symmetry, with a source current $I/2$ at $X = X_i$, and a matching sink current $-I/2$ at $X = -X_i$ (compare earlier Fig. 2 B and Eqs. 8 and 9), similar treatment of this problem yields the input resistance

$$R_{c,\,\text{clp}}(X_i, L, R_\infty) = R_\infty \cosh (L - X_i) \sinh X_i/\cosh L, \qquad (\text{A 2})$$

for a cylinder of length L, which is clamped $(V = 0)$ at $X = 0$, and insulated at $X = L$, with steady input current injected at X_i. This input resistance reduces to Eq. 9 when $X_i = L$.

By making use of the insight contained in earlier Eq. 15 and the physical interpretation given in the paragraph following it, the corresponding superposition for the present problem provides the solution for the injection of steady current I at the point $X = X_i$, in only one of N equal cylinders coupled at $X = 0$. For the range, $0 \leq X \leq X_i$ of the input cylinder, this solution can be expressed

$$V(X) = IR_{T\infty} \cosh (L - X_i) \left\{ \frac{\cosh X}{N \sinh L} + \frac{(N - 1) \sinh X}{N \cosh L} \right\}. \quad (A\,3)$$

At the origin, this simplifies to

$$V(O) = (I/N)R_{T\infty} \cosh (L - X_i)/\sinh L$$

$$= IR_N \cosh (L - X_i)/\cosh L, \quad (A\,4)$$

where the second form makes use of Eq. 11 for R_N. This result remains unaffected by the branching considerations that follow; it is used later to obtain an expression for a generalized attenuation factor.

When we set $X = X_i$ in Eq. A 3, the result can be expressed $V(X_i) = IR_{NC}$, where R_{NC} represents the input resistance for this case. This input resistance can be expressed

$$R_{NC}(X_i, L, N, R_{T\infty}) = R_{T\infty} \cosh (L - X_i)$$

$$\cdot \left\{ \frac{\cosh (X_i)}{N \sinh L} + \frac{(N - 1) \sinh (X_i)}{N \cosh L} \right\}, \quad (A\,5)$$

for current injection at $X = X_i$ to only one of N equal cylinders coupled at the origin. This input resistance reduces to Eq. 14 when $X_i = L$; it also reduces to Eq. 11 when $X_i = 0$.

Next, consider one order of symmetric dendritic branching, with $X_i > X_1$. Then the odd symmetry for $I/2$ applied at X_i of the input branch, with a matching $-I/2$ applied at X_i of the sister branch, is responsible for a contribution corresponding to Eq. 18 but modified as suggested by a comparison of Eq. A 2 with Eqs. 8 and 9. Here, this contribution can be expressed

$$V(X) = (I/2)(2R_{T\infty}) \cosh (L - X_i) \sinh (X - X_1)/\cosh (L - X_1), \quad (A\,6)$$

and a similar contribution is provided by each order of branching for which the branch point occurs at an electrotonic distance less than X_i from the origin. Let k_i represent the order of the branch which receives the input current. The solution in the input branch, for $X_{k_i} \leq X \leq X_i$, can be written as

$$V(X) = IR_{T\infty} \cosh (L - X_i)$$

$$\cdot \left\{ \frac{\cosh X}{N \sinh L} + \frac{(N - 1) \sinh X}{N \cosh L} + \sum_{k=1}^{k_i} 2^{(k-1)} \frac{\sinh (X - X_k)}{\cosh (L - X_k)} \right\}, \quad (A\,7)$$

which differs from Eq. 20 (for input branch) in two respects: the factor $\cosh (L - X_i)$, and the fact that the summation runs to $k = k_i$ rather than to $k = M$. Clearly, Eq. A 7 reduces to this earlier result when $X_i = L$, with $k_i = M$. By setting $X = X_i$ in Eq. A 7 and dividing by I, we obtain the corresponding expression for input resistance

$$R_{BX} = R_{T\infty} \cosh (L - X_i)$$

$$\cdot \left\{ \frac{\cosh (X_i)}{N \sinh L} + \frac{(N - 1) \sinh (X_i)}{N \cosh L} + \sum_{k=1}^{k_i} 2^{(k-1)} \frac{\sinh (X_i - X_k)}{\cosh (L - X_k)} \right\}, \quad (A 8)$$

which may be compared with previous Eq. 22.

Effects of Unequal Trunks and Branches

There is no difficulty in treating trunks and branches of unequal diameter, provided that all of the trees satisfy the equivalent cylinder constraint (preservation of $\sum d^{3/2}$ with successive branching). This is simplest when these trees all have the same electrotonic length L. In our derivation, the importance of N was that it represented the ratio of the summed $d^{3/2}$ value (for all trunks of the neuron model) to the $d^{3/2}$ value of the trunk of the input tree, alone; when the trunk diameters are unequal, this ratio of $d^{3/2}$ values can be designated[9] as γ. Then, also the ratio of the $d^{3/2}$ sum for the "other" cylinders to that for all cylinders can be expressed as $(\gamma - 1)/\gamma$, corresponding to $(N - 1)/N$ of the previous derivations.

Similarly, for first-order branches of unequal diameter, we use γ_1 to designate the ratio of trunk $d^{3/2}$ to the $d^{3/2}$ value of the input receiving branch. The equivalent cylinder constraint implies that the corresponding ratio for the sister branch is $\gamma_1/(\gamma_1 - 1)$ because the reciprocal of this plus the reciprocal of γ_1 must sum to unity. Referring to Fig. 3 A, but with unequal branch diameters, we can see that the input current would not be represented as two equal source currents of $I/2$, but rather, a source current of I/γ_1 in the input branch, together with a different source current of $(\gamma_1 - 1)I/\gamma_1$ in the sister branch. Then, the source-sink pair of Fig. 3 B must be chosen to be currents of plus and minus$(\gamma_1 - 1)I/\gamma_1$, in order to obtain a zero slope at the sister terminal after superposition, corresponding to Fig. 3 C. This means that the product, $(I/2)$ times $(2R_{T\infty})$, in Eq. 18 or A 6 for the source branch of the previous derivation, must be replaced by the product, $(\gamma_1 - 1)I/\gamma_1$ times $(\gamma_1 R_{T\infty})$, which equals $(\gamma_1 - 1)IR_{T\infty}$; it should be noted that $\gamma_1 R_{T\infty}$ is the R_∞ value of this branch cylinder. Superposition of this source-sink current with the source current of I/γ_1 in the input branch results in a total source current of I in the input branch. Thus, with the next order of branching, we are led to a source-sink current of $(\gamma_2 - 1)I/\gamma_2$ multiplied by a R_∞ value of $\gamma_1\gamma_2 R_{T\infty}$ for the input branch; this product equals $\gamma_1(\gamma_2 - 1)IR_{T\infty}$. With kth-order branching, this product becomes $\gamma_1\gamma_2 \ldots (\gamma_k - 1)IR_{T\infty}$ instead of the product, $(I/2)(2^k R_{T\infty}) = 2^{(k-1)}IR_{T\infty}$ of previous Eq. 19.

Now, referring to Eqs. 20 and A 7, we are ready to write the generalized expression for the distribution of steady potential in the input branch, allowing both for X_i different from L and for unequal trunk and branch diameters. This result can be expressed,

$$V(X) = IR_{T\infty} \cosh (L - X_i)$$

$$\cdot \left\{ \frac{\cosh X}{\gamma \sinh L} + \frac{(\gamma - 1) \sinh X}{\gamma \cosh L} + \sum_{k=1}^{k_i} p_k \frac{\sinh (X - X_k)}{\cosh (L - X_k)} \right\}, \quad (A 9)$$

---

[9] The ratio γ takes the more general form shown below in Eq. A 10 when dendritic trees can have unequal L values as well as unequal diameters.

where $p_1 = (\gamma_1 - 1)$, $p_2 = \gamma_1(\gamma_2 - 1), \ldots p_k = \gamma_1\gamma_2 \ldots (\gamma_k - 1)$, with γ_1, $\gamma_2 \ldots \gamma_k$ defined as in the preceding paragraph, and where γ is defined by Eq. A 10 below; also, $R_{T\infty}$ and L refer here specifically to the input receiving tree.

Effect of Including Trees with Unequal L Values. In order to find the effect of unequal L values, we refer to the analysis associated with Figs. 2 D, E, F and Eqs. 12–15, where the superposition of unbranched cylinders was presented. There the component source currents and sink currents were all of equal magnitude; here these component currents must be chosen unequal in order to obtain the required superposition result. Corresponding to the even-type symmetries of Fig. 2 D, we choose unequal source currents which satisfy the previous condition at the origin, namely, $dV/dX = 0$ with a common value of V. Then, corresponding to the odd-type symmetries of Fig. 2 E, we choose unequal source-sink combinations which satisfy the following conditions: each sink current (cf., Fig. 2 E) is chosen to cancel exactly the source current (cf., Fig. 2 D) at the terminal of one of the $(N - 1)$ other cylinders; also, at the origin, $V = 0$ and the current is continuous. The result of the complete superposition is to find that γ, in Eq. A 9, represents the following generalized ratio,

$$\gamma = \left(\sum_j d_j^{3/2} \tanh L_j \right) / (d_i^{3/2} \tanh L_i), \qquad (A 10)$$

where d_i and L_i refer to the input receiving cylinder, and where the summation is taken over all N cylinders, including the input cylinder. This ratio has a simple physical interpretation: it is the ratio of the combined input conductance of all cylinders (from their common origin) to the input conductance of the input cylinder alone (taken from this origin). When all L_j are equal, γ reduces to the $d^{3/2}$ ratio noted earlier, and when all d_j are also equal, $\gamma = N$.

More General Input Resistance Ratio and Attenuation Factor

We can now obtain a more general input resistance R_B by setting $X = X_i$ in Eq. A 9, and dividing by the input current I. If we also note that Eq. 11 for R_N should be generalized by replacing N with γ, we can write our general result as the input resistance ratio,

$$\frac{R_B}{R_N} = \cosh(L - X_i) \left\{ \frac{\cosh(X_i)}{\cosh L} + \frac{(\gamma - 1)\sinh(X_i)}{(\coth L)(\cosh L)} \right.$$

$$\left. + \frac{\gamma}{\coth L} \sum_{k=1}^{k_i} p_k \frac{\sinh(X_i - X_k)}{\cosh(L - X_k)} \right\}. \quad (A 11)$$

Also, the more general attenuation factor can be expressed in two useful forms,

$$AF_{BX/0} = (R_B/R_N)(\cosh L)/\cosh(L - X_i)$$

$$= \cosh(X_i) + \frac{(\gamma - 1)\sinh(X_i)}{\coth L}$$

$$+ \gamma \sinh L \sum_{k=1}^{k_i} p_k \frac{\sinh(X_i - X_k)}{\cosh(L - X_k)}. \quad (A 12)$$

It can be seen that when $X_i = L$, $\gamma = N$, and $p_k = 2^{(k-1)}$, Eqs. A 11 and A 12 reduce to previous Eqs. 23 and 26.

Generalization to AC Steady-State Impedance and Attenuation

The same superposition scheme can be used for the AC steady state. Current and voltage become complex quantities; conductances and resistances are replaced by complex admittances and impedances. For a sinusoidal angular frequency, $\omega = 2\pi f$, the ratio of membrane admittance per unit area to membrane conductance per unit area can be expressed,

$$Y_m/G_m = 1 + j\omega\tau = q^2.$$

The cable equation for AC steady states in nerve cylinders can be expressed

$$d^2V/dX^2 - q^2V = 0, \tag{A 13}$$

which may be compared with Eq. 1 of the earlier derivation. The corresponding general solution can be expressed

$$V(X, \omega) = A \sinh (qX) + B \cosh (qX), \tag{A 14}$$

where we note that differentiation with respect to X will introduce the complex factor q into the expressions for slope and for core current.

Following the previous consideration of the even and odd symmetries in Figs. 2 A and 2 B, we obtain the corresponding impedances,

$$Z_{CL,ins} = (R_\infty/q) \coth (qL), \tag{A 15}$$

and

$$Z_{CL,clp} = (R_\infty/q) \tanh (qL). \tag{A 16}$$

It may be noted that for zero frequency, $q = 1$, and these impedances reduce to the corresponding resistances of Eqs. 7 and 9.

In the same way, the whole neuron impedance at the origin of the model with N equivalent cylinders or trees, can be expressed

$$Z_N = (R_{T\infty}/qN) \coth (qL)$$

$$= (R_N/q) \tanh L \coth (qL). \tag{A 17}$$

Also, by noting previous Eqs. 14 and 15 together with Eqs. 22 and 23, we can write down the corresponding expression for the ratio of branch terminal input impedance to Z_N, as follows

$$Z_{BL}/Z_N = 1 + (N - 1)[\tanh (qL)]^2$$
$$+ N \tanh (qL) \sum_{k=1}^{M} 2^{(k-1)} \tanh [q(L - X_k)]. \tag{A 18}$$

Similarly, the attenuation factor from the input terminal to the origin (soma) of the model can be expressed as the modulus of V_{BL}/V_0, as follows

$$|V_{BL}/V_0| = |Z_{BL}/Z_N| |\cosh (qL)|. \tag{A 19}$$

In order to obtain the real and imaginary parts of these complex impedances and ratios, we make use of the definitions of a, b, and r (see list at beginning of Appendix) as the real part, imaginary part, and the squared modulus, respectively, of q, together with the following two identities:

$$\tanh (qL) = (\sinh \alpha + j \sin \beta)/(\cosh \alpha + \cos \beta),$$

$$\coth (qL) = (\sinh \alpha - j \sin \beta)/(\cosh \alpha - \cos \beta),$$

where $\alpha = 2aL$, and $\beta = 2bL$. Making use of these definitions and identities, we can express the real and imaginary parts of Z_N as

$$\Re(Z_N) = \frac{R_N(\tanh L)(a \sinh \alpha - b \sin \beta)}{r(\cosh \alpha - \cos \beta)},$$

$$\Im(Z_N) = \frac{R_N(\tanh L)(-b \sinh \alpha - a \sin \beta)}{r(\cosh \alpha - \cos \beta)},$$

and the modulus can be expressed as

$$|Z_N| = \frac{R_N(\tanh L)(\sinh^2 \alpha + \sin^2 \beta)^{1/2}}{(r)^{1/2}(\cosh \alpha - \cos \beta)}.$$

Also, the ratio of the imaginary to the real part provides the tangent of the phase angle.

A similar treatment of the impedance ratio Z_{BL}/Z_N can be carried out, where we also define $\alpha_k = 2a(L - X_k)$ and $\beta_k = 2b(L - X_k)$. Then

$$\Re(Z_{BL}/Z_N) = 1 + \frac{(N - 1)(\sinh^2 \alpha - \sin^2 \beta)}{(\cosh \alpha + \cos \beta)^2}$$
$$+ N \sum_{k=1}^{M} 2^{(k-1)} \left[\frac{\sinh \alpha \sinh \alpha_k - \sin \beta \sin \beta_k}{(\cosh \alpha + \cos \beta)(\cosh \alpha_k + \cos \beta_k)} \right],$$

$$\Im(Z_{BL}/Z_N) = \frac{(N - 1)(2 \sinh \alpha \sin \beta)}{(\cosh \alpha + \cos \beta)^2}$$
$$+ N \sum_{k=1}^{M} 2^{(k-1)} \left[\frac{\sinh \alpha \sin \beta_k + \sinh \alpha_k \sin \beta}{(\cosh \alpha + \cos \beta)(\cosh \alpha_k + \cos \beta_k)} \right].$$

These results can then be used to compute the modulus, $|Z_{BL}/Z_N|$, and then the AC attenuation factor defined by Eq. A 19.

REFERENCES

AITKEN, J., and J. BRIDGER. 1961. *J. Anat.* 95:38.

ARSHAVSKII, Y. I., M. B. BERKINBLIT, S. A. KOVALEV, V. V. SMOLYANINOV, and L. M. CHAILAKHYAN. 1965. *Dokl. Biophys.* 163:994.

BARRETT, J. N., and W. E. CRILL. 1971. *Brain Res.* 28:556.

BOK, S. T. 1936. *Proc. K. Ned. Akad. Wet. Ser. B Phys. Sci.* 39:1209.

BOK, S. T. 1959. *Histonomy of the Cerebral Cortex*. Elsevier, Amsterdam.

BURKE, R. E. 1967 *a*. *J. Physiol. (Lond.)*. **193**:141.

BURKE, R. E. 1967 *b*. *J. Neurophysiol*. **30**:1114.

BURKE, R. E., and G. TEN BRUGGENCATE. 1971. *J. Physiol. (Lond.)*. **212**:1.

COOMBS, J. S., J. C. ECCLES, and P. FATT. 1955. *J. Physiol. (Lond.)*. **130**:291.

CREUTZFELDT, O. D., H. D. LUX, and A. C. NACIMENTO. 1964. *Pflügers Arch. Gesamte Physiol. Menscher Tiere*. **281**:129.

ECCLES, J. C., B. LIBET, and R. R. YOUNG. 1958. *J. Physiol. (Lond.)*. **143**:11.

FRANK, K., and M. G. F. FUORTES. 1956. *J. Physiol. (Lond.)*. **134**:451.

GELFAN, S., G. KAO, and D. S. RUCHKIN. 1970. *J. Comp. Neurol*. **139**:385.

HUMPHREY, D. R. 1968. *Electroencephalogr. Clin. Neurophysiol*. **25**:421.

JACK, J. J. B., S. MILLER, R. PORTER, and S. J. REDMAN. 1970. *In* Excitatory Synaptic Mechanisms. P. Andersen, and J. K. S. Jansen, editors. Universitets Forlaget, Oslo. 199.

JACK, J. J. B., S. MILLER, R. PORTER, and S. J. REDMAN. 1971. *J. Physiol. (Lond.)*. **215**:353.

JACK, J. J. B., and S. J. REDMAN. 1971. *J. Physiol. (Lond.)*. **215**:321.

JACOBSON, S., and D. A. POLLEN. 1968. *Science (Wash. D. C.)*. **161**:1351.

KATZ, B. 1966. Nerve, Muscle and Synapse. McGraw-Hill Book Company, New York.

KATZ, B., and R. MILEDI. 1963. *J. Physiol. (Lond.)*. **168**:389.

KATZ, B., and S. THESLEFF. 1957. *J. Physiol. (Lond.)*. **137**:267.

KERNELL, D. 1966. *Science (Wash. D. C.)*. **152**:1637.

KOIKE, H., Y. OKADA, T. OSHIMA, and K. TAKAHASHI. 1968. *Exp. Brain Res*. **5**:173.

KUNO, M. 1971. *Physiol. Rev*. **51**:657.

KUNO, M., and R. LLINAS. 1970. *J. Physiol. (Lond.)*. **210**:807.

KUNO, M., and J. T. MIYAHARA. 1969. *J. Physiol. (Lond.)*. **201**:465.

LUX, H. D., and D. A. POLLEN. 1966. *J. Neurophysiol*. **29**:207.

LUX, H. D., P. SCHUBERT, and G. W. KREUTZBERG. 1970. *In* Excitatory Synaptic Mechanisms. P. Andersen, and J. K. S. Jansen, editors. Universitets Forlaget, Oslo. 189.

MACGREGOR, R. J. 1968. *Biophys. J*. **8**:305.

MANNEN, H. 1966. *Prog. Brain Res*. **21A**:131.

MARTIN, A. R. 1955. *J. Physiol. (Lond.)*. **130**:114.

NELSON, P. G., and H. D. LUX. 1970. *Biophys. J*. **10**:55.

RALL, W. 1959. *Exp. Neurol*. **1**:491.

RALL, W. 1960. *Exp. Neurol*. **2**:503.

RALL, W. 1962. *Ann. N. Y. Acad. Sci*. **96**:1071.

RALL, W. 1964. *In* Neural Theory and Modeling. R. F. Reiss, editor. Stanford University Press, Stanford, Calif. 73.

RALL, W. 1967. *J. Neurophysiol*. **30**:1138.

RALL, W. 1969 *a*. *Biophys. J*. **9**:1483.

RALL, W. 1969 *b*. *Biophys. J*. **9**:1509.

RALL, W. 1970. *In* Excitatory Synaptic Mechanisms. P. Andersen, and J. K. S. Jansen, editors. Universitets Forlaget, Oslo. 175.

RALL, W., R. E. BURKE, T. G. SMITH, P. G. NELSON, and K. FRANK. 1967. *J. Neurophysiol*. **30**:1169.

RALL, W., and G. M. SHEPHERD. 1968. *J. Neurophysiol*. **31**:884.

RAMON-MOLINER, E. 1962. *J. Comp. Neurol*. **119**:211.

RAMON-MOLINER, E. 1968. *In* The Structure and Function of the Nervous System. G. H. Bourne, editor. Academic Press, Inc., New York. **1**:205.

SCHEIBEL, M. E., and A. B. SCHEIBEL. 1970. *Int. Rev. Neurobiol*. **13**:1.

SHOLL, D. A. 1953. *J. Anat*. **87**:387.

SHOLL, D. A. 1956. The Organization of the Cerebral Cortex. John Wiley and Sons, Inc., New York.

SPENCER, W. A., and E. R. KANDEL. 1961. *J. Neurophysiol*. **24**:260.

TAKAHASHI, K. 1965. *J. Neurophysiol*. **28**:908.

WUERKER, R. B., A. M. MCPHEDRAN, and E. HENNEMAN. 1965. *J. Neurophysiol*. **28**:85.

8.3 Transient Response in a Dendritic Neuron Model for Current Injected at One Branch (1974), *Biophys. J.* 14:759–790

John Rinzel and Wilfrid Rall

ABSTRACT   Mathematical expressions are obtained for the response function corresponding to an instantaneous pulse of current injected to a single dendritic branch in a branched dendritic neuron model. The theoretical model assumes passive membrane properties and the equivalent cylinder constraint on branch diameters. The response function when used in a convolution formula enables one to compute the voltage transient at any specified point in the dendritic tree for an arbitrary current injection at a given input location. A particular numerical example, for a brief current injection at a branch terminal, illustrates the attenuation and delay characteristics of the depolarization peak as it spreads throughout the neuron model. In contrast to the severe attenuation of voltage transients from branch input sites to the soma, the fraction of total input charge actually delivered to the soma and other trees is calculated to be about one-half. This fraction is independent of the input time course. Other numerical examples, which compare a branch terminal input site with a soma input site, demonstrate that, for a given transient current injection, the peak depolarization is not proportional to the input resistance at the injection site and, for a given synaptic conductance transient, the effective synaptic driving potential can be significantly reduced, resulting in less synaptic current flow and charge, for a branch input site. Also, for the synaptic case, the two inputs are compared on the basis of the excitatory postsynaptic potential (EPSP) seen at the soma and the total charge delivered to the soma.

INTRODUCTION

To understand the passive integrative behavior of a neuron, we feel it is important to study the contribution made by individual input events. The steady-state aspect of such problems in an extensively branched neuron model was presented in a previous paper (Rall and Rinzel, 1973), hereafter referred to as RR-I. Symmetry, idealized branching, and linearity were exploited there to obtain analytical expressions for the steady membrane potential distribution in a branching neuron model for steady current input at a single dendritic branch site. These results were used to calculate the input resistance at branch terminal input sites and also to determine the steady-state voltage attenuation factor from a branch terminal input site to the soma. Here, we use the same superposition methods as in RR-I to solve the corresponding transient problem for arbitrary current injection at a single dendritic branch site. An explicit expression for the response function is obtained. We illustrate our results by calculating the transient potential at several locations in the neuron model for a particular transient current applied to a branch terminal. In addition, we discuss the reduction of synaptic driving potential associated with dendritic synaptic conductances and also the distribution of total charge dissipation for a transient current injection. More general response functions are derived in an appendix. We have also applied the results presented here in a theoretical study of dendritic spine function. This work will appear in a subsequent paper.

The applicability of this model to experimental neurons was discussed in RR-I. There we reviewed experimental evidence to show that cat spinal motoneurons satisfy the assumptions of the model to a reasonable approximation. The case for pyramidal tract neurons was also reviewed.

Previous transient solutions for dendritic neuron models have usually dealt with dendritic branches by lumping them together to avoid treating them individually. Those of Rall (1960) were obtained by using Laplace transform methods to treat dendritic cylinders of infinite length. Those of Rall (1962, 1969) defined a class of dendritic trees that can be treated as equivalent to cylinders of finite length, and used the classical method of separation of variables to treat a variety of initial conditions and boundary conditions. Studies of Jack and Redman (1971 *a,b*) have extended the application of Laplace transform methods to several difficult problems involving both cylinders of infinite length and cylinders of finite length. Recently, Redman (1973) has obtained the transient potential distribution in a neuron model which receives current in only some of its dendritic trees. Even these solutions, however, do not treat input at only a single branch of a tree. Transient results providing for segregation of input between four portions of the dendritic periphery were obtained in computations with compartmental models (Rall, 1964, Fig. 9). These results demonstrated that the membrane potential time course is the same at the soma (but not in the branches) for any apportionment of simultaneous current injection amongst the dendritic terminals, and that the amplitude at the soma depends only upon the total amount of this current. This property follows, of course, from the linearity of the system. Transient problems, for dendritic neuron models and membrane cylinders have also been treated by Lux (1967), MacGregor (1968), Barnwell and Cerimele (1972), and Norman (1972); transient input to a single location, with explicit treatment of branching, has been considered by Barrett and Crill (1974), and Butz and Cowan (personal communication).

Assumptions

We make the same assumptions here as in our previous paper (RR-I). Since a detailed discussion of these assumptions was provided there we will only summarize them here. Our neuron model is composed of N identical dendritic trees each of which exhibits M orders of symmetric branching. We assume that all branchings are symmetric bifurcations and that they satisfy the 3/2-power law, that is, each daughter branch diameter raised to the 3/2-power is equal to one-half times the 3/2-power of the parent branch

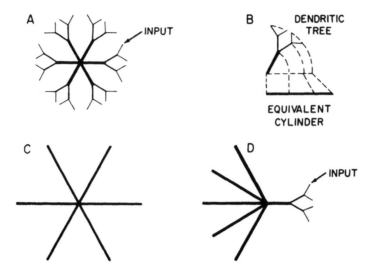

FIGURE 1   Diagrams illustrating features of the idealized neuron model. A represents the neuron model composed of six identical dendritic trees. B indicates the relation of a dendritic tree to its equivalent cylinder. C represents the same model as A, with each dendritic tree replaced by an equivalent cylinder. D represents the same model as A and C, with dendritic branching shown explicitly only for the tree which receives input current injected into the terminal of one branch; the five other trees of the model are represented by their equivalent cylinders, here shown gathered together. In diagrams A, C, and D, the point of common origin of the trees or equivalent cylinders is regarded as the neuron soma. Same as Rall and Rinzel (1973).

diameter. Hence, each tree is mathematically equivalent to a single membrane cylinder (Rall, 1962, 1964). Fig. 1 illustrates our branching neuron model with $N = 6$, $M = 2$ and the equivalent cylinder concept. Fig. 1 D should convey the following idea. When input is delivered to only one branch terminal in a single tree, the branching details of the other trees, which do not receive input directly, are unimportant. In the Appendix, we present solutions for problems with relaxed geometric assumptions.

Each trunk and branch segment in the neuron model is considered to be a cylinder of uniform passive membrane. The extracellular medium is taken to be isopotential; then, with the usual core conductor assumptions, we can treat each cylinder as a one dimensional, finite length, electrotonic cable. The membrane potential is continuous and core current is conserved at all branch points. The dendritic terminals, which do not receive applied current directly, are assumed to be sealed; that is, the membrane potential has zero slope with respect to axial distance at such terminals.

SYMBOLS

For Membrane Cylinders

$V_m = V_i - V_e$ Membrane potential, as intracellular minus extracellular electric potential; (volt).

$V = V_m - E_r$ Electrotonic potential, as deviation of membrane potential from its resting value E_r; (volt).

R_i Resistivity of intracellular medium; (ohm centimeter).

R_m Resistance across a unit area of membrane; (ohm centimeter^2).

C_m Capacity of a unit area of membrane; (farad centimeter^{-2}).

d Diameter of membrane cylinder; (centimeter).

$r_i = 4R_i/(\pi d^2)$ Core resistance per unit length; (ohm centimeter^{-1}).

$r_m = R_m/\pi d$ Resistance across a unit length of membrane; (ohm centimeter).

$c_m = \pi d C_m$ Membrane capacity per unit length; (farad centimeter^{-1}).

$\tau = R_m C_m$ Passive membrane time constant; (second).

t Time; (second).

$T = t/\tau$ Dimensionless time variable.

p Laplace transform variable for transform with respect to T.

$q = \sqrt{p + 1}$.

$\bar{F}(p)$ Laplace transform of $F(T)$.

$\lambda = [(R_m/R_i)(d/4)]^{1/2}$ Characteristic length of membrane cylinder, when extracellular resistance is neglected; (centimeter).

x Actual distance along a cylinder axis; (centimeter).

$\Delta X = \Delta x/\lambda$ Increment of electrotonic distance; (dimensionless).

$X = \int_0^x (1/\lambda)\,dy$;   Electrotonic distance from origin; in a tree, λ changes at each branch point; (dimensionless).

L Electrotonic distance from origin ($X = 0$) to the end of finite length cylinder ($X = L$).

$R_\infty = \lambda r_i = (2/\pi)(R_m R_i)^{1/2}(d)^{-3/2}$ Input resistance at origin of membrane cylinder of semi-infinite length; (ohm).

$K_{\text{ins}}(X, L, T)$ Response at time T and location X in a cylinder of length L *insulated* ($\partial V/\partial X = 0$) at the origin for instantaneous point charge placed at the end $X = L$.

$K_{\text{clp}}(X, L, T)$ Response at time T and location X in a cylinder of length L *clamped* ($V = 0$) at the origin for instantaneous point charge placed at the end $X = L$.

I Transient current applied outward across membrane at $X = L$; (ampere).

For Idealized Neuron Model

N Number of equivalent dendritic trees (or their equivalent cylinders) that are coupled at $X = 0$.

L Electrotonic length of each of those trees or equivalent cylinders.

M Number of orders of symmetric branching, specifically in the dendritic tree which receives the input.

X_1 Electrotonic distance from the origin to the first point of branching.

X_k Electrotonic distance from the origin to the kth-order branch points.

$R_{T\infty}$ Input resistance for a dendritic *trunk* cylinder when extended for infinite length away from soma; (ohm).

R_N Whole *neuron* input resistance at the point ($X = 0$) of

	common origin of the N trees or equivalent cylinders; (ohm).
R_{BL}	Input resistance at the end $(X = L)$ of one terminal *branch* of the neuron model, for current applied as in Figs. 1 A and D; (ohm).
X_{in}	Electrotonic distance from the origin to the point of current injection.
I	Transient current applied outward across membrane at X_{in}; (ampere).
$K(X, T; X_{in})$	Response at time T and location X in the neuron model for instantaneous point charge placed at location X_{in}.

For the Discussion

I_p	Peak value of transient input current; Eq. 35; (ampere).
$V_{X;X_{in}}$	Transient depolarization at location X due to current injection at location X_{in}; (volt).
$W(X)$	Time integral of potential at location X; Eq. 40; (volt-second).
Q_{in}	Total input charge for a transient current injection; (coulomb).
$i_l(X, T)$	Current per unit length flowing across membrane leakage resistance; (ampere-centimeter^{-1}).
$q(X)$	Charge dissipation per λ length; (coulomb).
$Q(X_a, X_b)$	Total charge dissipated by membrane leakage in branch section from X_a to X_b; (coulomb).
V_{in}	Transient synaptic depolarization at some synaptic site, X_{in}; (volt).
g_ϵ	Synaptic excitatory conductance at this synaptic site; (ohm^{-1}).
$V_\epsilon = E_\epsilon - E_r$	Synaptic excitatory equilibrium potential, being the difference between the excitatory emf and the resting emf; (volt).
$(V_\epsilon - V_{in})$	Effective driving potential for excitatory synaptic current; (volt).
I_ϵ	Synaptic excitatory current; (ampere).

THEORY

For the usual assumptions of one dimensional cable theory, transient distributions of membrane potential along the length of a passive membrane cylinder must satisfy the partial differential equation:

$$\partial^2 V/\partial X^2 = (\partial V/\partial T) + V, \tag{1}$$

where X, T, and $V = V(X, T)$ are explicitly defined in the list of symbols. Our basic assumption is that this partial differential equation is satisfied in every trunk and branch cylinder of the idealized neuron model illustrated in Fig. 1.

The initial-boundary value problem for the injection of a time varying current, $I(T)$, to a single branch terminal (Fig. 1 A and D), can be broken down into component problems (RR-I, Figs. 2 and 3). The overall problem consists of Eq. 1 together with an initial condition:

$$V(X, 0) = 0 \qquad (2)$$

for all trunks and branches, and with boundary conditions analogous to those of the steady-state problem. These boundary conditions can be stated as follows: $V(X, T)$ is continuous at the common origin and at all branch points ($X = X_k$); also there is conservation of current (Kirchhoff's law) at the origin and at all branch points; for the input branch, the terminal boundary condition can be expressed:

$$\partial V / \partial X = 2^M R_{T\infty} I(T), \qquad \text{at } X = L, \qquad (3)$$

where $2^M R_{T\infty}$ represents the R_∞ value (input resistance for semi-infinite length) of an Mth order branch (assuming symmetric branching which satisfies the equivalent cylinder constraint); for all other branch terminals, the boundary condition is simply:

$$\partial V / \partial X = 0, \qquad \text{at } X = L \qquad (4)$$

which represents a sealed end.

Solution as a Convolution of $I(T)$ with a Response Function

Because we are dealing with a linear system, we know that the solution, $V(X, T)$ for $I(T)$ injected at one branch terminal can be formally expressed and also computed numerically in terms of the response function, $K(X, T; L)$, which is a function of T corresponding to the response at the location X, for an instantaneous point charge delivered at $T = 0$ at the input site, $X = L$, of one branch. The Appendix treats also other input sites, $X = X_{in}$, for which the response function is $K(X, T; X_{in})$. Here we express the transient solution, for $I(T)$ injected at $X = L$ of one branch, as the convolution:

$$V(X, T) = \int_0^T I(s) K(X, T - s; L) \, ds. \qquad (5)$$

The corresponding formula in the Laplace transform space is the product:

$$\tilde{V}(X, p) = \tilde{I}(p) \tilde{K}(X, p; L) \qquad (6)$$

where $\sim$ indicates Laplace transform with respect to T, and p is the transform variable. For examples and discussion, see Chapters XII and XIV of Carslaw and Jaeger (1959).

It is useful to comment on the relation between the response function and an instantaneous point charge represented in terms of the Dirac delta functions, $\delta(T)$ and $\delta(X)$. Consider an instantaneous point charge, Q_0 coulombs, applied at the terminal,

$X = L$, of one branch at $T = 0$. This can be treated as an input function:

$$I(T) = (Q_0/\tau)\delta(T) \tag{7}$$

which is applied at $X = L$ of one branch. Then from Eq. 5, the resulting response can be expressed:

$$V(X, T) = (Q_0/\tau)K(X, T; L). \tag{8}$$

It may be noted that Q_0/τ is in amperes, $K(X, T; L)$ is in ohms, and $V(X, T)$ is in volts; also, the factor (Q_0/τ) in Eq. 7, satisfies the condition that

$$\int_0^\infty I(t/\tau)\,dt = \tau \int_0^\infty I(T)\,dT = Q_0.$$

Normalization by setting $Q_0/\tau = 1$ A, means that $V(X, T)$ in volts has the same magnitude and dependence upon X and T as $K(X, T; L)$ in ohms. For an initial boundary value problem, we can alternatively set $I(T) = 0$ and regard the instantaneous point charge as an initial condition involving $\delta(X)$; if the instantaneous initial charge is Q_0 coulombs at the point $X = L$ of one branch, the initial condition in that branch can be expressed:

$$V(X, 0) = (Q_0/\lambda c_m)\delta(X - L)$$
$$= (2^M R_{T_\infty} Q_0/\tau)\delta(X - L). \tag{9}$$

Here it may be noted that λc_m is the membrane capacity per λ length of the terminal branch, and this times $V(X, 0)$, when integrated over X, yields Q_0 as the total initial charge. Also, the second expression follows from the first because

$$(\lambda c_m)^{-1} = (r_m/\lambda)/\tau, \text{ and } (r_m/\lambda) = 2^M R_{T_\infty}$$

represents the input resistance for a semi-infinite length of the terminal branch cylinder, as in Eq. 3.

For the present problem, the required response function consists of a sum of several component response functions, where each of these components corresponds to one of the components of the steady-state problem, as presented in (RR-I, Figs. 2 and 3). The correspondence between these components is made most apparent when the component initial-boundary value problems are expressed in the Laplace transform space, as illustrated in the next section.

Case of Cylinder Insulated at the Origin

For the single cylinder with current applied at $X = L$ and zero slope at $X = 0$ (see RR-I, Fig. 2 A), the initial-boundary value problem consists of Eqs. 1 and 2 together with:

$$\partial V / \partial X = R_{\infty} I(T), \qquad \text{at } X = L \tag{10}$$

and

$$\partial V / \partial X = 0, \qquad \text{at } X = 0. \tag{11}$$

Laplace transformation of Eq. 1 yields:

$$d^2 \tilde{V} / dX^2 = (p + 1) \tilde{V}, \tag{12}$$

which is an ordinary differential equation whose general solution can be expressed:

$$\tilde{V}(X, p) = A(p) \sinh(qX) + B(p) \cosh(qX), \tag{13}$$

where $q = (p + 1)^{1/2}$. Laplace transformation of Eq. 11 yields the boundary condition:

$$\partial \tilde{V} / \partial X = 0, \qquad \text{at } X = 0, \tag{14}$$

and this requires that $A(p) = 0$ in Eq. 13. It remains to determine $B(p)$ from the other boundary condition.

Laplace transformation of Eq. 10 yields the boundary condition:

$$\partial \tilde{V} / \partial X = R_{\infty} \tilde{I}(p), \qquad \text{at } X = L. \tag{15}$$

This, together with Eq. 13 and $A(p) = 0$, yields the solution:

$$\tilde{V}(X, p) = \frac{\tilde{I}(p) R_{\infty} \cosh(qX)}{q \sinh(qL)} \tag{16}$$

in the Laplace transform space, for this particular case.

Either by comparing Eq. 16 with Eq. 6, or by setting $I(T) = \delta(T)$, implying that $\tilde{I}(p) = 1$, we obtain the Laplace transform of the response function for this component problem, namely,

$$\tilde{K}_{\text{ins}}(X, L, p) = \frac{R_{\infty} \cosh(qX)}{q \sinh(qL)}. \tag{17}$$

Here, subscript "ins" designates this case of the cylinder insulated at the origin; also X designates the point where the response is observed, p is the complex variable of the Laplace transform domain, and L designates the electrotonic length of the component cylinder; it is assumed that current is injected at the end, $X = L$. When the point of observation is also set at $X = L$, then Eq. 17 simplifies to

$$\tilde{K}_{\text{ins}}(L, L, p) = (R_{\infty} / q) \coth(qL).$$

This particular Laplace transform has a formal correspondence with the input resistance, $R_{CL,\text{ins}}$, and the input impedance, $Z_{CL,\text{ins}}$, of the steady-state presentation (RR-I, Eqs. 7 and A 15).

Case of Cylinder Clamped at the Origin

The other important special case will be presented more briefly. This is the case of a cylinder with $I(T)$ applied at $X = L$, and clamped at the origin ($V = 0$ at $X = 0$) corresponding to Fig. 2 B of the steady-state presentation. Here, Eqs. 1, 2, and 10 apply as before, and the clamped boundary condition at the origin requires that $B(p) = 0$ in Eq. 13. Then the boundary condition (Eq. 15) leads to the following Laplace transform of the response function for this component problem:

$$\tilde{K}_{\text{clp}}(X, L, p) = \frac{R_\infty \sinh(qX)}{q \cosh(qL)}. \tag{18}$$

This result for the clamped origin may be contrasted with Eq. 17 for the insulated origin. When $X = L$, this result corresponds formally to $R_{CL,\text{clp}}$ and the input impedance, $Z_{CL,\text{clp}}$, of the steady-state presentation (RR-I, Eqs. 9 and A 16). The next step is to combine these component results by means of superpositions corresponding to those of the steady-state presentation.

Result for Input Restricted to One Dendritic Branch Terminal

Given the two component results above, and reviewing the superpositions leading to (Eqs. 12 and 13 of RR-I) for N coupled cylinders and to (Eqs. 18–20 of RR-I) for the M orders of branching, we obtain the following general expression for the Laplace transform of the response function, for input restricted to one dendritic branch terminal,

$$\tilde{K}(X, p; L) = N^{-1} \tilde{K}_{\text{ins}}(X, L, p) + A N^{-1} \tilde{K}_{\text{clp}}(X, L, p)$$

$$+ \sum_{k=1}^{M} 2^{(k-1)} B_k \tilde{K}_{\text{clp}}(X - X_k, L - X_k, p), \tag{19}$$

where A and B_k are simple constants whose values are specified according to location, as follows:

in the input tree	$A = N - 1$;
in the input branch	$B_k = 1$, for all k from 1 to M;
in the sister branch	same, except $B_M = -1$;
in the parent branch	same, except $B_M = 0$;
in the first cousin branches	same, except $B_M = 0$, and $B_{M-1} = -1$;
in grandparent branch	same, except $B_M = 0$, and $B_{M-1} = 0$;
$\cdots$	
in the input trunk	$B_k = 0$, for all k;
in the other trees,	$\begin{cases} A = 1, \text{ assuming, } X < 0, \text{ and} \\ B_k = 0, \text{ for all } k. \end{cases}$

In this expression, all component response functions (Eqs. 17 and 18) have R_∞ set equal to $R_{T\infty}$.

Response Functions in the Time Domain

In the time domain, the response function, $K(X, T; L)$ for input restricted to one dendritic branch terminal is equal to the corresponding linear combination of component response functions. Thus, corresponding to Eq. 19 and using the notation introduced there, we have

$$K(X, T; L) = N^{-1} K_{\text{ins}}(X, L, T) + A N^{-1} K_{\text{clp}}(X, L, T)$$

$$+ \sum_{k=1}^{M} 2^{k-1} B_k K_{\text{clp}}(X - X_k, L - X_k, T). \tag{20}$$

This means that we can have a completely explicit expression for $K(X, T; L)$ as soon as we have explicit expressions for the two types of response functions, $K_{\text{ins}}(X, L, T)$ and $K_{\text{clp}}(X, L, T)$, in the time domain. These explicit expressions can be obtained by two quite different approaches. One is to invert the two Laplace transforms defined by Eqs. 17 and 18. These inverse transforms can be found in Roberts and Kaufmann (1966) expressed in terms of theta functions. The functional relations satisfied by the theta functions immediately give two representations for each response function. The other approach is to solve the component problems directly in the time domain. The response functions can again be represented in two ways. One way corresponds to solving the problem by separation of variables and the other by the method of images. The equivalence of the two representations is seen through an application of Poisson's summation formula (e.g., Carslaw and Jaeger, 1959).

The method of separation of variables has been previously applied to membrane cylinders by Rall (1969). To find the component response functions, we use his equations 17 and 30–32 with the initial condition $F(X) = R_\infty \delta(L - X)$ and obtain

$$K_{\text{ins}}(X, L, T) = R_\infty \frac{e^{-T}}{L} \left\{ 1 + 2 \sum_{n=1}^{\infty} (-1)^n \cos(n\pi X/L) \exp[-(n\pi/L)^2 T] \right\}, \tag{21}$$

and

$$K_{\text{clp}}(X, L, T) = R_\infty \frac{2e^{-T}}{L} \sum_{n=1}^{\infty} (-1)^{n-1} \sin\left(\frac{(2n-1)\pi}{2L} X\right) \exp\left[-\left(\frac{(2n-1)\pi}{2L}\right)^2 T\right]. \tag{22}$$

These infinite series representations converge rapidly for large values of T. For small values of T, we make use of different representations which are based upon the fundamental solution

$$V(X, T) = [Q_0 R_\infty / \tau(\pi T)^{1/2}] \exp[-(T + X^2/4T)] \tag{23}$$

for an instantaneous point charge Q_0 placed at $X = 0$ of a semi-infinite $(0 \leq X \leq \infty)$ membrane cylinder. It may be noted that $Q_0 R_\infty / \tau = Q_0 / (\lambda c_m)$, because $\tau = r_m c_m$ and $R_\infty = r_m / \lambda$. For the case of a cylinder which extends infinitely in both directions from $X = 0$, half of the charge spreads in each direction, and the expression above is divided by 2; then this agrees with Hodgkin, as cited in Appendix I of Fatt and Katz (1951). The required representations, for small T, can be constructed by using the method of images (e.g., Carslaw and Jaeger, 1959). To satisfy the boundary condition, $\partial V / \partial X = 0$ at $X = 0$, equal instantaneous point charges are placed simultaneously, along an infinite line, at locations, $X = (2n - 1)L$ for all integer values of n. This superposition yields the response function,

$$K_{\text{ins}}(X, L, T) = R_\infty \frac{e^{-T}}{(\pi T)^{1/2}} \sum_{n=-\infty}^{\infty} \exp\{-[L(2n - 1) + X]^2/4T\}. \qquad (24)$$

Also, one obtains $V = 0$ at $X = 0$ by using instantaneous point charges of alternating signs at successive odd multiple locations, $X = (2n - 1)L$, along an infinite line; this superposition yields the response function,

$$K_{\text{clp}}(X, L, T) = R_\infty \frac{e^{-T}}{(\pi T)^{1/2}} \sum_{n=-\infty}^{\infty} (-1)^n \exp\{-[L(2n - 1) + X]^2/4T\}. \qquad (25)$$

These (small T) representations of the two response functions can be shown to be equivalent to the expressions derived and used by Jack and Redman (1971 a), provided one notes that their X corresponds to our $L - X$ (for the electrotonic distance between the input site and the point of observation), and that their summation of two expressions, over $n = 0$ to $n = \infty$, is equivalent to our summation of one expression over $n = -\infty$ to $n = +\infty$; then their Eq. 11 agrees with our Eq. 24, and their Eq. 14 agrees with our Eq. 25. While these two infinite series converge well for small values of T, they converge poorly for large values of T.

We have used the large time and small time representations to advantage in our calculations switching from one to the other in order to minimize computational effort. When $X = 0$ or $X = L$, the errors made in truncating the alternate representations for $K_{\text{ins}}(X, L, T)$ and $K_{\text{clp}}(X, L, T)$ are easily bounded. For example, with $X = L$, by neglecting all terms with $|n| > 1$ in Eqs. 24 and 25 when $T \leq 0.1$ for $L = 0.5$ and when $T \leq 0.5$ for $L = 1.5$, a relative error of no greater than 10^{-5} is committed. For the large time representations, Eqs. 21 and 22, the use of at least four terms when $T > 0.1$ for $L = 0.5$, and six terms when $T > 0.5$ for $L = 1.5$, will guarantee the same relative accuracy. We observe here that the number of terms needed for a given relative accuracy depends on the length L. In this sense, the small T representations can be also thought of as large L representations and similarly the large T representations can be thought of as small L representations.

ILLUSTRATIVE RESULTS AND DISCUSSION

Asymptotic Behavior of the Response Function at the Input Terminal

Useful physical intuitive insight can be obtained by considering the response function at the input terminal, in the time domain. When an instantaneous point charge, Q_0 coulombs, is placed at $X = L$ of the input branch, the earliest spread of charge occurs only within that one branch. During this very early time (before charge spreads into the parent branch and the sister branch) the voltage transient at the terminal must be identical with the early transient for Q_0 placed at the end of a semi-infinite cylinder whose R_∞ value is $2^M R_{T\infty}$. This early transient can be expressed (compare Eq. 23) as:

$$V(L, T) \sim (R_{T\infty} Q_0/\tau) 2^M \frac{e^{-T}}{(\pi T)^{1/2}} \text{ as } T \to 0, \qquad (26)$$

where $\sim$ means "is asymptotic to."

As time goes on, the charge spreads and decays. If the membrane resistivity were infinite, there would be no dissipative charge decay, and the original charge Q_0 would spread and become distributed uniformly over the entire surface of the N dendritic trees of Fig. 1 A. The total membrane capacity of those trees equals that of the N equivalent cylinders (Fig. 1 C) and is $NL\lambda c_m$ where c_m is the membrane capacity per unit length of a trunk cylinder. Thus, the final uniform voltage (without dissipative decay) would be $Q_0/(NL\lambda c_m)$. However, because of finite membrane resistance, the charge redistribution is concurrent with charge decay (dissipative leak across membrane resistance). For very large values of time, the decaying voltage at the input terminal approaches that at all other locations; that is, for all X:

$$V(X, T) \sim \frac{Q_0}{NL\lambda c_m} e^{-T} = \left(\frac{R_{T\infty} Q_0}{\tau}\right) \frac{e^{-T}}{NL} \text{ as } T \to \infty \qquad (27)$$

where the second expression makes use of'the fact that $R_{T\infty} = r_m/\lambda$ and $\tau = r_m c_m$ together imply $R_{T\infty}/\tau = (\lambda c_m)^{-1}$. These physical intuitive considerations tell us that $V(L, T)$ begins as expression 26, but with spread of charge into other branches it departs from this transient function, and with further spread into all of the trees, it must finally approach expression 27; the complete solution must define the stages of transition from the early limiting case (26) to the final decay (27). This will now be shown to be the case.

If we set $X = L$ in Eqs. 20, 24, and 25, the response function at the terminal (for small T) is found to be:

$$\frac{K(L, T; L)}{R_{T\infty}} = \frac{e^{-T}}{N(\pi T)^{1/2}} \sum_{n=-\infty}^{\infty} \exp(-n^2 L^2/T)$$

$$+ \frac{(N-1)e^{-T}}{N(\pi T)^{1/2}} \sum_{n=-\infty}^{\infty} (-1)^n \exp(-n^2 L^2/T)$$

$$+ \frac{e^{-T}}{(\pi T)^{1/2}} \sum_{k=1}^{M} 2^{k-1} \sum_{n=-\infty}^{\infty} (-1)^n \exp[-n^2(L - X_k)^2/T]. \qquad (28)$$

For each of the three infinite series in this expression, only the term for $n = 0$ does not vanish as $T \rightarrow 0$; then, noting that

$$\left(\frac{1}{N} + \frac{N-1}{N} + \sum_{k=1}^{M} 2^{k-1}\right) = 2^M,$$

we can write

$$\frac{K(L, T; L)}{R_{T_\infty}} \sim \frac{2^M e^{-T}}{(\pi T)^{1/2}} \text{ as } T \rightarrow 0. \tag{29}$$

This is seen to agree with the previous physical intuitive result (26) when normalized by setting $Q_0/\tau = 1.0$ A in Eq. 8.

To find the large time behavior of the response function at the terminal, we use the other representation. With $X = L$ in Eqs. 20–22, we have

$$\frac{K(L, T; L)}{R_{T_\infty}} = \frac{e^{-T}}{NL}\left\{1 + 2\sum_{n=1}^{\infty} \exp[-(n\pi/L)^2 T]\right\}$$

$$+ \frac{(N-1)e^{-T}}{NL} 2\sum_{n=1}^{\infty} \exp\left[-\left(\frac{(2n-1)\pi}{2L}\right)^2 T\right]$$

$$+ \frac{e^{-T}}{L}\sum_{k=1}^{M} 2^{k-1} \sum_{n=1}^{\infty} \exp\left[-\left(\frac{(2n-1)\pi}{2(L-X_k)}\right)^2 T\right]. \tag{30}$$

First, we note that these series fail to converge as $T \rightarrow 0$, because then each exponential term under each summation approaches unity. Then we note that as $T \rightarrow \infty$, each exponential term under each summation approaches zero. Therefore we can write

$$\frac{K(L, T; L)}{R_{T_\infty}} \sim \frac{e^{-T}}{NL} \text{ as } T \rightarrow \infty. \tag{31}$$

This agrees with the corresponding physical intuitive result (Eq. 27) when normalized by setting $Q_0/\tau = 1.0$ A in Eq. 8. Moreover, the same limit is obtained at any point X in the tree. This limit corresponds to the zero order ($n = 0$) term of a Fourier (cosine) series (see p. 1492 of Rall, 1969) and is independent of X; in other words, it corresponds to a component of potential that is uniformly distributed over the entire surface of the neuron model.

When T is neither too small nor too large, numerical computations with both representations (Eqs. 28 and 30) give identical results, to many significant figures. Fig. 2 illustrates this response function with the solid curve, for $M = 3$, $X_1 = 0.25$, $X_2 = 0.5$, $X_3 = 0.75$, $L = 1.0$, and $N = 6$. These parameters correspond to those used in the steady-state example of RR-I, Fig. 4. The upper dashed curve represents Eq. 29

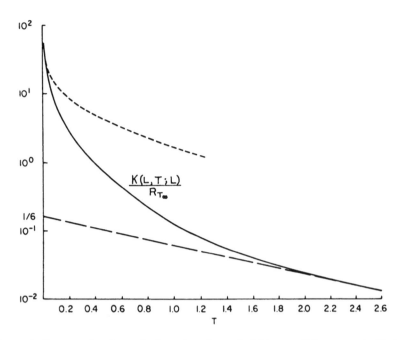

FIGURE 2   Response function at the input branch terminal (shown solid), compared with two asymptotic cases (shown dashed); ordinates are plotted on a logarithmic scale. The solid curve represents the response function defined by Eqs. 28 and 30 for $M = 3$, $X_1 = 0.25$, $X_2 = 0.5$, $X_3 = 0.75$, $L = 1.0$, and $N = 6$. The lower dashed curve is a straight line representing uniform decay and representing the asymptotic behavior of the response function as $T \rightarrow \infty$ (Eq. 31); its left intercept represents a value of $1/6$ because $NL = 6$. The upper dashed curve represents the asymptotic behavior as $T \rightarrow 0$ (Eq. 29); this also represents the response for a semi-infinite length of terminal branch. For any combination which makes $Q_0 R_{T_\infty} / \tau = 1$ mV, the values of the functions plotted here would correspond to V in millivolts; see Eqs. 26 and 27.

extended to all values of T. This full time course is valid for the limiting special case in which the length of the input branch is increased indefinitely. The earliest deviation of the solid curve from this dashed curve is due, physically, to the fact that when the spread of charge reaches the parent node $X = X_3$ its further spread is facilitated by the lower resistance provided by the parallel combination of the parent branch and the sister branch.

The lower dashed line in Fig. 2 represents Eq. 31, and it can be seen that the later decay of the solid curve agrees with this. The complications of spread over the entire surface of the neuron model, and the complications of the various infinite series in Eqs. 28 and 30 govern the precise way in which the solid curve transient passes from early agreement with the upper dashed curve to late agreement with the lower dashed curve.

The Response Function at $X = 0$

Here we state briefly the alternate representations in the time domain of the response function at the soma ($X = 0$) for input to a dendritic branch terminal. We recall that for locations in the trunk of the input tree, the branching terms in Eq. 20 do not apply, and furthermore, when $X = 0$, the K_{clp} term must vanish. Therefore,

$$K(0, T; L) = (1/N) K_{ins}(0, L, T).\tag{32}$$

For small values of T, we have the representation

$$K(0, T; L) = \frac{R_{T_*} e^{-T}}{N(\pi T)^{1/2}} \sum_{n=-\infty}^{\infty} \exp\{-[L(2n - 1)]^2/4T\}\tag{33}$$

which vanishes in the limit, as $T \rightarrow 0$. For T not too small, we have the representation

$$K(0, T; L) = \frac{R_{T_*} e^{-T}}{NL} \left\{ 1 + 2 \sum_{n=1}^{\infty} (-1)^n \exp[-(n\pi/L)^2 T] \right\}\tag{34}$$

which agrees with Eq. 31 in the limit, as $T \rightarrow \infty$, as expected intuitively from Eq. 27.

It is important to realize that the response function evaluated at the origin is independent of the manner in which the input current $I(T) = \delta(T)$ is distributed among the branch terminals. More generally, for arbitrary current injections, the solution at $X = 0$ does not depend upon the way in which the input current is shared by locations which are electrotonically equidistant from the soma.

Illustrative Transients Computed by Convolution

Figs. 3–5 illustrate voltage transients computed according to the convolution formula (5) for several different locations in the neuron model, when one particular current transient was applied to a single branch terminal. The neuron model parameters were $N = 6, M = 3$, and with all of the same branch lengths as in RR-I, Fig. 4. The input current, $I(T)$, had a time course of the form

$$I(T) = I_p \alpha T e^{(1 - \alpha T)}\tag{35}$$

with $\alpha = 50$. This input function has a smooth time course, starting from $I = 0$ at $T = 0$, reaching a peak value of I_p at $T = (1/\alpha) = 0.02$, returning halfway down at about $T = 2.7/\alpha = 0.054$, and being effectively zero from $T = 0.15$ onwards. The graph of Eq. 35 with $I_p = 1$ A, appears in Fig. 3. This function is the same as the "fast input transient" used previously (Rall, 1967). This family of input transients has also been used extensively by Jack and Redman (1971 *a, b*). As mentioned previously, we have employed both the small time and large time component response functions in our calculations. To evaluate convolutions of Eq. 35 with the small time representations, we used a technique described by Jack and Redman (1971 *a;* pp. 312–313).

In Fig. 3, the upper dashed curve shows the input current time course and the solid curve shows the resulting voltage transient at the input branch terminal. Here, a linear voltage amplitude scale has been used, and the attenuated soma voltage transient

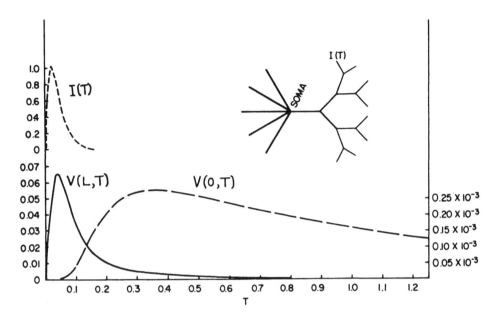

FIGURE 3   Computed voltage time course at the input receiving branch terminal (solid curve) and at the soma (lower dashed curve) for a particular time course, $I(T)$, of injected current (upper dashed curve). $I(T)$ is given by Eq. 35 with $\alpha = 50$ and shown here as $I(T)/I_p$.   The neuron model is shown upper right and the parameters used were $N = 6$, $M = 3$, $X_1 = 0.25$, $X_2 = 0.5$, $X_3 = 0.75$, and $L = 1$.   The ordinate values for the solid curve, using scale at left, represent dimensionless values of $V(L, T)/(2^M R_{T\infty} I_p e)$ where $V(L, T)$ was obtained using Eqs. 5, 28, 30, and 35.   The soma response (lower dashed curve) has been amplified 200 times; the ordinate values, using scale at right, represent dimensionless values of $V(0, T)/(2^M R_{T\infty} I_p e)$ where $V(0, T)$ was obtained using Eqs. 5, 33, 34, and 35.   The factor $2^M R_{T\infty} I_p e$ equals $8 \times (4.56\, R_N) \times (I_p e)$ which is approximately equal to 100 times the product R_N and I_p.   For example, if $R_N = 10^6\,\Omega$ and $I_p = 10^{-8}$ A, the above factor is approximately 1 V; then the left-hand scale can be read in volts for $V(L, T)$ and the right-hand scale can be read in volts for $V(0, T)$.

(lower dashed curve) has been amplified 200 times to aid visual comparison of these voltage response shapes.   In Fig. 4, the same two voltage transients have been re-plotted to a log amplitude scale, together with transients at other locations.   This permits comparison for successive locations along the main line from the input branch terminal (BI), to the parent node (P), to the grandparent node (GP), to the greatgrand-parent node (GGP), and to the origin ($X = 0$, or soma) of the model.   Also included is the further attenuated and delayed transient predicted for the branch terminals of the five other trees (OT) which do not contain the input branch.   It can be seen that with increasing electrotonic distance from the input terminal, the time of the peak be-comes increasingly delayed and the peak amplitude becomes increasingly attenuated. These peak times, amplitudes and attenuation factors have been collected in Table I. Each transient attenuation factor represents the ratio of peak $V(L, T)$ to the peak V at the location in question; these transient attenuation factors are all greater than those for the steady-state problem, which are included in the bottom row of Table I, for comparison.   It should be emphasized that these particular values depend upon

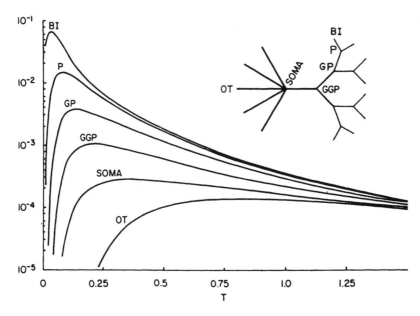

FIGURE 4   Semi-log plots of transient membrane potential versus T at successive sites along the mainline in the neuron model for transient current injected into the terminal of one branch. BI designates the input branch terminal while P, GP, and GGP designate the parent, grandparent, and great grandparent nodes, respectively, along the mainline from BI to the soma. The response at the terminals of the trees not receiving input directly is labeled OT. The model parameters, neuron branching diagram, and current time course are the same as in Fig. 3. Also as in Fig. 3, the ordinate values represent dimensionless values of $V(X, T)/(2^M R_{T_\infty} I_p e)$ where $V(X, T)$ was obtained as the convolution of $I(T)$ with $K(X, T; L)$ defined by Eqs. 5, 20, and 35 using 21, 22, 24, and 25.

the particular values of $N = 6$, $M = 3$, $L = 1$ with $\Delta X = 0.25$, and the particular input transient used. A faster input transient would result in larger transient voltage attenuation factors, while a slower input transient would result in smaller factors, with the steady-state values as a lower limit; see Fig. 3 of Redman (1973) for an illustration of this point. In Table I, the transient attenuation factor of 235 (from BI to soma) is nearly 10 times the factor, 23.9, for the steady-state case.

It may be noted that both of these attenuation factors can be attributed partly to electrotonic distance and partly to branching. This can be demonstrated by comparison with results obtained without branching (or with input current divided equally

TABLE I

TRANSIENT ATTENUATION FACTORS AND PEAK TIMES FROM FIGS. 4 AND 5,
AND STEADY-STATE ATTENUATION FACTORS FROM (RR-I, FIG. 4)

Location:	BI	P	GP	GGP	Soma	BS	BC-1	BC-2	OT
Peak time	0.04	0.085	0.135	0.21	0.35	0.12	0.27	0.46	0.84
Peak value $\times 10^3$	64.8	14.5	3.75	1.05	0.276	12.8	2.54	0.557	0.135
Transient attenuation factor	1.0	4.5	17.3	62	235	5.1	25	116	479
Steady-state attenuation factor	1.0	2.3	5.3	12.0	23.9	2.4	6.0	15.5	34.0

among the eight branch terminals of one tree). Then, for the same input current time course (α = 50 in Eq. 35) the response at the soma is the same as before, but the voltage at the input terminals is reduced. .The transient attenuation factor is reduced to 30.3 and the steady-state factor is reduced to 6.02; these reduced values represent attenuation attributable solely to electrotonic distance, and not to branching.

Transients at All Branch Terminals.

In Fig. 5, all of the voltage transients correspond to branch terminals (X = L), and the comparison is between the input branch terminal (BI), its sister branch terminal (BS), the first and second cousin branch terminals (BC-1) and (BC-2) of the same dendritic tree (see diagram of neuron model), as well as all terminals of the other dendritic trees (OT). It can be seen that the sister transients (BI and BS) become effectively identical from T = 0.25 onward; also this joint transient later becomes effectively identical with the transient (BC-1) from T = 0.75 onwards. These effects can be intuitively understood as due to rapid equalizing electrotonic spread between neighboring branches.

Also, it can be seen in Figs. 4 and 5, and verified in Table I, that both the peak time and the attenuation factor of the sister terminal (BS) exceed the values for the parent node (P), as should be expected from the intuitive consideration that the spread of charge must reach the parent node before it can spread into the sister branch. It is

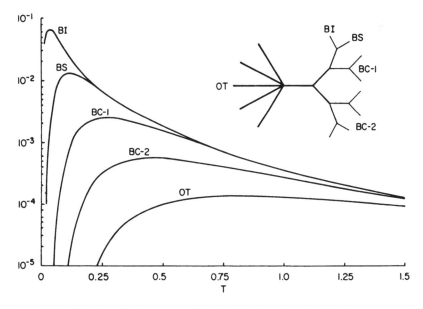

FIGURE 5   Semi-log plots of voltage versus T at all of the branch terminals in the neuron model for transient current injected into the terminal of one branch. Refer to Fig. 3 for model parameters and input current parameters. BI and BS designate the input branch terminal and the sister branch terminal. BC-1 and BC-2 designate the terminals of the two first cousin and the four second cousin branches in the input tree, while OT designates the branch terminals of the other five trees. The transients are computed and scaled as indicated in Fig. 4.

noteworthy that in both the transient and in the steady state, the attenuation from BI to P is much greater than that from P back out to BS. In the steady-state results (RR-I, Fig. 4) this is an obvious result of the fact that the zero slope boundary condition at the sister terminal (BS) tends to minimize attenuation, while the relatively large current flows at the parent node (P) permit steep gradients and large attenuation. Similar statements can be made about the first cousin terminals (BC-1) following the grandparent node (GP), and about (BC-2) following (GGP), and (OT) following soma.

Transient Peak Depolarization Not Proportional to Input Resistance

This section is concerned with current injection only; additional complications associated with synaptic membrane conductance are treated in a separate section. We will compare the case of membrane depolarization at a dendritic branch terminal when current is injected only there, with the reference case of membrane depolarization at the soma when the same current is injected only at the soma. For steady current, it follows from the definition of input resistance, that the ratio of the steady depolarizations obtained in these two cases must equal the ratio, R_{BL}/R_N, of the input resistances at these two sites. However, for brief transient input current, it is not the two input resistances but the response functions at the two input sites that must be considered; this has been noted earlier in RR-I and Redman (1973). It is the convolution of $I(T)$ with the response function $K(L, T; L)$ for the case of branch terminal input, which is to be compared with the reference case provided by convolution of the same $I(T)$ with the response function $K(0, T; 0)$ at the soma for input at the soma.

Such a comparison is illustrated by the solid curves of Fig. 6, which were computed for the same neuron model parameters and the same brief current transient as before (see figure legend for specifics). Here, the ratio of the peak depolarizations, peak $V_{L;L}$/peak $V_{0;0}$, is equal to 46.3; this is nearly three times the ratio of the input resistances, $R_{BL}/R_N = 15.5$, that was calculated for the same model parameters (RR-I, p. 667). It should also be emphasized that $V_{L;L}(T)$ and $V_{0;0}(T)$ have no overall constant of proportionality because of their difference in time course; this is seen by means of the dashed curves in Fig. 6, which rescale the amplitude of $V_{0;0}(T)$ by the factor, 15.5 for the lower dashed curve, and by the factor, 48, for the upper dashed curve. It can be seen that the half-width of this soma response time course is more than 3/2 that of $V_{L;L}(T)$. The more rapid response at a branch terminal can be understood in terms of the rapid equalization between neighboring branches.

To understand why the peak depolarizations at the two input sites scale as they do, we consider the asymptotic behavior (as $T \to 0$) of the corresponding response functions. The small time expression for the response function at a terminal input location $K(L, T; L)$ is given by Eq. 28 and its asymptotic form (as $T \to 0$) is expressed by Eq. 29. For the soma, the small time expression for $K(0, T; 0)$ is given by Eq. (54) in the Appendix, and its asymptotic form can be expressed

$$\frac{K(0, T; 0)}{R_{T\infty}} \sim \frac{e^{-T}}{N(\pi T)^{1/2}} \text{ as } T \to 0. \tag{36}$$

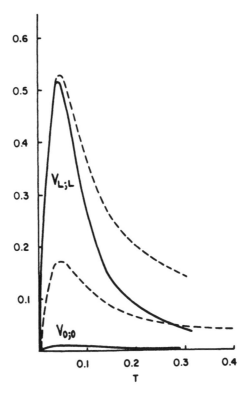

FIGURE 6   Voltage transients (shown solid) versus T at two different sites of current injection. The upper solid curve $V_{L;L}(T)$ is the voltage transient at $X = L$ for current injection to that branch terminal; it is obtained as the convolution of $I(T)$ with $K(L, T; L)$, given by Eqs. 28 and 30. The lower solid curve $V_{0;0}(T)$ is the response at the soma when the same current is applied there; it is obtained as the convolution of $I(T)$ with $K(0, T; 0)$, given by Eqs. 53, 54, and 21. The model neuron parameters and current time course agree with those used in Fig. 3. The ordinate values represent dimensionless values of $V/(I_p e \, R_{T_\bullet})$. The lower dashed curve is $V_{0;0}(T)$ times 15.5 which is the ratio, R_{BL}/R_N of the input resistance at the branch terminal to that at the soma. The upper dashed curve is $V_{0;0}(T)$ times 48 which is equal to $N2^M$ for $N = 6$, $M = 3$.

Because 29 and 36 have the same time dependence, we can express the limiting ratio of these response functions simply as

$$\lim_{T \to 0} \left\{ \frac{K(L, T; L)}{K(0, T; 0)} \right\} = N2^M. \qquad (37)$$

This ratio equals 48 for our example ($N = 6$ with $M = 3$). It follows from Eq. 37 that for very small values of T, $V_{L;L}(T)/V_{0;0}(T) \sim N2^M$, for the case of a branch terminal input site compared with a soma input site. When $I(T)$ is very brief, this makes the peak values of $V_{L;L}(T)$ and $V_{0;0}(T)$ occur early, and it follows that the ratio, peak $V_{L;L}$/peak $V_{0;0}$ will also be close to $N2^M$. This explains the peak ratio of 46.3 in Fig. 6 being close to the limiting value of 48. For slower $I(T)$, the peak values of $V_{L;L}(T)$ and $V_{0;0}(T)$ occur later, Eq. 37 does not apply, and the peak ratio is expected to be smaller; for very slow $I(T)$, the ratio, $V_{L;L}/V_{0;0}$, approaches the steady-state ratio, R_{BL}/R_N, of 15.5 for this case. The physical intuitive explanation of Eq. 37 is that at very early times, both input locations respond like the origin of a semi-infinite cylinder, and it may be noted that the response function of a semi-infinite cylinder scales as $d^{-3/2}$. The branch terminal $d^{3/2}$ value is 2^{-M} times that of a trunk of this model, while at the soma, the N trunks provide a combined $d^{3/2}$ value which is N times that of a single trunk; this implies a $d^{3/2}$ ratio of $N2^M$ which agrees with the limiting response function ratio of Eq. 37.

Before leaving this subject, we note that here we have compared different input sites which have response functions of quite different time course. If, instead, we compare input sites at the somas of two neurons or neuron models of different size but having equal L (and equal ρ if the lumped soma is considered), then the two response functions have the same time course and their relative magnitudes correspond to their input resistance ratio. Similarly, input sites on two different cylinders of infinite length ($\pm\infty$) would also have response functions whose relative magnitudes correspond to their input resistance ratio; cf., Katz and Thesleff (1957); also, Katz and Miledi (1963). But for the general case of different input sites having different response functions (of different time course), it is clear that the early portions of the responses to brief input will not exhibit the input resistance ratio.

Comment Contrasting This Ratio with Attenuation Factor

In the preceding section, we considered the voltage peak ratio, peak $V_{L;L}/$peak $V_{0;0}$ which had a value of 46.3 in the example illustrated in Fig. 6. This peak ratio should be distinguished from the transient attenuation factor (from branch terminal to soma), the ratio, peak $V_{L;L}/$peak $V_{0;L}$, and which has a value of 235 in Figs. 3 and 4, and Table I. It should be noted that for a given $I(T)$, the numerator, peak $V_{L;L}$, is the same in both ratios, but the denominators are different: peak $V_{0;L}$ is the delayed and attenuated peak at the soma for input at the dendritic terminal, while peak $V_{0;0}$ is the early peak at the soma for a separate input at the soma.

Ratios of Time Integrals of Voltage Transients

It is well known that when the applied current, $I(T)$, is prolonged and approaches a steady current, then the relative voltage amplitudes at different locations approach their relative steady-state voltage values. It is less well known, but it has been noted both by Redman (1973) and by Barrett and Crill (1974) that these steady-state relative values also hold for the time integrals of brief voltage transients, provided that these are produced by the same transient $I(T)$. To be completely explicit, this means for the present study, that

$$\frac{\int_0^\infty V_{L;L}(T)\,dT}{\int_0^\infty V_{0;0}(T)\,dT} = \frac{R_{BL}}{R_N}, \tag{38}$$

and that

$$\frac{\int_0^\infty V_{L;L}(T)\,\mathrm{d}T}{\int_0^\infty V_{0;L}(T)\,\mathrm{d}T} = \frac{R_{BL}\cosh L}{R_N}. \tag{39}$$

The last ratio represents the steady-state attenuation factor (from branch terminal to soma) of our previous paper (RR-I, Eqs. 24–26).

The easiest way to justify these assertions about the ratios of time integrals of voltage for transient $I(T)$ will also serve to prepare the way for the next section which deals with the distribution and dissipation of membrane charge over the neuron model.

We define the time integral of $V(X, T)$ as

$$W(X) = \tau \int_0^\infty V(X, T)\,\mathrm{d}T. \tag{40}$$

If $I(T)$ has a finite duration, such that $V(X, T) = 0$ at $T = 0$ and at $T = \infty$, it follows that integration of $\partial V/\partial T$ from $T = 0$ to $T = \infty$ must equal zero because $V = 0$ at both limits of integration. This means that integration of each term in the partial differential equation (Eq. 1) from $T = 0$ to $T = \infty$ yields the ordinary differential equation

$$\mathrm{d}^2 W/\mathrm{d}X^2 - W = 0. \tag{41}$$

This means that $W(X)$ satisfies the corresponding steady-state problem in all branches of the neuron model, and it follows that Eqs. 38 and 39 above must hold. The boundary condition at the input terminal can then be expressed

$$\mathrm{d}W/\mathrm{d}X = 2^M R_{T\infty} Q_{in} \text{ at } X = L, \tag{42}$$

where

$$Q_{in} = \tau \int_0^\infty I(T)\,\mathrm{d}T \tag{43}$$

is the total input charge delivered by the transient input current.

Distribution of Charge Dissipation in the Dendritic Model

The total input charge is dissipated by leakage across the passive membrane resistance of the entire neuron model, because portions of this charge spread from the terminal along the dendrites to the soma and into the other dendritic trees of the model during the time that charge dissipation takes place. Questions about how this charge dissipation is distributed over dendrites and soma have been posed and discussed by Redman (1973), Iansek and Redman (1973), and by Barrett and Crill (1974). Here we present the results obtained for our particular neuron model.

At any location in the model, charge is dissipated by the leakage current

$$i_l = V/r_m \qquad \text{amperes per centimeter,}$$

which represents a current density per unit length of the cylinder in question. For a location in a kth order branch of the model, the charge dissipation current per λ length, can be expressed

$$\lambda i_l = \lambda V/r_m = V/(2^k R_{T_\infty}) \qquad \text{amperes per } \lambda, \qquad (44)$$

where $(2^k R_{T_\infty})^{-1} = \lambda/r_m$ is the membrane conductance per λ length in a kth order branch.

The time integral of this current provides $q(X)$, the total charge dissipation per λ length, at the location X; using Eqs. 40 and 44, this can be expressed

$$q(X) = \tau \int_0^\infty \lambda i_l dT = \frac{W(X)}{2^k R_{T_\infty}} \qquad \text{coulombs per } \lambda. \qquad (45)$$

It may be noted that $q(X)$ can also be expressed

$$q(X) = \lambda c_m \int_0^\infty V(X, T) \, dT \qquad (46)$$

where λc_m represents the membrane capacity per λ length of the cylinder in question; because $\lambda \propto d^{1/2}$ and $c_m \propto d$, it follows that $\lambda c_m \propto d^{3/2}$, and for symmetric branching with the equivalent cylinder constraint $d_k^{3/2} \propto 2^{-k}$, implying that $\lambda c_m \propto 2^{-k}$ in Eq. 46, in agreement with Eq. 45.

Because the scaling factor in Eq. 45 depends on position X in the neuron model, we see that the dependence of $q(X)$ upon X is different from that of $W(X)$ and, hence, different from that of a steady-state potential distribution. To be completely explicit, this means, for brief $I(T)$ injected at a dendritic terminal, the ratio of $q(L)$ at the terminal to $q(0)$ at the soma (per λ length of one dendritic tree trunk) can be expressed

$$q(L)/q(0) = (R_{BL} \cosh L)/(2^M R_N). \qquad (47)$$

For our specific example ($N = 6, M = 3, L = 1, \Delta X = 0.25$), this means that the steady-state attenuation factor (Eq. 39) of 23.9, is divided by 8 to obtain a value slightly less than 3 for the charge dissipation ratio of Eq. 47. The physical intuitive reason why the charge dissipation ratio (Eq. 47) is smaller than the voltage ratio (Eq. 39) is that the terminal branch has a smaller membrane capacity per λ length than does the dendritic trunk; see Eq. 46 and comments attached to it.

Total Charge Dissipation in Each Branch

The amount of total charge dissipation in a segment of a kth order branch, from X_a to X_b, can be expressed,

$$
\begin{aligned}
Q(X_a, X_b) &= \int_{X_a}^{X_b} q(X) \, dX \\
&= (2^k R_{T_\infty})^{-1} \int_{X_a}^{X_b} W(X) \, dX \\
&= (2^k R_{T_\infty})^{-1} \left(\frac{dW}{dX} \bigg|_{X_b} - \frac{dW}{dX} \bigg|_{X_a} \right),
\end{aligned}
\tag{48}
$$

where use has been made of Eq. 45 and the integration makes use of Eq. 41. The last expression represents exactly the difference between the total charge which has flowed into the cylinder at X_a and out of the cylinder at X_b, i.e., the difference of the core currents integrated over time. As a consequence of Eq. 41 we see that $Q(X_a, X_b)$ can be determined merely by evaluating derivatives of W. It is important to realize that $q(X)$, and hence any integral of $q(X)$, is independent of the time course of the transient input current. Moreover, the fraction of total input charge dissipated in the segment X_a to X_b is given by the ratio, $Q(X_a, X_b)/Q_{in}$. This fraction exhibits no dependence upon input time course, provided that $V(X,0) = 0 = V(X, \infty)$; in other words, it depends only upon geometric and electrotonic parameters. Also, at the soma and in the dendritic trunks, $q(X)$ is independent of the way in which $I(T)$ might be distributed among one or more sites at the same electrotonic distance from the soma in that tree. Redman (1973) and Iansek and Redman (1973) have made a similar observation regarding the amount of charge which reaches the soma in their theoretical model.

For illustrative purposes, we have computed the fraction of total input charge dissipated in various portions of our neuron model when input is restricted to a single branch terminal. The results of our calculations are displayed in Fig. 7 as percentages. We find that the portion of charge dissipated along the mainline from the input site to the origin is 7.6 + 6.6 + 5.7 + 5.3, or about 25%. The portion dissipated in the side branches off the mainline is 4.5 + 7.4 + 9.1, or about 21%. Thus, combining the mainline with the side branches, the entire input tree dissipates about 46% of the total input charge. The portion dissipated in the other trees (5 × 10.8) equals 54% of the total. These figures account for 100% of the charge dissipation; however, if we designate a finite soma surface area composed of six initial length increments, $\Delta X = 0.1$, one from each dendritic trunk, it follows that this soma surface dissipates about 8.5% of the total input charge.

At first, it may seem surprising that half of the total input charge spreads from the input tree through the soma into the other trees, to be dissipated there. This may seem

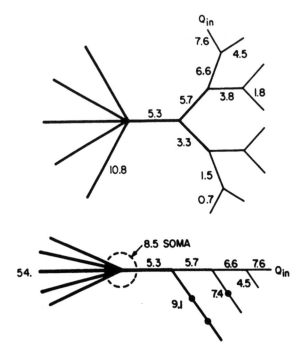

FIGURE 7 Diagrams illustrating percentages of total input charge Q_{in} dissipated in different branches of the neuron model for transient current injection at a single branch terminal. The model neuron parameters agree with those of Fig. 3. The upper diagram indicates the distinct percentages dissipated in various branches of the input tree. For those branches which dissipate equal percentages of Q_{in}, that percentage is indicated only once, e.g., each second cousin branch claims 0.7% of Q_{in}. The lower diagram shows the percentage of Q_{in} dissipated in the various side paths which leave the mainline from the input site to the origin. Also indicated is the percentage 8.5% of Q_{in} dissipated in a soma which corresponds to the segment of $X = 0$ to $X = 0.1$ of each trunk. The percentages are calculated using Eq. 48 and (RR-I, Eq. 20 where V and I are replaced by W and Q_{in}, respectively).

to conflict with the large transient peak attenuation factors; 235 from input terminal to soma, and 479 from input terminal to other trees (see Fig. 4 and Table I). One must remember, however, that charge dissipation at different locations is quite different from the transient voltage peaks for two reasons: (*1*) it is not the voltage peak but the time integral of voltage that is important here, and these $W(X)$ values relate to steady-state voltage attenuation (see Eqs. 40 and 41); (*2*) the relative values of membrane capacity per λ length further reduce the steady-state voltage ratios to give total charge dissipation ratios. It may be noted that the ratio of capacity per λ length of $(N - 1)$ other trees to that of the terminal branch equals $(N - 1)2^M$, or 40 in our example of $N = 6, M = 3$, (see Eqs. 45–47).

Which is most important, the low charge dissipation ratio, the moderate steady-state voltage attenuation factor, or the larger transient voltage peak attenuation factor? It depends upon the situation and the focus of concern. When one is concerned about the nonlinear effects of combining several synaptic inputs treated as synaptic conductance changes the voltage at the input sites is very important; attempts to estimate this from observations at the soma involve estimation of the transient voltage peak attenuation factor. On the other hand, when such nonlinear effects are shown or assumed to be unimportant, and one wishes to compare contributions of synapses at different locations, it can be useful to do this in the context of several input charges, and total charge dissipation. However, one must add the caution that such considerations of total charge dissipation completely disregard temporal considerations such as input time course and relative timing of several inputs; see (Rall, 1964, Fig. 7) for an illustration.

Synaptic Membrane Conductance Change as Input

In our previous paper (RR-I), we pointed out that synaptic depolarization at the input site should not be expected, in general, to be proportional to the input resistance at the synaptic site, and a steady-state illustration was provided. Here we will give the promised illustration and discussion for transients. There are two important factors.

One factor is often referred to as synaptic nonlinearity; when there is significant synaptic depolarization of different amounts at two synaptic sites, equal conductance transients do not produce equal synaptic current; this is explained and illustrated below. The other factor is the difference between the response functions at different input sites; this has been discussed above with Eq. 37 and Fig. 6.

For a transient excitatory membrane conductance, $g_\epsilon(T)$, the synaptic current $I_\epsilon(T)$ is given by

$$I_\epsilon(T) = g_\epsilon(T)[V_\epsilon - V_{in}(T)], \tag{49}$$

where V_ϵ is the synaptic equilibrium potential, assumed constant, and $V_{in}(T)$ is the transient depolarization at the input site X_{in}. Explanation and discussion of how this equation relates to the membrane equivalent circuit can be found in earlier papers (Rall, 1962, 1964); there G_ϵ was used to represent g_ϵ per unit area. The important point to notice is that membrane depolarization (increase of V_{in} from its zero resting value) reduces the effective synaptic driving potential, $V_\epsilon - V_{in}$, during the temporal variation of g_ϵ; consequently, less synaptic current flows than would have flowed if V_{in} did not change in Eq. 49.

The solution in all parts of the neuron model can be expressed in terms of the response function $K(X, T; X_{in})$ for current input at X_{in}. In particular, the solution at X_{in} satisfies

$$V_{in}(T) = \int_0^T I_\epsilon(s)K(X_{in}, T - s; X_{in}) \, ds.$$

The convolution on the right defines V_{in} explicitly only when I_ϵ does not depend upon V_{in}; however, substitution of Eq. 49 yields

$$V_{in}(T) = \int_0^T g_\epsilon(s)[V_\epsilon - V_{in}(s)]K(X_{in}, T - s; X_{in})\,ds. \tag{50}$$

This is a linear Volterra integral equation for $V_{in}(T)$. The equivalent steady-state equation is the linear algebraic equation appearing immediately before Eq. 32 in RR-I.

Solutions of Eq. 50 for particular transient $g_\epsilon(T)$ at particular locations must be obtained numerically. Barrett and Crill (1974) have computed such solutions. Equivalent computations for a compartmental model have been illustrated (Rall, 1967, Fig. 4). Here we summarize results obtained by numerical solution of Eq. 50 for the two cases of soma synaptic input location and dendritic terminal synaptic input location in our neuron model.

Our computations used the same neuron parameters as in the calculations for Figs. 3–7; here, we set $R_N = 1$ MΩ. The synaptic conductance time course was of the form given by Eq. 35 with $\alpha = 50$ and I_p replaced by 10^{-7} mho; hence the maximum conductance, attained at $T = 0.02$, was equal to 10^{-7} mho. When this $g_\epsilon(T)$ was applied to the soma, it resulted in a peak depolarization, peak $V_{in} \approx 0.0138\ V_\epsilon$ at the soma. Note that for $V_\epsilon = 70$ mV, this peak $V_{in} \approx 1$ mV, which lies near the upper end of the experimental size range for a unitary (single terminal) somatic EPSP of cat spinal motoneurons (Iansek and Redman, 1973; see also Burke, 1967, and Kuno 1971). The fact that this peak V_{in}/V_ϵ is much smaller than unity implies that the synaptic driving potential remains also constant. Thus, the peak value of $I_\epsilon(T)$ was found to be 99% of the reference value obtained when V_{in} is replaced by zero in Eq. 49. Similarly, for this case, peak V_{in} was 99% of the reference value obtained when V_{in} is replaced by zero on the right in Eq. 50.

Greater effects were found when the same $g_\epsilon(T)$ was applied to a branch terminal. There, peak $V_{in} = 0.411\ V_\epsilon$, which implies a very significant reduction of the synaptic driving potential, varying with time. The resulting synaptic current had its peak value reduced to 68.2% of its reference value; however, its time integral (the total input charge) was reduced to 67.2% of its reference value obtained when $V_{in} = 0$ in Eq. 49. The difference between the 68.2 and the 67.2% figures results from a slight distortion of the current time course; this is indicated also by a synaptic current peak time, $T = 0.014$, compared with a reference value of 0.02 for the input transient with $\alpha = 50$. It may be noted that with larger membrane depolarization at the input site, larger distortions of synaptic current should be expected to produce large discrepancies between the reduction in the current peak and the reduction in the total input charge.

The resulting EPSP at the soma for the above synaptic current at a dendritic terminal was computed by means of the response function at the soma for current injection at a branch terminal (Eqs. 33 and 34). This EPSP had a peak value of 0.00184 V_ϵ, which was 67.2% of its reference value, in agreement with the reduction of total input charge.[1] When this EPSP peak at the soma is compared with the peak $V_{in} = 0.411\ V_\epsilon$ at the

---

[1] It is useful to know that the EPSP peak at the soma remains proportional to the total input charge at the branch terminal, even for slight changes in brief input time course.

branch terminal synaptic site, one obtains a peak voltage attenuation factor of 224 for this case. For those quantitatively inclined, one asks why this attenuation factor is 5% less than the factor of 235 found for the reference case of current injection. The answer is to be found in the fact that peak V_{in} (of 0.411 V_e) at the branch terminal was only 63.9% of its reference value, even though the time integral of $V_{in}(T)$ was 67.2% of its reference value. The difference between these 63.9 and 67.2% values results from a distortion of voltage time course that is revealed also by a voltage peak time, T = 0.036, at the branch terminal, compared with T = 0.04 for the reference case. When the input charge and the soma peak were both reduced to 67.2%, while the input peak was reduced to 63.9%, the attenuation factor becomes reduced from 235 to (63.9/67.2) (235) = 224.

It is instructive to briefly recapitulate this example of the several factors that effect the EPSP at the soma when a brief synaptic conductance transient is shifted from the soma to a branch terminal. Although the input resistance ratio, R_{BL}/R_N, is 15.5, the ratio of the voltage peaks at these two synaptic sites would be 46.3 (Fig. 6) if the input were current injection; however, because of synaptic conductance, this ratio of voltage peaks is reduced to about 30. Then the transient attenuation factor of 224 from the branch terminal to the soma results in an EPSP at the soma whose peak is less than one-seventh of that obtained with the same synaptic input at the soma.

Next, if we compare the charge delivered to and dissipated by the soma membrane in these two cases, the difference appears smaller. We have already noted that the synaptic conductance transient at the branch terminal delivered only 67.2% of the reference input charge. From Fig. 7, we are reminded that 8.5% of the actual input charge will be dissipated at the soma designated there; the result is (8.5) (0.672) = 5.7% of the reference input charge. For synaptic input at the soma, 99% of the reference input charge was delivered, and of this, 12.7% can be shown to be the portion dissipated at the same designated soma; this is about 12.6% of the reference input charge. Therefore, the ratio, 5.7/12.7 $\simeq$ 0.45 tells us that the amount of charge dissipated at the soma for the synaptic input at the branch terminal is almost half that dissipated at the soma for the synaptic input at the soma. This is in general agreement with estimates that Barrett and Crill (1974) obtained for their example. There is no contradiction between the charge dissipation ratios and the voltage peak ratios; the difference results from the fact that the EPSP for somatic input has an earlier and larger voltage peak, while that for distal dendritic input is slower with a later, more flattened and lower voltage peak (cf. illustrations in Rall 1962, 1964, 1967).

We conclude with a simple example illustrating nonlinear summation of transient EPSPs. This phenomenon results from the reduction in driving potential caused by the proximity in time and/or spatial location of multiple synaptic events. The consequence for simultaneous dendritic conductance inputs is that the EPSP seen at the soma does indeed depend on how the synaptic conductance transient is distributed between the branches. This is not the case for current inputs. Consider the above example. If the synaptic conductance g_e is shared equally by the eight branch terminals of one tree, the peak g_e is 1.25×10^{-8} mho for each terminal and very little reduction in synaptic driving potential is found. The peak value of I_ϵ is 94% of its reference value. The resulting EPSP at the soma is also reduced to 94% of the reference value.[1] This contrasts with the previous example of EPSP reduction to 67% when the synaptic input (conductance transient) was all placed on a single branch. This provides one more specific illustration of this transient phenomenon which has been previously discussed and illustrated (Rall, 1964, 1967, 1970). Nonlinear summation of synaptic input occurs when the individual synapses cause significant membrane depolarization (reduction of synaptic driving potential) at the time and place of the other synaptic inputs. Questions related to this phenomenon have also been addressed by Iansek and Redman (1973).

SUMMARY

(a) Analytic expressions are obtained for the response function corresponding to an instantaneous pulse of current injected to a single dendritic branch in a branched dendritic neuron model. In the main text these results are derived under strict assumptions of symmetry; more general results are provided in the Appendix. The dendritic membrane is assumed passive and the branching satisfies the 3/2-power law. The response function is obtained by a superposition technique using component response functions. This technique was described for the corresponding steady state problem in (Rall and Rinzel, 1973). Each component response function has two different series representations: one converges better as $T \to \infty$; the other as $T \to 0$. These alternate representations are used to analyze the small time and large time behavior of the response function.

(b) The voltage transients at various points in the dendritic tree for a brief current injection at a terminal branch were computed using the response function in a convolution formula (Eq. 5); these transients are illustrated in Figs. 4 and 5. The attenuation and delay characteristics of the depolarization peak as it spreads throughout the neuron model are summarized in Table I.

(c) Because the system is linear, the transient depolarization seen at the soma is independent of the way in which a given current input might be shared among several branches provided the input locations are (electrotonically) equidistant from the soma.

(d) In general, the peak depolarization for a given current injection is not proportional to the input resistance at the injection site. An example, which compares a branch terminal site with a soma site, is presented to illustrate this point. For this case, the ratio of depolarization peaks, for a brief current input, very nearly equals $N2^M$, the ratio of the input resistance of the input branch extended as a semi-infinite cylinder to the input resistance of the parallel combination of all the dendritic trunks extended as semi-infinite cylinders.

(e) While there is severe attenuation of voltage transients from branch input sites to the soma, the fraction of total input charge actually delivered to the soma and other trees is about one-half. This fraction is independent of the input time course. The calculation of the fraction of charge dissipated in various portions of the dendritic tree is outlined and an example is illustrated by Fig. 7.

(f) When synaptic input is represented as a conductance change, it is important to consider the reduction in the effective synaptic driving potential caused by membrane depolarization at the input site. This is taken rigorously into account by Eqs. 49 and 50. For any given input site and given synaptic conductance time course, one can compute both a reference voltage transient (assuming $V_{in} = 0$ in Eq. 50, right-hand side), and the actual reduced voltage transient defined by Eq. 50. An illustrative example showed the peak synaptic current at the branch terminal reduced to 68% of the reference value, the total input charge reduced to 67% of reference, the local voltage peak reduced to 64% of reference, and the EPSP peak at the soma reduced to 67% of reference. In contrast, the same synaptic conductance input at the soma resulted in 99% of reference synaptic current and 99% of reference EPSP.

APPENDIX

Generalizations

In the Appendix of RR-I we provided the steady-state solutions to a variety of problems with relaxed assumptions of symmetry and input location. Here we consider some analogous transient problems. In each case we give the Laplace transformed response functions. For Eqs. 51–53, 55, and 56, the appropriate time domain expressions can be found by using the addition formulas for the hyperbolic functions along with the component response function inversions (Eqs. 21, 22, 24 and 25). We do not present derivations of the solutions to the problems considered below. Rather, we obtain the Laplace transformed response functions for a given problem from the corresponding steady-state solution for maintained unit current injection, $I = 1$, as follows. We replace the argument Z of any hyperbolic function by qZ and then multiply the entire steady-state solution by q^{-1}. This formal procedure is based on the observation that under the change of variable $Y = qX$, the transformed transient problem for the response function becomes a steady-state problem with steady current source q^{-1}. If one prefers to derive these results, the discussion which accompanies the solution of the steady-state problems in RR-I is applicable here also.

Effect of Input Site Not Restricted to $X = L$

Suppose the site of current injection is located at a distance X_{in} from the origin on a branch of order k_i so that $X_{k_i} \leq X_{in} \leq X_{k_{i+1}}$. Then the response function $K(X, T; X_{in})$ is obtained from RR-I, Eq. A 7, by following the above recipe. If we use the component response functions 17 and 18, we can express the solution in the input branch, for $X_{k_i} \leq X \leq X_{in}$, as

$$\tilde{K}(X, p; X_{in}) = \cosh[q(L - X_{in})]\left[N^{-1}\tilde{K}_{ins}(X, L, p)\right.$$

$$\left. + (N - 1)N^{-1}\tilde{K}_{clp}(X, L, p) + \sum_{k=1}^{k_i} 2^{(k-1)}\tilde{K}_{clp}(X - X_k, L - X_k, p)\right] \quad (51)$$

The response function, evaluated at $X = 0$, takes the reduced form

$$\tilde{K}(0, p; X_{in}) = N^{-1}\cosh[q(L - X_{in})]\tilde{K}_{ins}(0, L, p). \quad (52)$$

In the special case when $X_{in} = 0$, this can be written (using Eq. 17)

$$\tilde{K}(0, p; 0) = N^{-1} \tilde{K}_{\text{ins}}(L, L, p).\tag{53}$$

Thus, for example, the small T representation follows from Eq. 24 as

$$K(0, T; 0) = \frac{R_{T_\bullet} e^{-T}}{N(\pi T)^{1/2}} \sum_{n=-\infty}^{\infty} \exp[-(2nL)^2/4T].\tag{54}$$

Effects of Unequal Trunks and Branches

To treat the case in which the trunks and branches of the trees are not equal in diameter we refer to notation introduced in RR-I. The ratio of the summed $d^{3/2}$ value (for all trunks) to the $d^{3/2}$ value of the trunk of the input tree is denoted by γ. For a kth order branch point, γ_k is the ratio of the parent $d^{3/2}$ value to the $d^{3/2}$ value of the input carrying daughter branch. Now suppose all the trees have the same electrotonic length L. Then, in analogy with RR-I, Eq. A 9, the transformed response function for $X_{k_i} \leq X \leq X_{in}$ is

$$\tilde{K}(X, p; X_{in}) = \cosh[q(L - X_{in})][\gamma^{-1} \tilde{K}_{\text{ins}}(X, L, p)$$

$$+ (1 - \gamma^{-1}) \tilde{K}_{\text{clp}}(X, L, p) + \sum_{k=1}^{k_i} p_k \tilde{K}_{\text{clp}}(X - X_k, L - X_k, p)],\tag{55}$$

where $p_1 = \gamma_1 - 1, p_2 = \gamma_1(\gamma_2 - 1), \ldots, p_k = \gamma_1 \gamma_2 \ldots (\gamma_k - 1)$. At the origin we have

$$\tilde{K}(0, p; X_{in}) = \gamma^{-1} \cosh[q(L - X_{in})] \tilde{K}_{\text{ins}}(0, L, p).\tag{56}$$

In the case where the trees are not restricted to have the same length, the expressions 55 and 56 apply provided we replace γ by

$$\gamma = \left[\sum_j d_j^{3/2} \tanh(qL_j) \right] / [d_{in}^{3/2} \tanh(qL_{in})],\tag{57}$$

where the subscript "in" refers to the input tree. Implicit in the component response functions is a value for $R_\bullet$ which should be taken equal to the $R_{T_\bullet}$ value for the input tree.

The authors wish to thank Steven Goldstein, Maurice Klee, and Stephen Redman for helpful comments on the manuscript.

Received for publication 7 May 1974 and in revised form 23 July 1974.

REFERENCES

BARNWELL, G. M., and B. J. CERIMELE. 1972. *Kybernetik.* **10**:144.
BARRETT, J. N., and W. E. CRILL. 1974. *J. Physiol. (Lond.).* **239**:301, 325.
BURKE, R. E. 1967. *J. Neurophysiol.* **30**:1114.
CARSLAW, H. S., and J. C. JAEGER. 1959. Conduction of Heat in Solids. Oxford Press, London. 510.
FATT, P., and B. KATZ. 1951. *J. Physiol. (Lond.).* **115**:320.
IANSEK, R., and S. J. REDMAN. 1973. *J. Physiol. (Lond.).* **234**:665.
JACK, J. J. B., and S. J. REDMAN. 1971 *a. J. Physiol. (Lond.).* **215**:283.
JACK, J. J. B., and S. J. REDMAN. 1971 *b. J. Physiol. (Lond.).* **215**:321.
KATZ, B., and R. MILEDI. 1963. *J. Physiol. (Lond.).* **168**:389.
KATZ, B., and S. THESLEFF. 1957. *J. Physiol. (Lond.).* **137**:267.

KUNO, M. 1971. *Physiol. Rev.* **51**:657.

LUX, H. D. 1967. *Pflügers Arch.* **297**:238.

MACGREGOR, R. J. 1968. *Biophys. J.* **8**:305.

NORMAN, R. S. 1972. *Biophys. J.* **12**:25.

RALL, W. 1960. *Exp. Neurol.* **2**:503.

RALL, W. 1962. *Ann. N. Y. Acad. Sci.* **96**:1071.

RALL, W. 1964. *In* Neural Theory and Modeling. R. F. Reiss, editor. Stanford University Press, Stanford, Calif. 73.

RALL, W. 1967. *J. Neurophysiol.* **30**:1138.

RALL, W. 1969. *Biophys. J.* **9**:1483.

RALL, W. 1970. *In* Excitatory Synaptic Mechanisms. P. Anderson and J. K. S. Jansen, editors. Universitets Forlaget, Oslo. 175.

RALL, W., and J. RINZEL. 1973. *Biophys. J.* **13**:648.

REDMAN, S. J. 1973. *J. Physiol. (Lond.).* **234**:637.

ROBERTS, G. E., and H. KAUFMAN. 1966. Table of Laplace Transforms. Saunders, Philadelphia. 367.

9 EFFECTS OF CHANGING DIAMETER ON IMPULSE PROPAGATION

Introduction by John Rinzel and Idan Segev

Goldstein, S., and Rall, W. (1974). Change of action potential shape and velocity for changing core conductor geometry. *Biophys. J.* 14:731–757.

Nearly all neuroscientists are aware that Wil Rall's theorizing was fundamental to our current understanding of the functional significance of dendritic trees. Most of his work exploited the simplifying assumption that membrane potential remained below threshold level for activating voltage-dependent currents, that is, that the membrane was passive. Few may be aware that Wil had also studied action-potential propagation in branching geometries for active membrane cables, one of the subject areas of Goldstein and Rall 1974. More broadly, this work considers active propagation in regions of changing diameter and propagation toward cable (axon) termination.

As is typical of Wil's work, the problems are cast in a general framework. The model is formulated in an idealized way, retaining the barest essentials, thereby enabling conclusions with wide application. Both the active membrane model and the core conductor geometry are formulated with minimal detail.

The model of membrane excitability is qualitative, rather than quantitative; it originated with the Rall and Shepherd 1968 work (see that paper and Shepherd's commentary in section 5.1). It served adequately for the questions being addressed by Goldstein and Rall, for which particular gating properties of the conductance variables were thought unimportant. Additional motivation for this model included computational efficiency. Its nonlinearities are polynomial, rather than exponential, and so it can be integrated numerically more quickly than the Hodgkin and Huxley (1952) model. Moreover, the HH model had only been quantitatively determined for squid axon membrane, so its generality was limited.

Earlier, when Wil was developing a generalized definition of electrotonic length, he formulated a general cable equation that allowed for arbitrarily changing diameter with distance (Rall 1962a). A special case, the exponential taper, led to a particularly simple, modified cable equation. The only change was a convective term, $K\, dV/dZ$, added to the equation; here, Z is electrotonic distance, and K, the taper rate. As a consequence the velocity of a steadily propagating impulse was increased by an amount K in the direction of outward flare, or decreased by K in the opposite direction.

For one of us (John Rinzel), the mathematics in Rall's 1962 paper was magnetic, highly attractive. Here, a physiologist was carrying out mathematics similar to what I was seeing in my early graduate study in applied mathematics. I read this paper many times; my copy has numerous marginal notes and so many underlines that I probably should have underlined that which I wanted to skip over rather than read again. The work showed a unique combination of abstract formulation and mathematical analytic skill being brought to bear on identifiable physiology.

The Goldstein-Rall paper also reiterated Wil's general observation of 1962 that, if membrane and cytoplasmic properties are uniform in a branching tree, the treatment of propagation through branch points with impedance mismatch is equivalent to allowing a sudden change in diameter in an unbranched cable (assuming that effects of boundary conditions at terminals, or subsequent branching, could be ignored). As Wil had been pointing out for some time, impedances are matched if the parent diameter raised to the 3/2 power equals the summed daughter diameters each raised to the 3/2 power. A new corollary presented here was that if an action potential successfully propagated into one daughter branch, then it did so in every daughter. This meant under the stated assumptions that branching *per se* could not mediate selective filtering of action potentials, that is, routing of some impulses to, say, smaller or larger branches and not to others. Goldstein and Rall argued that branch points (and step change in axon diameter) can filter repetitive spikes but that this filtering would be the same for all postchange branches.

Experimentally it was, however, shown that differential filtering effects do occur at some branching axons (Grossman et al. 1979). The theoretical result of Goldstein and Rall thus forced many researchers to seek alternative explanations for this experimental observation. For example, differential channeling of action potentials into branches of the same axon could be explained when differences in membrane excitability or in the extracellular space (Parnas and Segev 1979) or in the axial resistivity of the daughter branches (Stockbridge 1989) were assumed (see reviews by Khodorov and Timin [1975]; Parnas [1979]; Swadlow et al. [1980]; and Waxman [1985]). A recent computational study (Manor et al. 1991a,b) on active propagation in axonal trees contains many references to related theoretical work on information channeling in geometrically nonuniform axons.

The equivalence of these two cases, the branching and the step change in diameter, meant that it was sufficient to study propagation in an unbranched cable in which the diameter jumped from one value to another at a location Z'. The quantity GR (geometrical ratio) was introduced to quantify the different cases of interest. GR equals the ratio of the two diameters raised to the 3/2 power (for a given direction of propagation, the diameter beyond the branch point appears in the numerator or, for branching, the sum of the daughter diameters each raised to the 3/2 power forms the numerator). Numerical solutions of the cable equations showed here that propagation fails if GR is much greater than one and succeeds when GR is less than a critical value, which exceeds one. (The case of failure was characterized analytically for an idealized problem by Pauwelussen [1982]). The reciprocal of GR (relative to its critical value) can be thought of as the physiologist's safety factor for this problem. From dimensional analysis, the asymptotic speed beyond the branch point must be either less or greater than the approach speed depending on whether GR < 1 or GR > 1, respectively. Goldstein and Rall showed, however, that impulse speed changed transiently near Z'; say for GR > 1, decelerating before and accelerating after encountering Z'. Overall, the action potential is delayed in this case as compared to the case with GR = 1.

The deceleration on approach to Z' for GR > 1 leads to an intermediate case for GR just less than the critical value. This paper showed that if the delay associated with this deceleration was substantial enough, the membrane behind Z' would recover from refractoriness. Then it could become reexcited by current spreading from the depolarization associated with the (delayed) impulse traveling successfully away from Z' in the forward direction. As a consequence, a second impulse was initiated that traveled in the backward direction, an echo or reflected wave. This phenomenon has been seen in some other models, although not very robustly for the HH model (Ramon et al. 1975). Some progress is being made to reveal for models such as Wil's the mathematical structure that underlies reflection (Rinzel 1990). Experimentally, the delay at axonal sites with low safety factor for propagation is reflected by a depolarizing hump on the falling phase of the action potential just before these sites. Typically this hump attenuates in the backward direction and does not succeed to elicit a second, full-blown, action potential (e.g., Khodorov and Timin 1975; Parnas and Segev 1979).

Goldstein and Rall also explored the case of an action potential traveling toward an axon termination where the sealed-end boundary condition was assumed. An interesting insight gained from this work is that this boundary condition is also satisfied, by even symmetry, at the point where two action potentials traveling towards each other along a uniform axon collide. As in the case of other nonuniformities, the action potential's velocity and shape are expected to change near the region of nonuniform properties. In the case of a sealed-end boundary (which is the limiting case for a sudden narrowing of the axon) the velocity and amplitude of the action potential increase.

This work was thought provoking for both experimentalists and theoreticians. It touches upon an important controversy (still unsettled) about axons. Does the axon function as a faithful transmission line, or should axons be treated as rather complicated processing devices where, under some conditions, spikes may differentially travel into one subtree and not to another? In this context, it has been speculated that branch-point failure may affect synaptic reliability and probability of release (Henneman et al. 1984). Goldstein and Rall's study shed some light on these issues and directed the experimentalists and theoreticians to further explore this topic. Theoretically, this work can also be viewed as part of the attempt, initiated by R. FitzHugh (1961), to develop reduced models of membrane excitability that can be explored analytically, using phase-plane techniques. Such reduced models of excitable membrane give important insights into the role of the various neuronal parameters in determining the repertoire of electrical activity of neurons (see Rinzel and Ermentrout 1989 for a review).

References

FitzHugh, R. (1961) Impulses and physiological states in models of nerve membrane. *Biophys. J.* 1:445–466.

Goldstein, S., and Rall, W. (1974) Change of action potential shape and velocity for changing core conductor geometry. *Biophys. J.* 14:731–757.

Grossman, Y., Parnas, I., and Spira, M. E. (1979) Differential conduction block in branches of a bifurcating axon. *J. Physiol.* 295:283–305.

Henneman, E., Luscher, H.-R., and Mathis, J. (1984) Simultaneously active and inactive synapses of single Ia fibres on cat spinal motoneurones. *J. Physiol. (Lond.)* 352:147–161.

Hodgkin, A. L., and Huxley, A. F. (1952) A quantitative description of membrane current and its application to conduction and excitation in nerve. *J. Physiol. (Lond.)* 117:500–544.

Khodorov, B. I., and Timin, E. N. (1975) Nerve impulse propagation along nonuniform fibers (investigation using mathematical models). *Prog. Biophys. Molec. Biol.* 30:145–184.

Manor, Y., Gonczarowski, Y., and Segev, I. (1991a) Propagation of action potentials along complex axonal tree: Model and implimentation. *Biophys. J.* 60: 1411–1423.

Manor, Y., Koch, C., and Segev, I. (1991b) Effect of geometrical irregularities on propagation delay in axonal trees. *Biophys. J.* 60:1424–1437.

Parnas, I. (1979) Propagation in nonuniform neurites: Form and function in axons. In *The Neurosciences: Fourth Study Program*, ed. F. O. Schmitt and F. G. Worden. Cambridge, MA: MIT Press.

Parnas, I. and Segev, I. (1979) A mathematical model of conduction of action potentials along branching axons. *J. Physiol.* 295:323–343.

Pauwelussen, J. (1982) One way traffic of pulses in a neuron. *J. Math. Biol.* 15:151–172.

Rall, W. (1962a) Theory of physiological properties of dendrites. *Ann. NY Acad. Sci.* 96:1071–1092.

Ramon, F., Joyner, R. W., and Moore, J. W. (1975) Propagation of action potentials in inhomogeneous axon regions, *Federation Proc.* 34:1357–1363.

Rinzel, J. (1990) Mechanisms for nonuniform propagation along excitable cables. In *Mathematical Approaches to Cardiac Arrhythmias*, ed. J. Jalife. *Ann. N.Y. Acad. Sci.* 591: 51–61.

Rinzel, J., and Ermentrout, G. B. (1989) Analysis of neural excitability and oscillations. In *Methods in Neuronal Modeling: From Synapses to Networks*, ed. C. Koch and I. Segev. Cambridge, MA: MIT Press.

Stockbridge, N. (1989) Theoretical response of a bifurcating axon with a locally altered axial resistivity. *J. Theor. Biol.* 137:339–354.

Swadlow, H. A., Kocsis, J. D., and Waxman, S. G. (1980) Modulation of impulse conduction along the axonal tree. *Ann. Rev. Biophys. Bioeng.* 9:143–179.

Waxman, S. G. (1985) Integrative properties and design principles in axons. *Int. Rev. Neurol.* 18:1–40.

9.2 Changes of Action Potential Shape and Velocity for Changing Core Conductor Geometry (1974), *Biophys. J.* 14:731–757

Steven S. Goldstein and Wilfrid Rall

ABSTRACT   The theoretical changes in shape and velocity of an action potential were computed in regions of changing core conductor geometry. Step decrease and step increase of diameter, branch points, and gradual taper or flare of diameter were studied. Results showed increase of both velocity and peak height as the action potential approaches a point of step decrease. A step increase causes decrease of both velocity and peak height with approach; propagation may either fail, succeed with brief delay, or, with longer delay, succeed in both forward and reverse directions. With branching, both the shape and the dimensionless velocity, $\tau\theta/\lambda$, remain unchanged when the $d^{3/2}$ values are matched. Without such matching, the changes of shape and dimensionless velocity of an action potential correspond to those found for step decrease or step increase of diameter. For regions of flare or taper, it was found (for a specific previously defined class) that velocity changed in proportion with the changing length constant. A simple formula was found to predict how this proportionality constant depends upon the amount of flare or taper.

INTRODUCTION

Theoretical and computational studies of action potentials have usually taken advantage of one or the other of the following simplifying assumptions: either space clamping conditions are assumed to prevent action potential propagation completely, or uniform properties and infinite length are assumed to provide propagation at constant velocity. Both assumptions offer the great computational advantage of permitting the partial differential equation (cable equation for spatio-temporal spread of membrane potential disturbances) to be reduced to an ordinary differential equation.

Here, neither simplifying assumption is permissible, because we wish to focus upon changes in the shape and the velocity of an action potential as it approaches a region of changing core conductor geometry. The specific kinds of change in geometry considered are illustrated in Fig. 1; included are sealed termination, step decrease or increase of diameter, taper or flare of diameter, and branching.

Depending upon the kind and the amount of the geometric change, action potential propagation can become faster, slower, or remain the same as it approaches the region of geometric change; also, it can fail to propagate beyond this region, or it can succeed with or without delay. Under certain conditions, it can propagate backwards as well as forwards from this region. Our purpose is to obtain information and gain biophysical understanding of such changing action potential behavior.

Relation of Shape and Velocity

In order to clarify the relation between action potential shape and velocity, we make use of Fig. 2. There each shape is shown as a function of distance (x/λ), and propagation is from left to right. The upper two shapes illustrate propagation of a constant shape at constant velocity; every point, such as A to A' or B to B', travels at the same velocity. In contrast, the lower two shapes illustrate propagation of a changing shape; then it can be shown that corresponding points, such as C to C', and D to D', travel neither at the same velocity nor at a constant velocity. What is more, with changing shape, even the definition of corresponding points presents a problem. Our choice has been to treat them as corresponding fractions of the changing peak voltage of the action potential in the distance domain (where the falling phase must be distinguished from the rising phase).

For the case of constant shape, there is no difficulty in characterizing the velocity. Given a

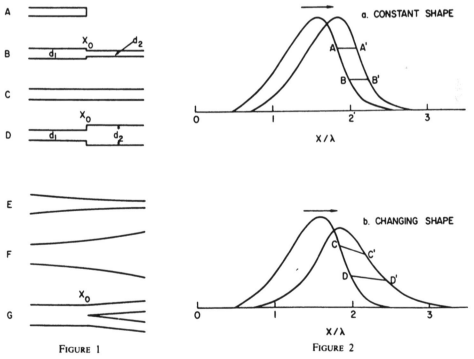

FIGURE 1

FIGURE 2

FIGURE 1   Summary of geometric regions considered, shown in longitudinal section.
FIGURE 2   Action potential propagation with constant and changing shape. The letters A, B, C, D represent points on the action potential at a given time. The corresponding points at a later time are A', B', C', D', respectively.

time increment, dt, every point advances by the same distance, dx, such as A to A', or B to B'; the propagation velocity, θ, is then unambiguously defined as this dx divided by this dt. Thus

$$\theta = (dx)/(dt) \qquad mm/ms, \tag{1}$$

and it can be shown that θ is not only the same for all pairs of corresponding points, but θ also remains constant as the action potential propagates to other locations along a uniform cylinder of infinite length. For such conditions it is well known that

$$\partial V/\partial t = -\theta(\partial V/\partial x), \tag{2}$$

where V represents the departure of membrane potential from its resting value. This equation has several implications: the action potential shape in the time domain is proportional to the shape in the distance domain, with $-\theta$ as the constant of proportionality; the peak in the time domain occurs at the same x and t as in the distance domain.

For the case of propagation with changing shape we cannot use Eq. 1 to define a unique velocity for such an action potential, and Eq. 2 does not apply. In order to be more explicit, we consider the total differential of V, which is defined as

$$dV = (\partial V/\partial x)dx + (\partial V/\partial t)dt. \tag{3}$$

For corresponding points, A to A' and B to B', $dV = 0$, and rearrangement of Eq. 3 with substitution of Eq. 1 yields Eq. 2. But which changing shape, as for corresponding points C to C' and D to D', $dV \neq 0$, and rearrangement of Eq. 3 yields

$$\partial V/\partial t = (dV)/(dt) - (\partial V/\partial x)(dx)/(dt). \tag{4}$$

With $dV \neq 0$, this equation has implications that contrast with those of Eq. 2: the action potential shape in the time domain is not proportional to the shape in the distance domain; the peak in the time domain (i.e., for a given $x = x_1$, the time at which $\partial V/\partial t = 0$ can be designated $t = t_1$) does not occur at the same x and t as in the distance domain (i.e., for $t = t_1$, the location where $\partial V/\partial x = 0$ cannot be $x = x_1$); also, corresponding points in the distance domain do not agree with corresponding points in the time domain.

Because the velocity of such an action potential is not defined, we have chosen to focus attention upon the changing velocity of the peak in the time domain. This velocity can be expressed

$$\theta_p = \lim_{\Delta t \to 0} [\Delta x/\Delta t]_p, \tag{5}$$

where it is understood that subscript p means that Δx and Δt are chosen as follows: $\partial V/\partial t = 0$ both at $x = x_1$, $t = t_1$, and at $x = x_1 + \Delta x$, $t = t_1 + \Delta t$.

In order to explore such velocity and shape changes in regions of changing geometry (Fig. 1) we simulated action potential propagation by means of a mathematical model.

THEORY AND METHODS

The specific mathematical model used in our computations is shown below as Eqs. 10–12. This model is a particular case of a general class of models defined and discussed by FitzHugh (1969); see also Evans and Shenk (1970). Because some theoretical considerations are common to this entire class, we present it first.

General Mathematical Model

This general model consists of the following system of partial differential equations:

$$(\partial^2 V/\partial X^2) - (\partial V/\partial T) = f(V, W_1, \ldots W_n) \tag{6}$$

$$(\partial W_j/\partial T) = f_j(V, W_1, \ldots W_n) \qquad \text{for } j = 1, \ldots n, \tag{7}$$

where V represents the departure of the transmembrane potential from its resting value (millivolts), $W_1, \ldots W_n$ are auxiliary variables defined by Eq. 7, and both X and T are dimensionless variables defined as follows: $X = x/\lambda$, where x is actual distance (millimeters) and λ is the length constant[1] (millimeters); $T = t/\tau$, where t is time (milliseconds), and τ is the passive membrane time constant[1] (milliseconds). Such systems have been shown to simulate propagating action potentials for suitable choice of f and f_j. The Bonhoeffer-van der Pol model of FitzHugh (1961, 1969) includes only one auxiliary variable and one f_j. The model of Hodgkin and Huxley (1952) includes three auxiliary variables (m, n, and h).

These equations apply to propagation in a uniform cylinder. When core conductor diameter changes with distance, Eq. 6 must be replaced by a more general expression (see section on tapering diameter below) in which the definition of $X = x/\lambda$ becomes generalized (see also Rall, 1962).

Velocity in Different Domains. Here we restrict consideration to the propagation of a single action potential in a uniform cylinder of infinite length. As others have done, we assume for this a constant velocity, θ; see Eqs. 1 and 2 above. It is well known that θ will have different values in different cylinders. Even for identical active membrane properties (f and f_j), θ will be different for different λ and different τ; however, this particular difference disappears in the dimensionless space of X and T, where Eq. 2 becomes transformed to

$$\partial V/\partial T = -(\tau\theta/\lambda)\partial V/\partial X. \tag{8}$$

The dimensionless velocity, $\tau\theta/\lambda$, is the same for all cylinders (regardless of diameter, λ or τ value) which have the same active membrane properties (f and f_j). This assertion follows immediately from the fact that Eqs. 6 and 7 are not dependent

---

[1] τ and λ are cable parameters defined in terms of *passive* cable properties; by definition, they remain unaffected by the permeability changes associated with active propagation.

upon the values of λ and τ; in other words, dimensionless propagation velocity in X, T space depends only upon f and f_j; see also FitzHugh (1973).

Distance Domain. When we compare constant propagation in two cylinders which differ only in their diameters, we know that both the shape and the velocity of the action potential are identical with respect to X, but they will be different with respect to x. If the two cylinders have diameters, d_1 and d_2, with characteristic lengths, λ_1 and λ_2, we know that $\tau\theta_1/\lambda_1$ equals $\tau\theta_2/\lambda_2$ and therefore, that

$$\theta_1/\theta_2 = \lambda_1/\lambda_2 = (d_1/d_2)^{1/2} \tag{9}$$

where the last expression represents the well-known dependence of λ upon the square root of diameter. (This implies the usual assumption of extracellular isopotentiality.)

For example, if d_1 is $4d_2$, not only the velocity in the x domain will be twice as great in cylinder 1 as in cylinder 2, but also the shape (V as a function of x for any particular t) is changed correspondingly. This is illustrated in Fig. 5, by comparing the shape at the far left (corresponding to d_1, λ_1, and θ_1) with the more contracted shape at the far right (corresponding to d_2, λ_2, and θ_2).[2] For any given distance (fraction of λ_1) in the left-hand shape, the corresponding distance (same fraction of λ_2) in the right-hand shape is half as great.

Time Domain. For two cylinders which differ only in their diameters, the action potential in the time domain has a shape (V as a function of t for any particular x) that is unchanged; in other words, different values of λ do not change the shape in the time domain. Nevertheless, propagation velocity is still governed by Eq. 9, as long as τ has the same value in both cylinders.

Specific Model

Simulations were performed with the following mathematical model:

$$(\partial^2\mathcal{V}/\partial X^2) - (\partial\mathcal{V}/\partial T) = \mathcal{V} - \mathcal{E}(1 - \mathcal{V}) + \mathcal{J}(\mathcal{V} + 0.1), \tag{10}$$

$$(\partial\mathcal{E}/\partial T) = k_1\mathcal{V}^2 + k_2\mathcal{V}^4 - k_3\mathcal{E} - k_4\mathcal{J}, \tag{11}$$

$$(\partial\mathcal{J}/\partial T) = k_5\mathcal{E} + k_6\mathcal{E}\mathcal{J} - k_7\mathcal{J}. \tag{12}$$

This is a particular case of the general model defined in Eqs. 6 and 7. Here $n = 2$, $W_1 = \mathcal{E}$, $W_2 = \mathcal{J}$ and f, f_1, and f_2 are the expressions on the right in Eqs. 10–12. Also, the variable voltage, V, has been replaced by a dimensionless variable, $\mathcal{V}$, which has been normalized to make $\mathcal{V}$ range from 0 to 1 as V ranges from 0 to the excitatory equilibrium potential; more detail on this normalization can be found on p. 79 of Rall (1964).

---

[2] With regard to Fig. 5, it may be noted that while the shapes are distorted near the origin (where the two cylinders are joined), those farthest from the origin are essentially the same as at greater distances.

TABLE I
VELOCITY OF MODEL ACTION POTENTIALS

	Kinetic parameters							Propagation velocities			
	k_1	k_2	k_3	k_4	k_5	k_6	k_7	$\tau\theta/\lambda$	θ(Squid)*	θ(Lobster)*	θ(Crab)*
									m/s	m/s	m/s
A	1,500	30,000	25	0.2	2.4	0.05	10	5.0	36	6.2	2.5
B	500	30,000	25	0.2	7.4	0.05	15	4.9	35	6.1	2.45
C	500	300,000	25	0.2	7.4	0.05	10	8.0	57	10	4.0
D	500	30,000	25	0.2	7.4	0.05	10	5.0	36	6.2	2.5
E	63	3,800	3.1	0.025	0.95	0.062	1.3	3.2	23	4.0	1.6

*Values, based on experimental τ and λ values from Katz (1966): $\lambda = 5$ mm $\lambda = 2.5$ mm $\lambda = 2.5$ mm
$\tau = 0.7$ ms $\tau = 2$ ms $\tau = 5$ ms

This particular model (Eqs. 10–12) was previously used to generate action potentials needed in a computational reconstruction of potentials in the olfactory bulb (Rall and Shepherd, 1968). For several different choices of $k_1, \ldots k_7$, such as those shown in Table I, we have obtained well-shaped propagating action potentials which can be regarded as mathematically stable (see Evans, 1972). Because the values of $k_1, \ldots k_7$ remain constant (independent of $\mathcal{U}$, X, and T), computation with this system is significantly simpler than with that of Hodgkin and Huxley (1952). In Table I, each set of $k_1, \ldots k_7$ is followed by the dimensionless velocity, $\tau\theta/\lambda$, found by numerical solution for constant propagation in a uniform cylinder of infinite length. To facilitate comparison with experimental velocities, these $\tau\theta/\lambda$ values are reexpressed in Table I as particular velocities, θ, for particular τ and λ values from the literature (see Katz, 1966).

Numerical Solutions. The set of partial differential equations (PDE) 10–12 was solved simultaneously using standard numerical techniques. The explicit method of solution was used (see Smith, 1965). The ratio of the time step, Δt, to the square of ΔX was 0.04.

The validity of this solution was tested for the case of constant propagation in the uniform cylinder. Here, we can make use of Eq. 8 to convert the system of partial differential equations (10–12) to the following system of ordinary differential equations (ODE):

$$(d^2\mathcal{U}/dX^2) + (\tau\theta/\lambda)(d\mathcal{U}/dX) = \mathcal{U} - \mathcal{E}(1 - \mathcal{U}) + \mathcal{J}(\mathcal{U} + 0.1), \quad (13)$$

$$-(\tau\theta/\lambda)(d\mathcal{E}/dX) = k_1\mathcal{U}^2 + k_2\mathcal{U}^4 - k_3\mathcal{E} - k_4\mathcal{E}\mathcal{J}, \quad (14)$$

$$-(\tau\theta/\lambda)(d\mathcal{J}/dX) = k_5\mathcal{E} + k_6\mathcal{E}\mathcal{J} - k_7\mathcal{J}. \quad (15)$$

This system of equations explicitly contains the dimensionless velocity, $\tau\theta/\lambda$. As was found originally by Hodgkin and Huxley (1952), we also found that an action potential solution of such a system of ODEs is extremely sensitive to a correct choice of velocity. The Runge-Kutta method of numerical solution was used. When the choice of velocity had been refined to eight significant figures, the shape of the rising phase and the peak of this action potential was found to at least three significant figures. When this solution (of Eqs. 13–15) was compared with that obtained by numerical solution of the PDEs 10–12 agreement to three significant figures was found for the rising phase and peak.

Clearly the ODEs 13–15 do not apply to regions where changing geometry causes changing shape and velocity. All such computations were necessarily made with the PDEs 10–12 (or 24–26 below). When performing such calculations, the initial condition was that $\mathcal{V} = \mathcal{E} = \mathcal{J} = 0$ for all X, except that a suprathreshold transmembrane potential ($\mathcal{V} = 0.9$) was imposed along a short length ($\Delta X = 0.2$) located 1.5 λ away from the region of interest. It was verified by our computations that the resulting action potential had constant shape and velocity before entering the region of interest. In the preparation of the figures, the after hyperpolarization portion of each action potential was omitted to avoid unnecessary confusion from overlaps.

Tapering Diameter

Here we consider noncylindrical core conductors which taper or flare continuously with distance. Such changing diameter implies a continuously changing λ. To emphasize this difference between a cylinder and a tapering core conductor we define a *generalized* length parameter, λ_{taper}, and a *generalized* electrotonic distance, Z, which are related to each other as follows:

$$\lambda_{taper} = \lambda_0 (r/r_0)^{1/2}[1 + (dr/dx)^2]^{-1/4}, \tag{16}$$

$$dx/dZ = \lambda_{taper}, \quad \text{or } Z_2 - Z_1 = \int_{x_1}^{x_2} (1/\lambda_{taper})\,dx, \tag{17}$$

where λ_0 is the length constant for a cylinder with a radius, r_0, taken as the radius at a reference location. The new variable, Z, replaces the previously used dimensionless distance, $X = x/\lambda$. The basis for these equations can be found on pp. 1078–1079 of an earlier publication (see Rall, 1962).

Our considerations are here restricted to a *particular* class of core conductors where the amount of flare or taper is determined by a single parameter, K, according to Eq. 18. Examples for several values of K are illustrated graphically in Fig. 11. For this class, the radius changes monotonically with distance according to the rule:

$$r^2 \propto (dx/dZ)\exp(KZ). \tag{18}$$

For some purposes it is desirable to express the dependence of r upon x rather than Z; this is provided by Eq. 22 below. Although this dependence is complicated in the most general case (see Appendix), it can be well approximated for most cases of interest, where $(dr/dx)^2$ is much smaller than unity.[3]   When this approximation is used, we can simplify Eq. 16 and 17 to

$$dx/dZ \simeq \lambda_0 (r/r_0)^{1/2}. \tag{19}$$

By substituting Eq. 19 into proportionality 18, we obtain

$$r \; \tilde{\alpha} \; \exp(2KZ/3), \tag{20}$$

where the proportionality constant is r_0.   When this r/r_0 is substituted into Eq. 19, integration yields

$$x/\lambda_0 \simeq (3/K)[\exp(KZ/3) - 1]. \tag{21}$$

Now substitution of $(r/r_0)^{1/2}$ for $\exp(KZ/3)$ in Eq. 21 yields an expression which can be rearranged to the following simple dependence of r upon x

$$r/r_0 \simeq ([Kx/3\lambda_0] + 1)^2. \tag{22}$$

This also implies

$$\lambda_{\text{taper}} \simeq \lambda_0([Kx/3\lambda_0] + 1). \tag{23}$$

For the class of taper or flare defined by Eqs. 16–18, it can be shown that the earlier model Eqs. 10–12, which apply to cylinders, become generalized to the following

$$(\partial^2 \mathcal{V}/\partial Z^2) + K(\partial \mathcal{V}/\partial Z) - (\partial \mathcal{V}/\partial T) = \mathcal{V} - \mathcal{E}(1 - \mathcal{V}) + \mathcal{J}(\mathcal{V} + 0.1) \tag{24}$$

$$\partial \mathcal{E}/\partial T = k_1 \mathcal{V}^2 + k_2 \mathcal{V}^4 - k_3 \mathcal{E} - k_4 \mathcal{E} \mathcal{J} \tag{25}$$

$$\partial \mathcal{J}/\partial T = k_5 \mathcal{E} + k_6 \mathcal{E} \mathcal{J} - k_7 \mathcal{J} \tag{26}$$

This assertion is based upon the demonstration (Rall, 1962) that $\partial^2 \mathcal{V}/\partial X^2$ for the cylindrical case becomes replaced by $\partial^2 \mathcal{V}/\partial Z^2 + K\partial \mathcal{V}/\partial Z$ for this class of taper. Also, it may be noted that the special case of zero taper, which implies $dr/dx = 0$ and $K = 0$, reduces Z to X and λ_{taper} to λ_0, with the result that the more general model (Eqs. 24–26) is reduced to the cylindrical model (Eqs. 10–12).

RESULTS

Case of Membrane Cylinder with Sealed End

Here we examine the changes in shape and velocity found for a computed action potential as it approaches a sealed (insulated) boundary.   By a sealed end (Fig. 1 A) we

---

[3] To verify that dr/dx is sufficiently small in any given case, one can evaluate the derivative of Eq. 22 below. For example, if $K = 3$, $r_0/\lambda_0 = 0.002$ and $x/\lambda_0 = 49$, then $dr/dx = 0.2$ and the factor $[1 + (dr/dx)^2]^{-1/4} = 0.990$ in Eq. 16.

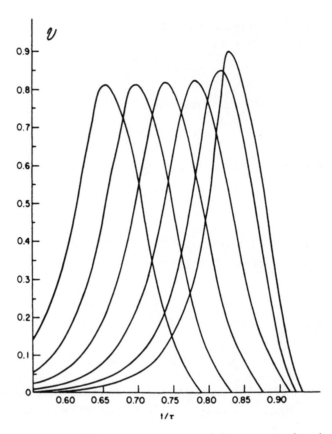

FIGURE 3   Action potential approaching a sealed end. Each shape represents the action potential (in the time domain) at six equally spaced ($\Delta X = 0.2\lambda$) locations along the cylinder. The leftmost curve corresponds to a location $X = 1$ from the sealed end.

mean that no current can leak across the membrane which closes the end of the cylinder; this corresponds to $\partial V/\partial X = 0$ at this boundary. The result, that both the peak and the velocity of the action potential increase as it approaches such a sealed boundary, is illustrated by the six curves in Fig. 3. These curves show temporal action potentials ($\mathcal{V}$ vs. T) at six equally spaced ($\Delta X = 0.2$) locations along the cylinder. The leftmost curve represents the action potential at a distance of λ away from the boundary; this curve has essentially the same shape and velocity as the action potential propagating in a cylinder of infinite length. From left to right, these curves show increasing peak height, narrowing half-width, and decreasing temporal displacement, as the action potential approaches the sealed boundary. With regard to velocity, the peak displacement at left is $\Delta T = 0.04$, implying a dimensionless velocity, $\tau\theta_p/\lambda = \Delta X/\Delta T = 5.0$; in contrast, the peak displacement at right is $\Delta T = 0.01$, implying $\tau\theta_p/\lambda = 20$, a fourfold increase.

In common with our other computed results, this figure shows that significant changes in shape and velocity occur only at locations less than λ from the boundary; the major effect occurs within $\lambda/2$.

It has been noted that when collision occurs between two action potentials propagating in opposite directions in a cylinder of infinite length, the conditions at the point of collision are equivalent to those at the sealed end (e.g., p. 467, Katz and Miledi, 1965). This is because symmetry implies $\partial V/\partial x = 0$ at the point of collision. It follows that peak height and velocity must increase just before collision and extinction.

In order to obtain biophysical understanding of such increase in peak height and velocity, we draw attention to the distribution of core current that flows downstream, ahead of the active membrane region. When the action potential is far from a boundary or point of collision, the leading core current is free to flow downstream for a considerable distance; it can leave the core over a large area of membrane at relatively low membrane current density. As the action potential approaches the point were $\partial V/\partial x = 0$, the core current cannot flow beyond this point, and must leave the core over a limited area of membrane at relatively high membrane current density. Such increased local current results in more rapid membrane depolarization, earlier attainment of threshold and peak (implying increased velocity); also the extra local current augments the amplitude of the peak.

Case of Step Reduction of Cylindrical Diameter (Fig. 1 B)

Fig. 4 shows an example of the changes in shape of an action potential as it traverses the region near a step reduction. The wave is viewed in the time domain at points labeled X_A, X_0, and X_B in the figure. Dotted curves show a reference action potential in a uniform cylinder of the initial diameter.

The behavior is qualitatively similar to the sealed end in that the peak is both earlier and higher, and the half-width is reduced as it approaches the boundary point, X_0. After the action potential passes X_0, it soon returns to its initial shape in the time domain, but its velocity becomes slower (as shown by the increased latency of the solid curve at X_B), as should be expected for the reduced diameter. The shape of an action potential is essentially stable when its peak is more than $X = 1$ distant from X_0 on either side.

Distance Domain.   Fig. 5 shows the same action potential in the distance domain. The curves are shown at equal time intervals. One notes immediately that the wave on the extreme right is narrower than the initial wave on the extreme left. Since these waves are propagating in cylinders of differing diameter, the half-width (in this distance domain) is reduced by the factor, λ_2/λ_1 (see Methods section, Distance Domain); also θ_2 is smaller than θ_1.

Transitional Shapes.   Fig. 5 shows that the action potential in the distance domain undergoes remarkable changes in shape at distances within λ of X_0. These changes include not only the previously noted increase in peak height as it approaches X_0, but also complicated changes of slopes and half-widths. It is important to realize that in this transitional region, different points of the wave travel at different velocities, depending upon how near and on which side of X_0 they are located. The increase of velocity with approach to X_0 from the left is revealed both by increasing distance between peaks and by increasing half-width; the latter results from the fact that the rising

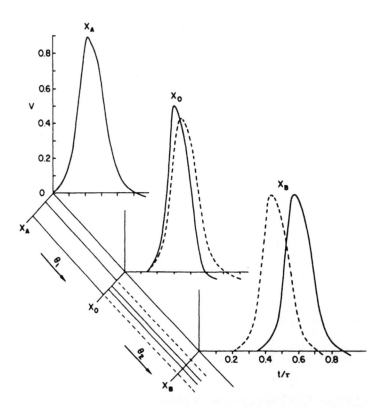

FIGURE 4   Action potential for a step reduction (at X_0) of cylindrical diameter. The shape (in the time domain) is shown at the points, X_A, X_0, and X_B. The dashed curves show the action potential as it would appear had no step reduction in diameter occurred. In this example $d_2/d_1 = 0.25$ and the kinetic parameters are shown in Table I (set A). X_A and X_B are $\Delta x = 0.6\lambda_1$ distant from X_0.

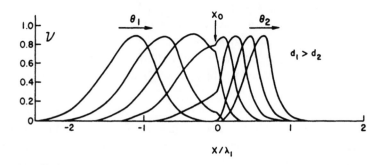

FIGURE 5   Action potential (in the distance domain) propagating in a region of step reduction (at X_0) of cylindrical diameter. Successive shapes from left to right illustrate the action potential at equal time intervals ($\Delta T = 0.1$). θ_1 = initial constant velocity; θ_2 = constant velocity attained in the smaller cylinder after passing X_0. In this example $d_2/d_1 = 0.25$ and the kinetic parameters are shown in Table I (set A).

phase (leading right-hand slope) is closer to X_0 and traveling faster than the falling phase. After passing X_0 (and entering the smaller diameter) decrease of velocity is revealed both by decreased distance between peaks and by decreased half-width. The contraction of the rising phase (in the distance domain to the right of X_0) can be understood either in terms of decreased velocity or in terms of decreased λ.

The discontinuity of slope at X_0 occurs because core resistance is discontinuous and continuity of current must be maintained. The core current, I_i, may be expressed:

$$I_i = -(\pi d_i^2/4R_i)\,[dV/dx]_{X_{0-}} = -(\pi d_2^2/4R_i)\,[dV/dx]_{X_{0+}} \tag{27}$$

where R_i is the intracellular specific resistance; X_{0-} and X_{0+} refer to points just to the left and right of X_0, respectively. In the example illustrated in Figs. 4 and 5 the ratio $d_1/d_2 = 4$.

Effect of Different Diameter Ratios upon θ_p. It is of interest to determine how velocity varies for different ratios of $d_2/d_1 \leq 1$. We will restrict attention to θ_p, the velocity of the peak in the time domain. The results of simulation are shown in Fig. 6. Here the ratio θ_p/θ_1, the ratio of the changing peak velocity to the stable velocity of

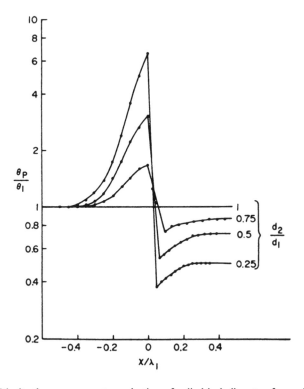

FIGURE 6   Velocity changes near a step reduction of cylindrical diameter for various diameter ratios, d_2/d_1. θ_p, the velocity of the peak of the action potential, is normalized by θ_1 the stable velocity in the initial large cylinder. The kinetic parameters are given in Table I (set B).

the initial cylinder is plotted versus distance. We note that velocity θ_p/θ_1, gradually begins to increase as the peak approaches within $x = 0.6\lambda_1$ of x_0; it reaches a maximum at X_{0-}, and falls sharply to a stable value (θ_2/θ_1) within a distance of $x = 0.3\lambda_2$ to the right of X_0. As d_2/d_1 decreases these effects are accentuated, i.e., velocity begins to increase farther from X_0, rises to a greater maximum value, and falls to a lower stable value. The following empirical relation has been found to give an approximate value for θ_p at X_0.

$$\theta_p(X_0) \approx \theta_1(d_1/d_2)^{3/2}. \tag{28}$$

In a personal communication, Dr. John Rinzel has shown that Eq. 5 can also be expressed, $\theta_p = -\partial^2 V/\partial t^2/(\partial^2 V/\partial x\partial t)$. At X_0, $\partial V/\partial X$ is discontinuous and θ_p is undefined.

Case of Step Increase of Cylindrical Diameter

Fig. 1 D illustrates the geometry of this case; here the ratio, $d_2/d_1 \geq 1$. As in the previous case, simulations were used to explore the changes in θ_p/θ_1 in the vicinity of X_0. In this case it was found that the velocity becomes slower as the peak approaches X_0. However, the effect of different d_2/d_1 values is more complicated than before: there are three different possibilities to be distinguished. Failure of propagation occurs when d_2/d_1 is large enough.[4] For smaller d_2/d_1, propagation continues in the larger cylinder. There is a third possibility, for intermediate d_2/d_1, where propagation not only continues in the larger cylinder but also reinvades the smaller cylinder, as will be explained more fully below with Fig. 10.

In Fig. 7, failure of propagation was found for $d_2/d_1 = 3.5$; the point of failure was judged to occur before the peak reached X_0, although a wave of subthreshold and decreasing amplitude did spread farther. Although the three curves to the left of X_0 in Fig. 7 show similar slowing of velocity over the range, -0.5 to -0.2 for x/λ_1, the two curves on the right show large increases of velocity. For large distance to the right of X_0, θ_p/θ_1 equals the stable ratio θ_2/θ_1 (i.e. Eq. 9); however, it is remarkable that θ_p/θ_1 is much larger than θ_2/θ_1 over the first quarter λ distance to the right of X. Further details of changing velocity and wave shape in the vicinity of X_0 are shown below in Fig. 8 for the time domain and Fig. 9 for the distance domain. Comparable results have been reported by others: one study (Pastushenko et al., 1969 a and b) is based upon analytical treatment of a square wave action potential; the other (Khodorov et al., 1969) is based upon computations with the Hodgkin and Huxley model.

Fig. 8 shows an example $(d_2/d_1 = 2)$ of our computed action potential as it propagated through the region in question. It shows the action potential in the time domain at three points. As the wave approaches the discontinuity the peak amplitude falls,

---

[4] A familiar example is antidromic propagation of an action potential along the axon toward the axon hillock-soma region (Brock et al., 1953 Fuortes et al., 1957); this has recently been simulated by Dodge and Cooley (1973); similar antidromic propagation was also simulated in computations for mitral cells by Rall and Shepherd (1968).

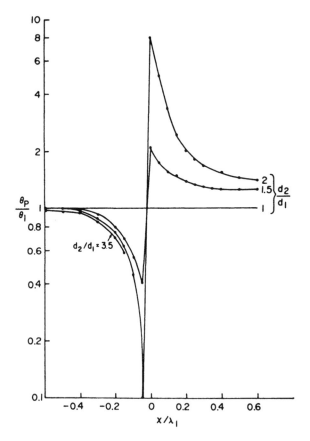

FIGURE 7   Velocity changes near a step increase of cylindrical diameter, for various diameter ratios, d_2/d_1. θ_p, the velocity of the peak is normalized by θ_1, the stable velocity in the initial small cylinder. Kinetic parameters are given in Table I (set B).

the half-width widens, and increased latency (relative to dashed control curve) reveals the slowed velocity. When the wave has reached X_2, the shape in the time domain has returned essentially to its original form. The increased velocity is revealed by decreasing latency (compare solid curves with dashed control curves at X_0 and X_2); in fact, the wave traveling at velocity, θ_2, will shortly overtake the control (dashed) wave which travels at velocity, θ_1, in the control cylinder.

Distance Domain.   Fig. 9 shows the same action potential in the distance domain. Each wave shown is the voltage distribution along the joined cylinders at a given instant of time. The time intervals are equal. The wave on the far left has the shape it would have in an infinite cylinder of diameter d_1. The wave on the far right has the shape it would have in an infinite cylinder of diameter, d_2; it is wider by the factor $\lambda_2/\lambda_1 = 1.414$ because $d_2/d_1 = 2$ (see Eq. 9). The smaller peak amplitude at X_0 can be seen in Fig. 9 as well as Fig. 8.

Transitional Shapes.   As was pointed out with Fig. 5, different points of such transitional shapes travel at different velocities; however, the changes in Fig. 9 con-

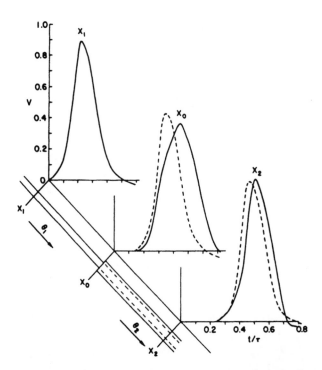

FIGURE 8   Action potential for a step increase (at X_0) of cylindrical diameter. The shape (in the time domain) is shown for three points X_A, X_0, and X_B. The dotted curves show the action potential as it would appear had no step increase in cylindrical diameter occurred. For this example $d_2/d_1 = 2.0$ and the kinetic parameters are shown in Table I (set A). X_A and X_B are $\Delta x = 0.6\lambda_1$ distant from X_0.

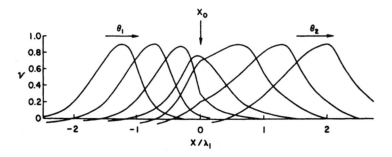

FIGURE 9   Action potential (in the distance domain) propagating in a region of step increase (at X_0) of cylindrical diameter. Successive shapes from left to right illustrate the action potential at equal time intervals ($\Delta T = 0.1$). θ_1 = initial constant velocity; θ_2 = constant velocity attained in larger cylinder after passing X_0. In this figure $d_2/d_1 = 2.0$ and the kinetic parameters are shown in Table I (set A).

trast with those in Fig. 5. The decrease of velocity with approach to X_0 from the left is revealed both by decreasing distance between peaks and by decreasing half-width; the latter results from the fact that the rising phase (leading right-hand slope) is closer to X_0 and traveling slower than the falling phase. After passing X_0 (and entering the large diameter) a large increase in velocity is revealed both by the increased peak distance and half-width of the fifth wave from the left. Although the distance between the last two peaks is not as great as this, it is still greater than that between the first two peaks; all this is consistent with the θ_p/θ_1 curve for $d_2/d_1 = 2$ in Fig. 7.

The unusual, somewhat flat-topped shape of the fifth curve from the left merits further comment. The almost flat top implies that a half λ length of the large cylinder peaked almost simultaneously. This can be partly understood as an indirect consequence of the slowing of propagation before the peak reached X_0; during this slowing, there is extra time for subthreshold electrotonic spread into the larger cylinder. The resulting distribution of subthreshold voltage becomes more uniform than usual; thus both threshold and peak are reached almost simultaneously over this length (about $\lambda/2$ in Fig. 9). This near simultaneity also accounts for the high peak velocity, just to the right of X_0, indicated by the curve labeled $d_2/d_1 = 2$ in Fig. 7.

At X_0, the shapes in Fig. 9 necessarily show discontinuities in their slopes, because of the discontinuity in core resistance; see Eq. 27. Here the slopes decrease by a factor of 4.

Forward and Reverse Propagation. Referring back to Fig. 7, we note that $d_2/d_1 = 3.5$ resulted in failure of propagation into the larger cylinder, while $d_2/d_1 = 2.0$ resulted in success. An intermediate example, for $d_2/d_1 = 2.5$, is illustrated in Fig. 10, where voltage vs. time shapes are shown for various locations; time is displayed horizontally; spatial locations are displaced vertically; X_0 locates the step increase of diameter, as before. The three action potentials at far left represent propagation toward X_0 in the smaller cylinder. The fourth shape from the left shows the delayed action potential occurring at X_0. Onward propagation in the larger cylinder is shown by the nine curves labeled "forward" toward lower right. Reverse propagation in the smaller cylinder is shown by the three shapes labeled "reverse" at upper right.

To understand how reverse propagation can occur, it is useful to contrast Fig. 10 with Fig. 8, where reverse propagation did not occur. The essential difference is the longer delay in achieving an action potential at X_0. At the time of peak at X_0, the membrane of the smaller cylinder is still refractory in Fig. 8, but with the longer delay of Fig. 10, this membrane is less refractory and thus able to propagate. Partial refractoriness is evidenced by the delay of this reverse propagation.

Reverse propagation was found before in computations (Rall and Shepherd, unpublished) which simulated antidromic propagation in a mitral cell axon to its junction with the soma and dendrites. This phenomenon has also been found computationally by Zeevi (personal communication) and an example of *decremental* reverse conduction is included in his Ph.D. thesis (Zeevi, 1972). Khodorov et al. (1969) also provide an example of reverse *decremental* conduction. Both expected that such decremental

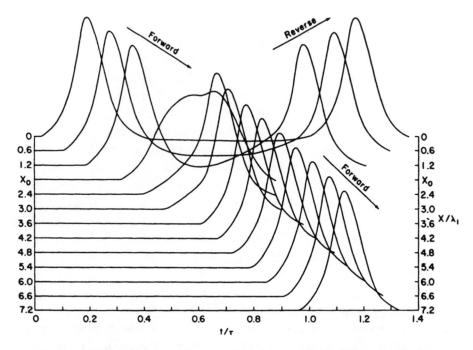

FIGURE 10   Forward and reverse propagation of the action potential in a region of step increase. The action potentials (in the time domain) are shown at successive locations indicated by the vertical scale with X_0 being the point of step increase. In this figure $d_2/d_1 = 2.5$; the kinetic parameters used are shown as set B in Table I.

reverse conduction might be converted to non-decremental reverse conduction if their calculations were redone with different parameters chosen to result in a shorter refractory period.

Returning to our computations with different values of d_2/d_1, we note that when d_2/d_1 is decreased from 2.5, delay in forward propagation is decreased. Thus an action potential which might propagate in reverse meets more refractory membrane. This can result in failure, i.e. reverse *decremental* conduction.

Case of Tapering Diameter.

Computations were carried out for different degrees of taper determined by choosing several values of the parameter K; see Methods and Fig. 11. For any particular taper the change of λ_{taper} with distance has already been defined by Eqs. 16–18. We expected that the velocity would also change as diameter and λ_{taper} change with distance, and our computations verified this. What is more, we found that the velocity, θ, is proportional to the changing λ_{taper}, which means that

$$\tau\theta/\lambda_{taper} = \text{constant} = \beta, \tag{29}$$

for a given taper (K) and given membrane kinetics $(k_1, \ldots k_7)$. It is noteworthy that this $\tau\theta/\lambda_{taper}$ represents a dimensionless velocity, and that its constancy means a con-

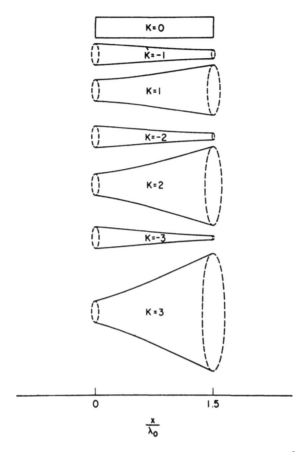

FIGURE 11   Longitudinal sections of core conductors whose radii obey the rule: $r^2 \ \alpha \ (dx/dZ) \exp(KZ)$, where K is a constant and Z a dimensionless distance; see also Eq. 22.

stant rate of propagation with respect to Z, the generalized electrotonic distance variable for taper. In addition this means that the shape of this action potential remains constant in the Z domain (but changes in the x domain). This also means that the shape remains constant in the time domain, as would be expected when the considerations embodied in Eq. 8 for cylinders are generalized from X to Z. In fact, such constancy of shape in the Z and T domains was explicitly verified in the computed results. It is to be emphasized that these results apply only when flare or taper obeys the rule given by Eq. 18.

Because Eq. 29 implies $\theta \ \alpha \ \lambda_{taper}$ and because an earlier equation (23) shows that λ_{taper} depends linearly upon x, it follows that the velocity, θ, also depends linearly upon x, for any given K; that is,

$$\theta \simeq (\beta\lambda_0/\tau)(1 + Kx/3\lambda_0). \tag{30}$$

It is an interesting result of our computations with different values of K, that β can be approximated as

$$\beta \simeq (\tau\theta_c/\lambda_0) - K, \qquad (31)$$

where θ_c represents the reference velocity of a cylinder ($K = 0$) with radius, r_0 and length constant, λ_0.

For a specific numerical illustration, we can choose a reference cylinder whose dimensionless $\tau\theta_c/\lambda_0$ value is 5. From Eq. 31, we see that $K > 5$ makes $\beta < 0$, which implies a failure of propagation; smaller values of K give larger values of β. For $K = 1, 2, 3, 4$, and 4.5, the implications of Eqs. 29–31 have been plotted in Fig. 12. The intercepts at left (for $x = 0$) correspond to the value of β for each K. The slope of each straight line (i.e. slope of $\tau\theta/\lambda_0$ vs. x/λ_0) is equal to $\beta K/3$ for each K value. In this

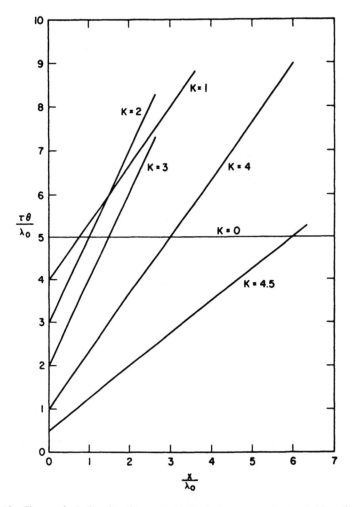

FIGURE 12   Change of velocity with distance (x/λ_0) in flaring core conductors (with radii defined by Eq. 22). It is assumed that Eqs. 30 and 31 are valid and that $\tau\theta/\lambda_0 = 5$.

example both $K = 2$ and $K = 3$ yield slopes of 2; the steepest possible slope (2.08), corresponds to $K = 2.5$, but is not shown in Fig. 12.

It seems desirable to elaborate some of the physical intuitive meaning of the results displayed in Fig. 12. It is simplest to consider all of these core conductors as having the same diameter and λ_0 value at $x = 0$ (see Eqs. 22 and 23). Then each velocity, θ, at $x = 0$, is proportional to the intercept at the left of Fig. 12. We note that increasing amounts of flare (associated with increasingly positive K values) cause progressively smaller values of velocity at the point ($x = 0$) where the diameters are all the same. An explanation of this fact can be based upon the reduced core resistance that results from flaring diameter; this increases the fraction of core current that flows downstream and decreases the fraction that depolarizes adjacent membrane. Because this decreasing current must depolarize an increasing membrane capacity per unit length (because of flare), the result is less rapid membrane depolarization, implying less rapid propagation of the impulse. It may be noted parenthetically that negative K values would yield increased velocity for the same core conductor diameter.

Next, we note that Fig. 12 shows that with positive K, the velocity in each case increases linearly with distance. At the point where each sloping line crosses the horizontal ($K = 0$) reference line, we can say that the effect of increased diameter on velocity has just compensated for the handicap associated with flare (i.e. dependence of β upon K in Eq. 31).

Referring back to Eqs. 30 and 31 we can see that flare (positive K) has two opposing effects on velocity in the x domain: one is an increase due to increasing λ_{taper} (see Eq. 23 in Methods), while the other is a decrease due to decreasing β (see Eq. 31). It is these two opposing effects that explain why the slopes in Fig. 12 increase from zero, for $K = 0$, to a maximum slope for $K = 2.5$, and then decrease to smaller slopes for larger values of K, until β falls to zero, implying failure of propagation.

The fact that Eq. 31 for β is only an approximate result of the computations is made clearer by Fig. 13. Here we plot (as ordinate) the dimensionless velocity, $\tau\theta/\lambda_{taper}$, vs. K. It should be noted that this dimensionless velocity in the Z domain is constant (independent of x and core diameter) for each value of K. The three solid lines present results computed with three different sets of kinetic parameters, $k_1, \ldots k_7$, as made explicit by the figure legend. In each case, the dashed line is a straight line defined by Eq. 31; each dashed line was chosen by setting $\tau\theta_c/\lambda_0$ in Eq. 31 equal to $\tau\theta/\lambda_{taper}$ of each solid curve at $K = 0$. In the case of the upper solid curve, the approximate relation provides an excellent fit for dimensionless velocities greater than 3. As K is increased from 4 to 6, the velocity deviates below the approximate values of the dashed line, and propagation of the computed action potential actually fails for $K = 6$, while the dashed line would imply failure for $K = 8$. This deviation can be seen to occur where the safety factor for propagation is low. Inspection of the computed results shows that the peak height of the action potential becomes significantly reduced over this range. It may be noted that this peak height decreased by only about 1% over the range ($\tau\theta/\lambda_{taper}$ from 10 to 3) where the solid line deviates negligibly from the dashed line.

388   Steven S. Goldstein and Wilfrid Rall

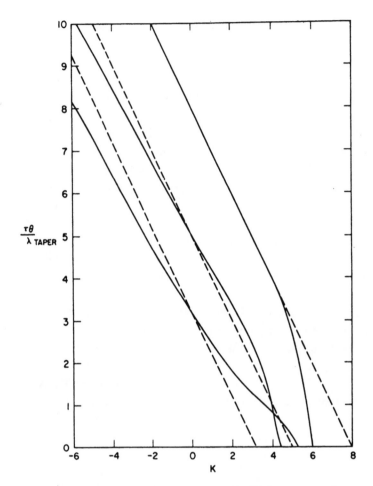

FIGURE 13   Change in dimensionless velocity, $\tau\theta/\lambda_{\text{taper}}$ with differing amounts of taper or flare. Kinetic parameters for the three solid curves shown are in Table I; the uppermost curve used set C; middle curve used set D; lowermost curve used set E.

Next we consider the deviation of the middle solid curve from its corresponding dashed straight line. For most of the dimensionless velocity range (10 to 2), there is a noticeable difference in slope, in contrast with the previous (upper) curve. This correlates well with the fact that the peak heights of the computed action potentials decreased from 0.88 to 0.75 as $\tau\theta/\lambda_{\text{taper}}$ decreases from 10 to 2. This change of peak height (approximately 15%) is much larger than that found with the upper curve. This result supports the conjecture that the dashed line represents a limiting case where action potential peak height remains unchanged. In fact, it can be demonstrated mathematically that the artificial assumption of a constant action potential shape (in the Z and T domains) would imply that Eq. 31 and the dashed straight lines follow exactly (see Appendix, Eqs. 37–42). The deviation of the lowermost solid curve from its corresponding dashed line also correlates with decreasing peak height: for the velocity range ($\tau\theta/\lambda_{\text{taper}}$ from 8 to 2) the peak height decreases from 0.96 to 0.90, or about 6%.

At low velocities, near the point of failure, all three curves deviated from their corresponding dashed lines. The lower solid curve differs from the others in being less steep and bending more gradually as K is increased toward failure. In fact, the fall is so gradual that it crosses the middle solid curve at $K = 4$. This result emphasizes the complex nature of the interaction of the active properties with the geometric properties of a core conductor at slow velocities. (It may be noted (see Table I) that the kinetic parameters corresponding to the lower curve are entirely different from the other sets. The kinetic parameters of the upper and middle curves differ only by one parameter, k_2).

Branching

Computations were used to explore the effects of core conductor branching upon action potential propagation. The assumption of extracellular isopotentiality insures that the angles between the branches can be neglected.

At a branch point, it is usual to distinguish anatomically between a parent branch and a pair of daughter branches, all of which may have different diameters. However, since we wish to consider action potential propagation in either direction in any branch, it becomes necessary to adopt additional branch designations. These distinguish between that branch along which the action potential *approaches* the branch point (regardless of whether this happens to be a parent or a daughter branch), and the *other* branches (along which no action potential approaches the common branch point). Propagation behavior near the branch point depends upon the value of the geometric ratio,

$$\text{GR} = \sum_j d_j^{3/2}/d_a^{3/2}, \tag{32}$$

where d_a represents the diameter of the branch along which propagation *approaches* the branch point, d_j represents the diameter of the j th *other* branch, and the summation is over all of these *other* branches. It may be helpful to note that this geometric ratio also equals the input conductance ratio (*other* branches/*approaching* branch) for branches of semi-infinite length.

For most of our computations, we assumed all branches to be at least several λ in length, with the result that propagation near the branch point, X_0, was not modified by any terminal or branching boundary conditions elsewhere. Then, the results were found to be clearly separable into three cases, determined by whether this geometric ratio, GR, is less than, equal to, or greater than unity.

Case of GR = 1. This case corresponds to the branching constraint (constancy of $\Sigma d^{3/2}$) which has been emphasized elsewhere (Rall, 1959, 1962, 1964) as permitting a dendritic tree to be transformed into an equivalent cylinder, for considerations of passive membrane electrotonus. Here, the *other* branches, together, correspond to an equivalent cylinder that has the same diameter as the *approaching* branch. This means that the partial differential equation in dimensionless X and T applies to a continuous equivalent cylinder region that extends in both directions (upstream and downstream) from the point X_0.

For active propagation, it should be noted that as long as the active membrane properties are the same per unit area in all branches (i.e. independent of λ) it can be shown that the shape and velocity of the propagating action potential (in the X and T domains) remain constant near X_0; a formal demonstration can be provided by the dimensional analysis considerations of FitzHugh (1973). This expectation was verified by computations with the $\mathcal{V} \, \mathcal{E} \, \mathcal{J}$ model and a pair of *other* branches (of unequal diameter) satisfying GR = 1. It should be added that with propagation into these *other* branches, the shape and velocity in the x domain of each branch change in proportion with each λ value, even though both remain unchanged in the X domain.

Case of GR < 1. Here, the *other* branches, together, correspond to an equivalent cylinder whose diameter is smaller than that of the *approaching* branch. Thus, the action potential shape and velocity in the X and T domains would be expected to undergo changes near the branch point, X_0, like those reported above for a step reduction of diameter (Figs. 4–6). Computations verified this expectation that the velocity and the peak amplitude both increase with approach to X_0. Also, in the *other* branches, the action potential shape and velocity soon return to their original values in the X domain, but, of course to changed values in their separate x domains.

Case of GR > 1. Here, the *other* branches, together, correspond to an equivalent cylinder whose diameter is larger than that of the *approaching* branch. We expected and we found changes near the branch point, X_0, like those reported above for a step increase of diameter (Figs. 7–10). Thus, the velocity and the peak amplitude both decrease with approach to X_0. When GR was made sufficiently large, propagation failed at X_0. Also, when GR was adjusted for propagation to succeed only after significant temporal delay at X_0, then, as in previous Fig. 10, there was retrograde propagation in the branch along which the impulse originally approached X_0, as well as onward propagation in all of the *other* branches. In none of these computations was propagation preferential between the *other* branches, i.e. it did not fail in one while succeeding in the others.

DISCUSSION

Additional implications of these results should be mentioned for the closely related cases of step diameter increase and of branching with GR > 1 (see Eq. 32). In situations when failure of propagation occurs at X_0, there is a short time during which the residual depolarization near X_0 may prevent failure of a second impulse. Consequently, at different repetition rates, every second, third, or fourth impulse could succeed in propagating past X_0. Thus geometry alone could filter the impulse repetition rate; in the application to branching, this filtering would be the same in all of the other branches.

In the situation where propagation succeeds at X_0 with sufficient delay to permit retrograde propagation, it should be noted that the retrograde impulse will collide with and thus extinguish a subsequent impulse that may approach X_0 at this time. Since collision could occur at any point along the approaching line, the timing of the second impulse would be less critical than in the previous example.

An interesting possibility arises when a long core conductor ends in enlargements at both ends (i.e. either a step increase in diameter or branches with GR > 1). Then under favorable conditions, successive retrograde propagations could be sustained (back and forth) between these two end regions. This possibility represents another design for a pacemaker, but we have not explored this further.

Next we consider two action potentials, one in each of two branches, both approaching X_0 simultaneously. All the previous considerations of failure or success at X_0 apply here, provided that $d_a^{3/2}$ in Eq. 32 is replaced by the sum of the $d^{3/2}$ values of these two ("*approaching*") branches.

When two action potentials, one in each of two branches, are not simultaneous in their approach to X_0, several possibilities arise; these have been explored computationally. If the action potential in the first branch is able to propagate onward into all other branches before the action potential in the second branch reaches X_0, a collision of the two action potentials will occur in this second branch. · If the first action potential is not able to propagate onward into the other branches, subthreshold current would spread in them passively. This would depolarize the membrane and result in an increasing velocity of the second action potential as it approaches X_0. A similar phenomenon has been noted independently by Pastushenko et al. (1969 *a* and *b*) using a square wave to simulate the action potential. We also observed that the possibility of retrograde conduction in the first branch is enhanced when the two waves do not reach X_0 simultaneously.

Preferential Propagation into Different Branches. The concept that preferential effects between large and small branches could contribute significant filtering of information in neural circuits has been advanced by several people; Lettvin presented this idea in several seminars and papers (Chung et al., 1970); additional references are given by Waxman (1972), and by Grossman et al. (1973). First, we emphasize that our computational and theoretical results provide no basis for such preferential effects. Then we note that this can be attributed to our simplifying assumptions: uniform membrane properties (both passive and active), extracellular isopotentiality, constant intracellular resistivity, implicitly constant ionic membrane equilibrium potentials. For example, if one were to assume that one branch is composed of more excitable membrane than the other, preferential effects could be expected. The recognition that some such additional factor is needed to explain preferential effects has been noted also by Zeevi (1972) and Grossman et al. (1973).

APPENDIX

Here we wish to examine the consequences of changing the taper rule to lesser and greater degrees of taper. We replace our earlier Eq. 22 by a more general expression

$$r/r_0 = \left(\frac{Kx}{3\lambda_0} + 1\right)^m \tag{33}$$

where $m = 0$ corresponds to a cylinder, $m = 1$ corresponds to a conical flare or taper, $m = 2$ corresponds to our special class, and $m > 2$ corresponds to flare or taper of higher degree.

Referring back to the general treatment of taper and branching (Rall, 1962, Eq. 20) we find that the coefficient of $\partial \mathcal{V}/\partial Z$ in the general partial differential equation can be expressed

$$\text{Coef} = (dx/dZ)(d/dx)\ln[r^{3/2}n(1 + (dr/dx)^2)]. \tag{34}$$

It is this coefficient which was shown to reduce to K for our special class. We set $n = 1$, because we are not here concerned with branching. Also, we restrict consideration to regions where $(dr/dx)^2$ is negligible[3] compared with unity; then Eq. 34 can be simplified to yield the approximate expression

$$\text{Coef} \simeq (3\lambda_0/2r_0)\left(\frac{r}{r_0}\right)^{-1/2}(dr/dx). \tag{35}$$

When Eq. 33 and its derivative with respect to x are substituted into Eq. 35, the result is

$$\text{Coef} \simeq \frac{mK}{2}\left(1 + \frac{Kx}{3\lambda_0}\right)^{(m-2)/2} \tag{36}$$

Now, when $m = 0$, this coefficient of $\partial V/\partial Z$ is zero, and the PDE reduces to the case of a cylinder, as expected. When $m = 2$, the exponent, $(m - 2)/2$, becomes zero, and the coefficient of $\partial V/\partial Z$ reduces simply to K, as in Eq. 24 and in the original presentation (Rall, 1962). However, now we can use Eq. 36 to learn the consequences of different taper classes obtained by setting $m = 1$ and $m > 2$.

For conical flare, $m = 1$, and the value of Eq. 36 becomes

$$\frac{K}{2}\left(1 + \frac{Kx}{3\lambda_0}\right)^{-1/2}$$

which equals $K/2$ at $x = 0$ and decreases with increasing x, when K is positive. As explained below, this would be expected to result in increasing dimensionless velocity, $\tau\theta/\lambda_{\text{taper}}$, with increasing x and positive K.

For greater degrees of flare, $m > 2$, it can be seen in Eq. 36 that the exponent is positive, which means that the coefficient of $\partial V/\partial Z$ increases with increasing x when K is positive. As explained below, this corresponds to decreasing dimensionless velocity, $\tau\theta/\lambda_{\text{taper}}$, with increasing x and positive K.

To understand the effect of this coefficient upon dimensionless velocity, we consider first our special class of taper which was found to result in constant dimensionless velocity, $\tau\theta/\lambda_{\text{taper}}$. For this class, we have the relation

$$\partial \mathcal{V}/\partial T = -(\tau\theta/\lambda_{\text{taper}})(\partial \mathcal{V}/dZ) \tag{37}$$

in analogy with Eq. 8 for cylinders. When this relation is substituted into Eqs. 24–26 we obtain the following

$$(\partial^2 \mathcal{V}/\partial Z^2) + (K + \tau\theta/\lambda_{\text{taper}})(\partial \mathcal{V}/\partial Z) = \mathcal{V} - \mathcal{E}(1 - \mathcal{V})$$
$$+ \mathcal{J}(\mathcal{V} + 0.1), \quad (38)$$

$$-\tau\theta/\lambda_{\text{taper}}(\partial\mathcal{E}/\partial Z) = k_1\mathcal{V}^2 + k_2\mathcal{V}^4 - k_3\mathcal{E} - k_4\mathcal{E}\mathcal{J}, \quad (39)$$

$$-\tau\theta/\lambda_{\text{taper}}(\partial\mathcal{J}/\partial Z) = k_5\mathcal{E} + k_6\mathcal{E}\mathcal{J} - k_7\mathcal{J}. \quad (40)$$

When we compare Eqs. 38–40 with the case of constant propagation in a cylinder (Eqs. 13–15), we note that the equations are quite similar. If the coefficients of $\partial\mathcal{V}/\partial Z$, $\partial\mathcal{E}/\partial Z$, and $\partial \mathcal{J}/\partial Z$ were all the same, the equations would be identical (assuming X replaced by Z) and the action potential shapes (in the time domain) would be identical. In particular, comparison of Eq. 38 with Eq. 13 suggests that one might expect the dimensionless velocity, $\tau\theta/\lambda$ in the cylinder, to correspond to the quantity, $K + \tau\theta/\lambda_{\text{taper}}$ in the taper; this suggests

$$\tau\theta/\lambda_{\text{taper}} = \tau\theta_c/\lambda_0 - K, \quad (41)$$

which agrees with Eq. 31, where $\beta = \tau\theta/\lambda_{\text{taper}}$. Our computations showed that this relation holds approximately (see discussion of Fig. 13). To understand why this relation is not exact (theoretically) we note the fact that the coefficients of $\partial\mathcal{E}/\partial Z$ and $\partial\mathcal{J}/\partial Z$ in Eqs. 39 and 40 differ from the coefficient of $\partial\mathcal{V}/\partial Z$ in Eq. 38, whereas the corresponding coefficients in Eqs. 13–15 are identical. Nevertheless, it can be appreciated, intuitively, that departures from Eq. 41 are least when the shape of the action potential in the time domain differs negligibly between the case of a cylinder and our special class of taper.

With different classes of taper, we do not expect constant dimensionless velocity. Nevertheless, in analogy with Eq. 41, we expect that the changing velocity can be at least roughly approximated by

$$\beta = \tau\theta/\lambda_{\text{taper}} \simeq \tau\theta_c/\lambda_0 - \frac{mK}{2}\left(1 + \frac{Kx}{3\lambda_0}\right)^{(m-2)/2} \quad (42).$$

where the coefficient, K in Eq. 41 has been replaced by the more general coefficient from Eq. 36. This relation implies that for the greater degrees of flare ($m > 2$, with positive K), the dimensionless velocity will decrease with increasing x. Also, for the lower degrees of flare ($m < 2$, with positive K), the dimensionless velocity would be expected to increase with increasing x. Only our special class of taper ($m = 2$), and the cylindrical case ($m = 0$) can be expected to have constant dimensionless velocity in the Z domain.

We would like to thank Maurice Klee and John Rinzel for their helpful comments upon reviewing the manuscript.

Received for publication 1 May 1974.

REFERENCES

BROCK, L. G., J. S. COOMBS, and J. C. ECCLES. 1953. *J. Physiol.* **122**:429.
CHUNG, S., S. A. RAYMOND, and J. Y. LETTVIN. 1970. *Brain Behav. Evol.* **3**:72.
DODGE, F. A., JR., and J. W. COOLEY. 1973. *IBM J. Res. Dev.* **17**:219.

EVANS, J. W. 1972. *Indiana Univ. Math. J.* **22**:577.

EVANS, J. W., and N. SHENK. 1970. *Biophys. J.* **10**:1090.

FITZHUGH, R. 1961. *Biophys. J.* **1**:445.

FITZHUGH, R. 1969. *In* Biological Engineering. H. P. Schwan, editor. McGraw-Hill Book Company, New York. 1–85.

FITZHUGH, R. 1973. *J. Theor. Biol.* **40**:517.

FUORTES, M. G. F., K. FRANK, and M. C. BECKER. 1957. *J. Gen. Physiol.* **40**:735.

GROSSMAN, Y., M. E. SPIRA, and I. PARNAS. 1973. *Brain Res.* **64**:379.

HODGKIN, A. L., and R. F. HUXLEY. 1952. *J. Physiol. (Lond.)* **117**:500.

KATZ, B. 1966. Nerve, Muscle, and Synapse. McGraw-Hill Book Company, New York.

KATZ, B., and R. MILEDI. 1965. *Proc. Ry. Soc. Lond. B. Biol. Sci.* **161**:453.

KHODOROV, B. I., Y. N. TIMIN, Y. VILENKIN, and F. B. GUL'KO. 1969. *Biofizika.* **14**:304.

PASTUSHENKO, U. F., V. S. MARKIN, and Y. A. CHIZMADAHEV. 1969 *a. Biofizika.* **14**:883.

PASTUSHENKO, U. F., V. S. MARKIN, and Y. A. CHIZMADAHEV. 1969 *b. Biofizika.* **14**:1072.

RALL, W. 1959. *Exp. Neurol.* **1**:491.

RALL, W. 1962. *Ann. N. Y. Acad. Sci.* **96**:1071.

RALL, W. 1964. *In* Neural Theory and Modeling. R. F. Reiss, editor. Stanford University Press, Stanford, Calif. 73–97.

RALL, W., and G. M. SHEPHERD. 1968. *J. Neurophysiol.* **31**:884.

SMITH, G. D. 1965. Numerical Solutions of Partial Differential Equations. Oxford University Press, London.

WAXMAN, S. G. 1972. *Brain Res.* **47**:269.

ZEEVI, Y. Y. 1972. Ph.D. Thesis, University of California, Berkeley.

10 DENDRITIC SPINES: PLASTICITY, LEARNING, AND ACTIVE AMPLIFICATION

10.1 Introduction by Gordon M. Shepherd with Supplemental Comments by John Miller

Rall, W. (1974). Dendritic spines, synaptic potency and neuronal plasticity.
In *Cellular Mechanisms Subserving Changes in Neuronal Activity*, ed. C. D. Woody,
K. A. Brown, T. J. Crow, and J. D. Knispel. Brain Information Service Research
Report #3. Los Angeles: University of California.

Miller, J. P., Rall, W., and Rinzel, J. (1985). Synaptic amplification by active
membrane in dendritic spines. *Brain Res.* 325:325–330.

Wil Rall has had a long love affair with dendritic spines. Few realize the
extent of his contributions to this area. Although a full account of the
development of concepts of spine function goes beyond the scope of the
present volume, it may be of interest to provide an orientation to the
specific areas in which Wil's contributions have been ground breaking.

Presynaptic and Postsynaptic Functions of Dendritic Spines

Rall's first contribution to the subject of dendritic spines was made in the
papers by Rall et al. (1966) and Rall and Shepherd (1968) (reprinted in this
volume). The idea that the granule cell might send its inhibitory synaptic
outputs through its dendritic spines onto the mitral cell dendrites arose
out of the previous work with Phillips and Powell (Shepherd 1963), in
which we envisaged the spines as functioning essentially like axon terminals for the axonless granule cell. The studies with Wil Rall supported this
output function for the granule cell spines, but Reese and Brightman's
work established that the granule cell processes are in fact dendritic in
their fine structure, and the spines are therefore dendritic despite having
presynaptic and postsynaptic relations. This effectively dissociated the
identification of a terminal as pre- or postsynaptic from the criteria for
identification of a terminal as axonal or dendritic, a lesson which is still
not understood by many. Parenthetically it may be noted that the term
gemmule was introduced to refer to these structures partly in order to
avoid confusion with spines that occupy only postsynaptic positions.

Although our biophysical models did not explicitly include the spines, it
was clear to us that the spines play a key role in the synaptic mechanisms.
The new ideas with regard to the spines were (1) the locally generated
EPSP in a spine activates the output inhibitory synapse from the same
spine to provide for recurrent inhibition of the mitral cell, and (2) spread
of the EPSP out of a spine and through the dendritic branch into neighboring spines provides for lateral inhibition of neighboring mitral cells.
We discussed this in the text and illustrated it with a diagram (figure 15,
Rall and Shepherd 1968) that shows the reciprocal and lateral actions
mediated by the spines. We noted that spread between spines would be
limited for spine stems that were unusually long or thin. This was the first
published observation by Wil or myself about the control of the spread of

activity between a spine head and its parent branch. It was essentially a restatement of Chang's (1952) inference concerning spines on cortical dendrites.

Over the subsequent quarter of a century there have been many speculations about the general properties of dendritic spines. An often-repeated claim is that spines have no interesting properties and serve "only to connect." The granule cell spines still stand as an often-ignored example of spines to which can be attributed specific functional operations of generally acknowledged significance for information processing.

Dendritic Spines and Learning

As with most of his work, Wil's interest in the possible role of dendritic spines in learning had deep roots. His first publication on this topic was in a "Comment on dendritic spines" at the end of his paper on "Cable properties of dendrites and effects of synaptic location," delivered at a meeting on "Excitatory Synaptic Mechanisms" held in Oslo in September of 1969 (Rall 1970). His comment was stimulated by a hypothesis that was brought forward at the meeting by Diamond, Gray, and Yasargil (1970), and which attracted wide attention at the time. They speculated that an intermediary "unit" in a reflex circuit under investigation was a spine whose activity was relatively isolated from other synaptic activity in the neuron by virtue of a high spine stem resistance. They speculated that the function of this isolation might be to reduce the noise level at the synapse; others speculated that it might linearize the summation of responses in neighboring spines. Wil comments in his paper from this meeting that his own preference is that "spine stem resistance might be used physiologically to change the relative weights of synaptic inputs from different afferent sources; this could provide a basic mechanism for learning in the nervous system." He notes that this is only a "slight extension" of his earlier suggestion in Rall 1962b that the relative weight contributed by dendritic synapses to summation at the soma "could be changed by changing the caliber (and hence the electrotonic decrement) of a dendritic subsystem," and that "this would be useful for learning."

In his comment, Wil notes that he has begun a theoretical exploration of this problem with his colleague John Rinzel. Anatomists were just beginning to make accurate measurements of spine dimensions, and Rall and Rinzel drew their data from the studies of Laatsch and Cowan (1966), Jones and Powell (1969), and Peters and Kaiserman-Abramof (1970) on dendritic spines of cortical pyramidal cells. These spines are exclusively postsynaptic in position and could be categorized into different types depending on their outward morphology. Jones and Powell had noted that spines with thin stems frequently arise from thin distal dendrites and spines with stubby stems from thick proximal dendrites. The key insight of Rall and Rinzel was that this anatomical correlation would have critical implications for the electrotonic relations between spines and dendrites, which in turn could have profound functional importance.

Their results were first contained in two abstracts (Rall and Rinzel 1971a,b), one presented to the IUPS Congress in the summer of 1971 and the other presented at the first meeting of the new Society for Neuroscience, held in Washington, D.C., in the fall of 1971. In these, Rall and Rinzel point out for the first time that the amount of spread of a synaptic potential from a spine to its parent branch is governed not just by the spine stem resistance alone but rather by the ratio of the spine stem resistance to the input resistance of the branch; in other words, one is dealing with an impedance matching problem. When this ratio is either very large or very small, changes in spine stem diameter (hence, spine stem resistance) have little effect on synaptic potential spread to the branch. In the middle range, however, where the ratio is near unity, a small change in spine stem resistance has a relatively large effect on the amount of spread. "Over this favorable range ... fine adjustments of the stem resistances of many spines, as well as changes in dendritic caliber ... could provide an organism with a way to adjust the relative weights of the many synaptic inputs received by such neurons; this could contribute to plasticity and learning of a nervous system" (Rall and Rinzel 1971b).

The reason that these abstracts are quoted here is that they were the only generally accessible publication of the hypothesis. The details of the study were published in the privately printed UCLA research report reproduced here (Rall 1974), and repeated and extended in an article in a festschrift volume for Archie McIntyre (Rall 1978). The hypothesis was first presented to a general readership in a book on synaptic organization (Shepherd 1974) in much the summary form given here, together with an extension to the concept of a microcompartment created within the spine head. As to why Wil did not publish this seminal work more fully, the answer is mainly to be found in his battle throughout the 1970s with cataracts and the consequences of cataract surgery. The fact that the study was well known among those working on the cellular basis of memory during that time was a further disincentive to more complete publication. Finally, there has always been enough of the mathematician in Wil for him to feel that "what is known is trivial," and that publishing a study once, however succinctly, should suffice for those who are interested. It is a luxury that few scientists nowadays can afford!

In the 1974 paper reprinted here, Wil shows how the anatomical dimensions of the different types of spines translate into simplified equations for impedance matching of the spine stem resistance to the branch input resistance. He explains that this approach builds on the theoretical method for estimation of branch input resistance presented fully in the study of Rall and Rinzel (1973); this paper is included in the present volume. He notes further that these results based on the assumption of steady-state electrotonic spread can be extended to the case of transient synaptic potentials with only qualitative differences.

From this study came several important concepts. First was the idea of an "optimal operating range" for the relation between a spine and its parent dendrite. Second was the idea of "synaptic potency." As is typical of Wil, he did not confine himself to spine stem length and diameter as the only possible mechanisms regulating synaptic potency. Among other candidates he mentions are synaptic contact area, amount of released chemical transmitter, duration of synaptic action, and changes in internal spine stem resistance. The possibility of changes in spine stem dimensions was soon examined in the experiments of Fifkova and van Harreveld (1977). Others of these suggestions were remarkably prescient. Later Bailey and Chen (1983) indeed found evidence in Aplysia for changes in synaptic contact area associated with activity. The prolonged duration of NMDA receptor actions in spine synapses and their possible relevance for learning mechanisms is another current example.

A notable quality of Wil's biophysical work has been his ability to generalize from biophysical property at the membrane or cellular level to the function of the system. We have already seen an example of this in the study of granule cell spines, where the reciprocal synapses were immediately seen to provide the mechanism for the system functions of recurrent and lateral inhibition underlying sensory processing. It is also seen in his 1974 paper in his inference, from adustable spine stems, of the larger functional view that "delicate adjustments of the relative weights (potency) of many different synapses" could be "responsible for changes in dynamic patterns of activity in assemblies of neurons organized with convergent and divergent connective overlaps." Thus, from these purely biophysical deductions, Wil essentially deduced the blueprint for neural networks consisting of nodes interconnected by synapses with adjustable weights. This general concept of course was not new; what was novel was directing attention to a critical site and suggesting some testable mechanisms.

This work had a large effect on investigators interested in the synaptic basis of learning and memory. During the 1970s and 1980s it provided one of the main organizing hypotheses for possible mechanisms of learning and memory. The fact that dramatic changes in spine size and shape were reported to be associated with sensory deafferentation as well as with specific types of mental disorders gave further credence to the hypothesis. With the rediscovery of Hebb and his learning rules around 1980, and the wealth of new data on the activity dependence of different types of membrane channels in the 1980s, interest has broadened to include these and other mechanisms in the basis of learning and memory. These can be seen as additions to the mechanisms previously suggested by Rall. They add to the complexity of spine synapses and the functional links between spine synapses, reinforcing the notion that they are likely to be critical to the integrative actions underlying higher cortical functions.

Active Dendrites and Dendritic Spines

No topic illustrates more clearly the common misconceptions about Rall's work than the question of nonlinear properties of dendrites in general and the active properties of dendrites and spines in particular. In the popular mind, Rall's contributions are regarded as lying entirely within the domain of passive cable properties of oversimplified dendritic trees. As such, they seem mainly to be of historical interest, because it is currently believed that active properties are the critical agents in dendritic integration. But the facts speak otherwise. They show that Rall led the way in analyzing the nonlinear properties of synaptic interactions, in incorporating active membrane into computational models of dendritic trees, in pointing out the logical possibilities of local active membrane in dendritic trees, in incorporating active membrane into models of dendritic spines, and in exploring the functional implications of populations of active dendritic spines. Let us consider each of these contributions.

Nonlinear Properties of Synaptic Interactions

This topic was first introduced into the literature in the landmark paper of Rall 1964, reproduced in this volume. As already pointed out in the introduction to that paper, the compartmental model presented in that paper enabled Rall to put synapses at different distances from each other in a dendritic tree and explore their interactions. A cardinal result from that analysis was that, contrary to the then-popular belief that excitation and inhibition sum algebraically (i.e., linearly), such summation was true only for summation of responses to injected current, in which the system was unperturbed. For the case of synaptic interactions, their summation was in general nonlinear, because the synaptic conductances perturbed the system. The nonlinear nature of these interactions was dependent on several key parameters. These included (1) the distance between two active synapses (i.e., the degree of shunting between them), (2) the relation of the membrane potential to the reversal potentials for the ions involved, and (3) the geometrical relations between the synapses within the branching structure of the dendritic tree (whether they were on different branches, on the same branch extending to the soma, and whether the excitatory or inhibitory synapse was proximal or distal in the on-line configuration).

At the time, these were recognized as new and fundamental insights into the nature of synaptic integration in dendrites. No longer could synapses be modeled by current injection, and no longer could dendrites with even purely passive membrane be regarded as linear systems. Unfortunately, there has been a tendency for people to forget this work and connect Rall with the exploration of only passive linear models of dendritic integration. The new generation of neural modelers has yet to rediscover the truths that Rall revealed some 30 years ago.

Active Membrane in Dendrites

The first experimental evidence that dendrites might contain sites of active membrane came from the studies of Eccles et al. (1958) on chromatolytic motoneurons and those of Spencer and Kandel (1961) on hot spots in pyramidal cell dendrites in the hippocampus. When in 1962 we began to construct our computational model of the mitral cell, it was clear to us that it would be essential to explore the functional consequences of active dendritic membrane. Our simulations therefore included either passive or active membrane in the mitral cell dendrites; the active properties could have either "hot" or "cold" kinetics. As reported in the initial abstract (Rall and Shepherd 1965) and the full papers (Rall et al. 1966; Rall and Shepherd 1968; see this volume), dendrites with active membrane facilitated antidromic invasion to the extent that we could rule out fast kinetics in large dendrites, because the near-simultaneous invasion would not produce sufficient longitudinal current flows to give the large amplitude extracellular field potentials that had been recorded experimentally. We concluded that the simulations were consistent with either antidromic invasion of thin dendrites by a relatively slowly propagating impulse, or passive invasion of relatively large dendrites (Rall and Shepherd 1968).

We also modeled active properties in the granule cell. For these we used only weakly active membrane, because active properties in the granule cell dendritic tree promoted rapid spread that, as in the mitral cell, reduced the field potential amplitudes unacceptably. A satisfactory result for the case of weakly active dendritic membrane could be obtained only if synaptic inhibition was applied to the deep granule cell processes at the same time as synaptic excitation was applied to the superficial processes. This was

probably the first computational neuronal model to contain all three basic
functional properties: active membrane and both synaptic excitation and
inhibition. Note that the model was heavily constrained in multiple ways:
the anatomy of the granule cells; the intracellular and extracellular unit
recordings; the time course of inhibitory synaptic output; the ratio of extracellular to intracellular current paths; and the time course, amplitude,
and depths of the extracellular field potentials. We concluded that the brief
repetitive impulse discharges that can be recorded from granule cells likely
are localized to their cell bodies, and that the spread of activity within the
granule cell dendritic tree and the activation of the output synapses from
the granule cell spines probably do not involve a prominent role for active
membrane. Subsequent studies of granule cell responses have been consistent with that interpretation, without, of course, ruling out that weak
voltage-sensitive inward currents could contribute to inhibitory synaptic
output, as originally suggested.

Given the explicit incorporation of active membrane properties in the
models of both mitral and granule cells, it seems past time to recognize
that Rall was a pioneer in analyzing active properties in compartmental
models of neuronal dendrites.

Functional Implications of Active Dendrites

In the same paper in which he first mentioned the idea of changes in spine
stem resistance underlying learning (Rall 1970), Rall also commented on
the more general functional implications of active membrane in dendrites
in relation to information processing:

Active dendritic membrane could result in unusual logical properties that have
interested a number of people (Lorente de Nó and Condouris, 1959; Richard
FitzHugh, personal communication, also Arshavskii et al., 1965). The notion is
that the excitation initiated in a dendritic branchlet will propagate centripetally
beyond each point of bifurcation only if it is aided at the right moment by excitation from several sibling branches along the way, and provided also that it does
not meet inhibition along the way. Such multiple possibilities of success or failure,
at many different points of bifurcation, could lead to elaborate sets of contingent
probabilities which would provide a single neuron (if it has suitable input patterns
over the dendritic branches) with a very large logical capacity.

Rall then went on to define some of the rules for these types of
interactions:

Even for passive dendritic membrane, localized dendritic synaptic excitation has
the property of being especially vulnerable to synaptic inhibitory conductance
which is delivered to the same dendritic location: the larger the amplitude of the
uninhibited local membrane depolarization, the larger is the reduction produced
by a locally superimposed inhibitory conductance. This is very nonlinear in that

the EPSP amplitude is reduced by much more than the amplitude of a control IPSP (which may be negligible). In contrast, when the inhibitory input is delivered to a different dendritic tree, the effect at the soma is simply a linear summation of the separate EPSP and IPSP observable at the soma; see Rall et al. (1967, pp. 1184–1185) for examples of both kinds. Synaptic inhibition delivered to the soma is effective against all excitatory inputs, provided the timing is correct, while synaptic inhibition delivered to a dendritic branch is selectively effective against excitatory inputs to the same branch.

These two comments taken together essentially set forth an agenda for specifying the rules of synaptic interaction in dendrites and relating them to the kinds of logical operations that they would support with the aid of active dendritic membrane properties. Much of this agenda was to be realized in the work of Christof Koch and Tomaso Poggio and their colleagues in the following decade, through detailed delineation of on-line excitatory and inhibitory synaptic actions, characterization of shunting versus summating synaptic inhibition (which constitute two extremes along the continuum of interactions Rall had explored), and modeling of explicit logic operations arising from excitatory and inhibitory synaptic interactions within a dendritic tree (Koch et al., 1982; see also Segev and Parnas 1983). The relevance of these properties for network models of cortical circuits underlying cognitive functions was addressed by Sejnowski, Koch, and Churchland (1988).

Active Dendritic Spines

The opportunity to explore more fully the question of the membrane properties of dendritic membrane came with the use of more powerful and flexible computational modeling programs. I had intended to pursue this question with Wil, but the problem with his cataracts made this impossible. I therefore began the collaboration with Robert Brayton that resulted in the more detailed simulation of the reciprocal dendrodendritic synaptic circuit (Shepherd and Brayton 1979). This simulation placed the Hodgkin-Huxley model in a proximal dendritic compartment of the mitral cell; the rest of the membrane in the mitral and granule cell dendritic models was passive.

By 1980 we had begun to explore the functional consequences of placement of active membrane at other dendritic sites in this model, including the granule cell spines. We also began to adapt our model to the case of the exclusively postsynaptic spines of cortical pyramidal cells, to deal with the question of whether active membrane would help to boost the responses of dendrites and spines in the most distal parts of the tree. We were especially interested in the case of pyramidal neurons in the olfactory cortex, where it is clear that the specific sensory information is conveyed from the input fibers (of the lateral olfactory tract) onto spines on the most distal dendrites. This placement is of course counterintuitive and against the common belief, still widely held, that synaptic inputs must be directed to the cell body of a neuron in order to transmit specific information in a rapid manner, distal synaptic inputs being believed to convey only slow background modulation. It should be clear from the previous discussion that we never believed that this could be a valid rule.

About this time John Miller joined Wil's laboratory to further the studies of dendritic integration. John and I met at a Winter Brain Conference, and I told him about the advantages of ASTAP for neural modeling. However, I soon learned, to my chagrin, that ASTAP was a proprietary IBM product that was not available for general use. This was a distinct disappointment, because I had become convinced that the use of large general-purpose circuit simulators, such as ASTAP, was the most effective way to make neural modeling more accessible for incorporation into experimental laboratories for parallel exploration of neuronal properties, in the same way that Wil had begun to develop the compartmental approach by adapting the general model of his colleague Mones Berman. However, in our 1979 paper Brayton had suggested that other more generally available circuit simulation programs such as SPICE could also be adapted for this purpose, so we recommended that John and Wil look into that. Doron Lancet was with me at the time, and he had several interactions with John in setting this up. Also, Wil and John came to IBM so that Brayton and I could demonstrate how ASTAP worked. We pointed out the advantage of being able to adjust the Hodkin-Huxley parameters from trial to trial, which was especially useful for exploring the values appropriate for active properties of thin dendritic branchlets and spines.

By 1984 John and Wil had successfully adapted SPICE for carrying out simulations of active properties of a single dendritic spine and the possible contribution to boosting the response of the spine to an excitatory synaptic input. A number of different lines of work then came to a head. Don Perkel and his son David had independently become interested in the same problem, using the neural modeling program MANUEL that Don had developed. The two groups were in touch with each other and agreed to submit companion papers to *Science*, consisting of Perkel and Perkel 1985 and the paper reproduced here (Miller et al. 1985). They were rejected as being of insufficient interest to a general audience, and were subsequently published in *Brain Research*. Brayton and I meanwhile had gotten our model of active dendritic spines going. We wanted especially to disprove the received wisdom that distal spines could mediate only slow background modulation, and chose first to show that interactions between active spines could provide for a kind of saltatory conduction that would convey distal active responses toward the soma. We kept in close touch with Wil and his team at NIH, which by then included not only John Miller but also John Rinzel and Idan Segev. We decided to submit a joint paper on our initial finding on the active boosting model; it was first rejected by *Nature* as being of insufficient interest but subsequently was sponsored by Ed Evarts in the *Proceedings of the National Academy* and accepted (Shepherd et al. 1985).

I have summarized this series of events to indicate that Wil not only pointed to the new era of investigation of active properties of dendrites with his earlier speculations, but he was also a driving force behind developing the first computational models that demonstrated these properties.

During this time Barry Bunow at NIH was working on adapting SPICE for more effective modeling of the nonlinear properties of the Hodgkin-Huxley equations. The problem was that the equations had to be simulated by a polynomial expansion, which made it cumbersome to manipulate the parameters. A great deal of effort went into this study (Bunow et al. 1985), and SPICE in this version played an important role during the latter part of the decade in providing a means for modeling complex dendritic systems. The studies of Robert Burke, involving detailed reconstructions of motoneuron dendritic trees, were among the best known (Fleshman et al. 1988). During this period Peter Guthrie wrote a version of SPICE specifically adapted for neuronal simulation, called NEUROS. At about this time Michael Hines was developing the program that became NEURON (Hines 1984, 1989), and shortly thereafter Matt Wilson and Jim Bower developed GENESIS (1989).

After developing the single active spine model, Wil teamed with Idan Segev to explore the functional implications of groups of active spines. This was again a natural step in going from the level of a single functional unit to the level of multiple units. They analyzed the rules governing the coincident activation of different subpopulations of active spines located on different dendritic branches (Rall and Segev 1987). These rules will likely govern the ways that subpopulations of spines control both the immediate responses of a neuron to synaptic inputs as well as the activity-dependent responses under conditions of long-term potentiation or depression. Rall has conceived of the properties governing spine potency very broadly; thus, the nonlinearities of spine responses may be due to active conductances in the spine heads, spine necks, or spine bases, as modeled in these studies; to changes in $Ca++$ concentration; to metabolic changes as might be mediated by protein kinases; and to effects mediated through the genome such as by immediate early genes. The importance of Rall's studies lies not only in the exploration of specifically electrical changes contributing to spine functions but also in the provision of a broader focus on nonlinear changes in synaptic potency by any or all of these mechanisms that endow the neuron with increased computational capacity, as indicated in the passages cited earlier. When these mechanisms can be correlated with specific logical or computational operations, we will have begun to solve one of the deepest and most perplexing problems in neuroscience: the specific contributions that neuronal dendrites make to brain functions.

References

Arshavskii, Y. I., Berkinblit, M. B., Kovalev, S. A., Smolyaninov, V. V., and Chailakhyan, L. M. (1965). The role of dendrites in the functioning of nerve cells. *Dokl. Akademii Nauk SSSR* 163:994–997. (Translation in *Dokl. Biophys. Consultants Bureau*, New York, 1965.)

Bailey, C. H., and Chen, M. (1983). Morphological basis of long-term habituation and sensitization in Aplysia. *Science* 220:91–93.

Bunow, B., Segev, I., and Fleshman, J. W. (1985). Modeling the electrical properties of anatomically complex neurons using a network analysis program: Excitable membrane. *J. Biol. Cyber.* 53:41–56.

Chang, H.-T. (1952). Cortical neurons with particular reference to the apical dendrites. *Cold Spring Harbor Symp. Quant. Biol.* 17:189–202.

Diamond, J., Gray, E. G., and Yasargil, G. M. (1970). The function of the dendritic spine: An hypothesis. In *Excitatory Synaptic Mechanisms*, ed. P. Andersen and J. K. S. Jansen, Jr. Oslo: Universitetsforlag.

Eccles, J. C., Libet, B., and Young, R. R. (1958). The behavior of chromatolyzed motoneurons studied by intracellular recording. *J. Physiol. London* 143:11–40.

Fifkova, E., and van Harreveld, A. (1977). Long-lasting morphological changes in dendritic spines of dentate granular cells following stimulation of the entorhinal area. *J. Neurocytol.* 6:211–230.

Fleshman, J. W., Segev, I., and Burke, R. E. (1988). Electrotonic architecture of type-identified α motoneurons in the cat spinal cord. *J. Neurophysiol.* 60:60–85.

Hines, M. (1984). Efficient computation of branched nerve equations. *Int. J. Bio-Med. Comp.* 15:69–76.

Hines, M. (1989). A program for simulation of nerve equations with branching geometries. *Int. J. Bio-Med. Comp.* 24:55–68.

Jones, E. G., and Powell, T. P. S. (1969). Morphological variations in the dendritic spines of the neocortex. *J. Cell. Sci.* 5:509–527.

Koch, C., Poggio, T., and Torre, V. (1982). Retinal ganglion cells: A functional interpretation of dendritic morphology. *Philos. Trans. R. Soc. Lond.* [B] 298:227–263.

Laatsch, R. H., and Cowan, W. M. (1966). Electron microscopic studies of the dentate gyrus of the rat. I. Normal structure with special reference to synaptic organization. *J. Comp. Neurol.* 128:359–396.

Lorente de No, R., and Condouris, G. A. (1959). Decremental conduction in peripheral nerve: integration of stimuli in the neuron. *Proc. Natl. Acad. Sci. USA* 45:592–617.

Miller, J. P., Rall, W., and Rinzel, J. (1985). Synaptic amplification by active membrane in dendritic spines. *Brain Res.* 325:325–330.

Perkel, D. H., and Perkel, D. J. (1985). Dendritic spines: Role of active membrane in modulating synaptic efficacy. *Brain Res.* 325:331–335.

Peters, A., and Kaiserman-Abramof, I. R. (1970). The small pyramidal neuron of the rat cerebral cortex: The perikaryon, dendrites and spines. *Am. J. Anat.* 127:321–356.

Rall, W. (1962b). Electrophysiology of a dendritic neuron model. *Biophys. J.* 2:145–167.

Rall, W. (1967). Distinguishing theoretical synaptic potentials computed for different soma-dendritic distributions of synaptic input. *J. Neurophysiol.* 30:1138–1168.

Rall, W. (1970). Cable properties of dendrites and effects of synaptic location. In *Excitatory Synaptic Mechanisms*, ed. P. Andersen and J. K. S. Jansen, Jr. Oslo: Universitatsforlag.

Rall, W. (1974). Dendritic spines, synaptic potency and neuronal plasticity. In *Cellular Mechanisms Subserving Changes in Neuronal Activity*, ed. C. D. Woody, K. A. Brown, T. J. Crow, and J. D. Knispel. Brain Information Service Research Report #3. Los Angeles: University of California.

Rall, W. (1978). Dendritic spines and synaptic potency. In *Studies in Neurophysiology*, ed. R. Porter. Cambridge: Cambridge University Press.

Rall, W., and Rinzel, J. (1971a). Dendritic spines and synaptic potency explored theoretically. *Proc. I.U.P.S. (XXV Intl. Congress)* 9:466.

Rall, W., and Rinzel, J. (1971b). Dendritic spine function and synaptic attenuation calculations. *Soc. Neurosci. Absts.* p. 64.

Rall, W., and Rinzel, J. (1973). Branch input resistance and steady attenuation for input to one branch of a dendritic neuron model. *Biophysic. J.* 13:648–688.

Rall, W. and Segev, I. (1987). Functional possibilities for synapses on dendrites and dendritic spines. In *Synaptic Function*, ed. G. M. Edelman, W. E. Gall, and W. M. Cowan. New York: Wiley.

Rall, W. and Shepherd, G. M. (1968). Theoretical reconstruction of field potentials and dendro-dendritic synaptic interactions in olfactory bulb. *J. Neurophysiol.* 31:884–915.

Rall, W., Shepherd, G. M., Reese, T. S., and Brightman, M. W. (1966). Dendro-dendritic synaptic pathway for inhibition in the olfactory bulb. *Exp. Neurol.* 14:44–56.

Segev, I., and Parnas, I. (1983). Synaptic integration mechanisms: a theoretical and experimental investigation of temporal postsynaptic interactions between excitatory and inhibitory inputs. *Biophys. J.* 41:41–50.

Sejnowski, T. J., Koch, C., and Churchland, P. S. (1988). Computational neuroscience. *Science* 241:1299–1306.

Shepherd, G. M. (1963). Neuronal systems controlling mitral cell excitability. *J. Physiol. Lond.* 168:101–117.

Shepherd, G. M. (1974). *The Synaptic Organization of the Brain*. New York: Oxford University Press.

Shepherd, G. M., and Brayton, R. K. (1979). Computer simulation of a dendrodendritic synaptic circuit for self- and lateral inhibition in the olfactory bulb. *Brain Res.* 175:377–382.

Shepherd, G. M., Brayton, R. K., Miller, J. F., Segev, I., Rinzel, J., and Rall, W. (1985). Signal enhancement in distal cortical dendrites by means of inter-actions between active dendritic spines. *Proc. Nat. Acad. Sci.* 82:2192–2195.

Spencer, W. A., and Kandel, E. R. (1961). Electrophysiology of hippocampal neurons. IV. Fast prepotentials. *J. Neurophysiol.* 24:272–285.

Wilson, M. A. and Bower, J. M. (1989). The simulation of large-scale neural networks. In *Methods in Neuronal Modeling: From Synapses to Networks*, ed. C. Koch and I. Segev. Cambridge, MA: MIT Press.

Supplemental Comments by John Miller

The paper on synaptic amplification by active membrane in dendritic spines that I authored with Wil and John Rinzel was cathartic, in several senses. From a scientific standpoint, it finally got down on paper some speculative ideas that Wil and John had been thinking about for a long time: that is, that spines might act as "current augmentation devices" to boost synaptic efficacy, if there were voltage-dependent conductance channels in the spine heads and the biophysical parameters of the spines were within appropriate ranges.

From a personal standpoint, the whole project represented a culmination of my education about neuronal integration that had begun in my first year of grad school. When asked by my advisor (Al Selverston) what I wanted to do with myself for the next few years, I replied that I wanted to "learn how nerve cells worked." His response was, "In that case, you'd better go read everything Rall has ever written." Having already glanced through the pile of abstruse-looking reprints by Rall that he was collecting, it was as if he had just whacked me upside the head with a giant integral sign ... one of those French ones with the big knobs on each end. Then he added, "You may as well read all of Rinzel's, too." Whack! Double integral. As it turned out, it was excellent advice, and I (and numerous others, I imagine) have repeated it many times over.

In reading through Wil's work and other related papers, many of which have been mentioned in the other notes in this volume, I became particularly intrigued by the few published passages about spines. The papers in *Excitatory Synaptic Mechanisms* by Diamond, Gray, and Yasargil and by Wil, noted in Gordon's preceding comments, attracted considerable attention, and I remember discussing spines at great length in one of our journal clubs. I was working in a lab that focused on the generation of motor patterns by neurons known to have voltage-dependent conductances out in the dendritic membrane, and I was drawn to speculations about how the functional characteristics of spines might change if they, too, had active membrane on their heads. (I also remember Selverston's astute tounge-in-cheek hypothesis: "Yeah, spines probably evolved to keep the neurons stuck together better so they wouldn't fall out of the cortex ... sort of like neuro-velcro.") Wil and John Rinzel visited Al's lab sometime later (1976) and I remember asking them about any thoughts they may have had about active membrane on spines. As I remember, Wil then and there anticipated the "gestalt" of most results we were later to obtain through our simulations, by either reconstructing his previous thoughts or realizing them on the spot.

Since I still had not quite figured out how nerve cells worked by the completion of my thesis work, Selverston thought it would be a good idea for me to do a postdoc in Rall and Rinzel's group. Many experimentalists at the time were realizing the necessity of transforming our qualitative hypotheses concerning synaptic integration into a more quantitative format and were inspired by the spectacular advances Pete Getting had made toward understanding one particular central pattern generator network using the compartmental modeling software developed by Don Perkel and colleagues. I had always been impressed by Wil's use of practical, well-thought-out simulations in his studies of complex neurons and subsystems to complement his analytical derivations in the "simpler" cases, and I thought that doing a postdoc with Wil would offer a unique opportunity to learn more about both analytical and compartmental modeling approaches.

Our interest in spines was actually very far from our minds for most of my stay at NIH but was brought to the surface again by several excellent papers on spine morphology, including one by Fifkova and Anderson (1981) and one by Charlie Wilson and colleagues (1983). Considering a slew of speculative papers that were appearing in the popular press about the possible involvement of "twitching" (but electrically passive) spines in synaptic plasticity, the time seemed ripe for a careful consideration of the functional implications of active spines. The basic idea of the "active spine" study was very simple, and our demonstration of the possibility of synaptic amplification should have come as no surprise.

There were really only two outcomes of the simulations that surprised us, at least, at the time. The first was the large magnitude of the augmentation effect that could be acheived within what we thought at the time to be the most reasonable estimates for spine dimensions: the net charge delivered to the dendrite at the base of an active spine could be as much as an order of magnitude greater than the charge delivered from a passive spine of the same dimensions. The second surprise was the extreme sensitivity of the augmentation effect to small variations in biophysical parameters of the spines: for any particular configuration of parameters determining the dendrite input resistance, spine head input resistance, and voltage-dependent conductance kinetics, there existed an extremely narrow "operating range" of spine stem resistance within which the synaptic augmentation could result. Thus, the degree of augmentation could be substantial, and could possibly be modulated dynamically over a wide range by fine "adjustments" of (for example) spine neck diameter.

Several other people including (at least) Gordon Shepherd, Idan Segev, Don Perkel, and Dave Perkel had been thinking along identical lines and had all arrived at essentially identical conclusions by the time we had completed our illustrative simulations. Wil, John, and I were aware of Gordon's thoughts; in fact, he had been extremely generous and encouraging to our pursuit of these simulations, and we discussed the ongoing work regularly. Indeed, the studies really grew out of the work on spines that Gordon had already done with Robert Brayton. As well as getting us on the right track conceptually, Gordon also steered us toward the use of large general-purpose network simulation programs such as SPICE.

When we were well into our own simulations, Wil, John, and I discovered that Idan had begun simulations very similar to ours. Idan and Wil went on to explore the functional significance of active spines in much greater detail, and they continue to pursue the functional possibilities.

After our studies were completed, we also discovered that Don and David Perkel had carried out essentially identical simulation studies. We did not find this out until the accidental scheduling of back-to-back presentations at a Neuroscience meeting symposium. It was this surprise and realization of mutual interest that led us to publish the two papers back-to-back (Perkel and Perkel 1985). This has always been an essential aspect of Wil's character: he is an innate "collaborator," not a "competitor." In this respect, the lessons he teaches us go far beyond dendritic electrotonus.

Supplemental References

Fifkova, E., and Anderson, C. L. (1981) Stimulation-induced changes in dimensions of stalks of dendritic spines in the dentate molecular layer. *Exp. Neurol.* 74:621–627.

Perkel, D. H. and Perkel, D. J. (1985) Dendritic spines: Role of active membrane in modulating synaptic efficacy. *Brain Res.* 325:331–335.

Wilson, C. J., Groves, P. M., Kitai, S. T., and Linder, J. C. (1983) Three dimensional structure of dendritic spines in the rat neostriatum. *J. Neurosci* 3:383–398.

10.2 Dendritic Spines, Synaptic Potency and Neuronal Plasticity (1974), in *Cellular Mechanisms Subserving Changes in Neuronal Activity*, ed. C. D. Woody et al., Brain Information Research Report #3, Los Angeles: University of California

Wilfrid Rall

Dr. Rall discussed a possible role of dendritic spines in neuronal plasticity. Dendritic spines were first reported by Ramón y Cajal in 1888 (*cf.* The Scheibels, 1968). The importance of dendritic spines as sites for synaptic inputs was first noted in 1897 by Berkley (1897). He observed that if a cell was sensitive to all other neighboring cells over its surface there would be chaos, that it was fortunate that the cells were covered with glia, that only the spines stuck out from the glia, and that only the spines would receive inputs, thereby avoiding chaos. In 1952, Chang made the additional observation that, because of their long thin stems, dendritic spines would provide high electrical resistance; this resistance would attenuate the effect of the synapse on the cell (Chang, 1952). He argued that because of this attenuation, a cell could be fired only by a large number of such inputs.

Synaptic inputs to cortical pyramidal cells are mostly by these spines. In 1959 Gray demonstrated synapses on the spines by electronmicroscopy (Gray, 1959). Subsequent studies were made by Colonnier (1968) and others (*cf.* The Scheibels, 1968). Diamond, Gray and colleagues (1970) pointed out that 95% of synaptic input to pyramidal cells is via the spines.

What then is the function of the spines? Presumably they must do something more than simply receive the synaptic input. It cannot be argued that the spines are there to increase receptive surface area since there is considerable surface area that is not occupied by synapses (*cf.* The Scheibels, 1968). With regard to large spine stem resistance, why would attenuation of synaptic potency be desirable? Some have postulated that this large resistance might ensure linear summation of synaptic effects by reducing the coupling between the synapses. One difficulty with this postulate is that extreme amounts of attenuation would be needed to get linear summation. A further possibility is that the dendritic spines could be used to provide a way of changing the relative contributions of different synapses. This could underlie or be a part of neuronal plasticity. This possibility, that spine stem resistance could be used to adjust the relative potency of different synapses on the cell, can be examined biophysically to see if it seems reasonable.

Consider the resistance to electric current flow through a spine stem (Figure 1), from the spine head to its point of attachment on a dendrite. This spine stem resistance is designated R_{ss}. With synaptic membrane

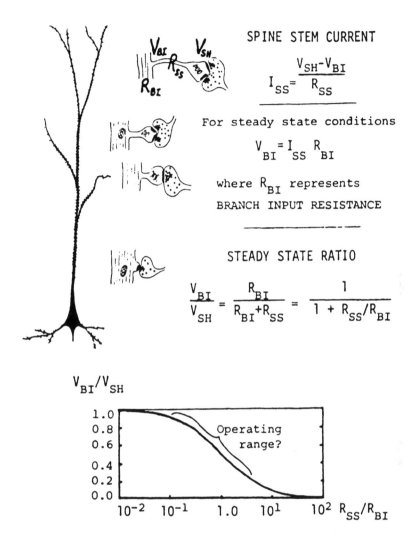

Figure 1
Diagram of the relation of spine stem currents to the resistances and voltages designated in the text.

PETERS AND KAISERMAN-ABRAMOF, 1970

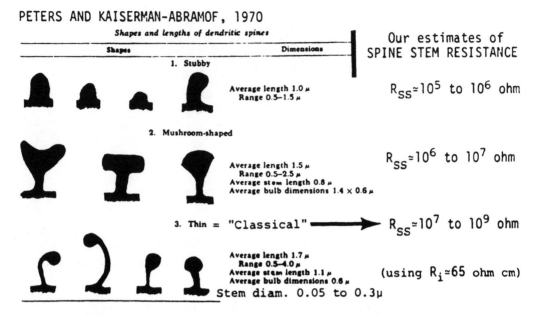

Figure 2
Variations of spine stems and their resistance values. (From Peters and Kaiserman-Abramof, 1970.)

depolarization at the spine head, intracellular current will flow through the spine stem in proportion to the potential difference between the voltage V_{SH} at the spine head and the voltage V_{BI} at the spine base. The potential difference divided by the spine stem resistance gives us the spine stem current I_{SS}, as indicated in Figure 1. For a steady depolarization at the spine head, I_{SS} becomes a steady current which also flows from the spine stem into what is known as the branch input resistance R_{BI} of the cell. This steady current is thus equal to several equivalent ratios:

$$I_{SS} = \frac{V_{BI}}{R_{BI}} = \frac{V_{SH} - V_{BI}}{R_{SS}} = \frac{V_{SH}}{R_{SS} + R_{BI}}$$

From these ratio and from Figure 1, it can be seen that if the spine stem resistance is equal to the branch input resistance, the voltage that is generated out at the synapse would be divided equally between the spine stem resistance and branch input resistance. That is, the voltage V_{BI}, at the branch would be half of that, V_{SH}, which is generated at the spine head. More generally, but still for steady states, the fraction of V_{SH} delivered to the dendrite (*i.e.*, the ratio V_{BI}/V_{SH}) depends upon the resistance ratio, R_{SS}/R_{BI}, as shown in the lower half of Figure 1. The sensitivity (or adjustment) of this relation can be seen to be greatest over the middle range. Can this be used as an operating range for adjusting synaptic potency?

What sort of value should be ascribed to the spine stem resistance? Figure 2 shows us why one must consider more than just one case. Peters and Kaiserman-Abramof (1970) classified the dendritic spines according to their various morphologies: stubby, thin, etc., and it can be seen that there is considerable variety in the dimensions and morphology (Figure 2).

Spine stem resistances can be estimated for these morphological types. Using the specific resistivity noted in Figure 2, we estimated the following ranges of values: for the stubby spines about 0.1 to 1 megohm, for the very thin spines about 10 to 1000 megohms, and for the mushroom shaped spines still other values. Jones and Powell (Jones and Powell, 1969; cf. Peters and Kaiserman-Abramof, 1970) noted that long thin spines are more frequent at distal dendritic locations. Near the cell body and the base of the apical dendrite they find more stubby spines. It seems strange that the long thin spine (which would be expected to cause more attenuation) is usually found at distal dendritic locations (which also cause attenuation). This seems paradoxical. Why should the synapse be doubly handicapped by such double attenuation?

Looking at the relationship of the spine stem resistance to the input resistance may provide a clue to this paradox. There seems to be an impedance matching involved here. If one takes seriously the hypothesis that the spines may be involved in adjusting the relative potency of synapses, then the lower half of Figure 1 provides a possible resolution of this apparent paradox. This graph indicates that as long as the spine stem resistance is no more than one per cent of the input resistance, the spine stem poses no disadvantage to synaptic effectiveness. Also, if the spine stem were used to adjust synaptic potency, one might expect the ratio R_{SS}/R_{BI} to lie in the range from 0.1 to 10, which could be regarded as an optimal operating range for such adjustment.

In order to estimate R_{SS}/R_{BI}, we must have estimates of branch input resistance as well as spine stem resistance. A theoretical method of estimating branch input resistance has recently been published in collaboration with John Rinzel (Rall and Rinzel, 1973). This paper provides full details of assumptions and methods, and many examples are tabulated in Table I (cf. Rall and Rinzel, 1973). There, the branch input resistance, R_{BI}, is expressed relative to the more familiar neuron (at the soma) input resistance, R_N, for many different amounts of branching and lengths of branches. For a distal branch of a pyramidal cell, one might have $R_{BI}/R_N \simeq 100$, and for a typical value of 10 megohms for R_N, this would imply 10^3 megohms for R_{BI}.

Also, when computations were generalized from simple steady state considerations to transient synaptic potentials, such as those illustrated in Figure 3 (top), Rall and Rinzel found that when the transient peak

VOLTAGE TRANSIENTS AT DIFFERENT LOCATIONS
FOR BRIEF INJECTION OF CURRENT AT ONE BRANCH

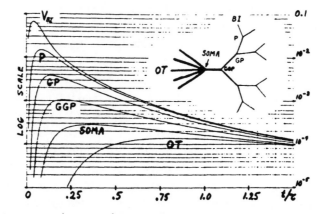

Attenuation of Peak Ampl.		(Compare Steady State)
P	1/4.6	(1/2.3)
GP	1/17	(1/5.3)
GGP	1/62	(1/12)
SOMA	1/232	(1/24)

SYNAPTIC INPUT TO SPINE,
EFFECT OF SPINE STEM RESISTANCE (R_{SS}/R_{BI})
UPON PEAK TRANSIENT VOLTAGES AT
SPINE HEAD (V_{SH}),

INPUT BRANCH (V_{BI}),

AND SOMA (V_{SOMA}).

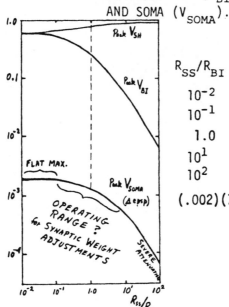

R_{SS}/R_{BI}	Peak V_{SOMA}
10^{-2}	~.002
10^{-1}	~.002
1.0	~.0013
10^{1}	~.0004
10^{2}	$<10^{-4}$

$(.002)(75mV) = 0.15mV$

amplitudes were plotted against R_{SS}/R_{BI} as in Figure 3 (bottom), the results (note log amplitude scale) were qualitatively similar to the steady state results of Figure 1. The attenuation from peak V_{SH} to peak V_{SOMA} is 500 or more, but that still can imply an EPSP amplitude of about 0.15 mV at the soma. It is important to notice the "flat maximum" at the soma for R_{SS}/R_{BI}, from 0.01 to 0.1; this means that adjusting the spine stem resistance to values smaller than one tenth of the branch input resistance would gain nothing in synaptic potency.

These results for the peak at the soma have been replotted in Figure 4. Peak V at the soma is plotted relative to its maximum value for that particular dendritic location, and this is plotted on an arithmetic scale (in contrast with the log scale of Figure 3). This also shows the flat maximum for R_{SS}/R_{BI} from 0.01 to 0.1, and the presumed optimal range, from 0.1 to 2 or 3, for adjusting the potency at the soma for the synapse on a spine at that particular dendritic location.

If we think in term of evolution, and conjecture that there is survival value in keeping the relative potency of many synapses adjustable, then one might expect to find that actual R_{SS}/R_{BI} values lie in this "optimal operating range". The lower half of Figure 4 summarizes the results of our order of magnitude estimates for the spine stem types most commonly found at three locations: distal dendritic, mid-dendritic, and somatic or proximal dendritic. The overall range of 10^7 to 10^9 ohms for R_{SS} of thin spines is separated into 10^8 to 10^9 ohms for the longer-thinner ones most frequent at distal locations, and 10^7 to 10^8 ohms for those most frequent at mid-dendritic locations. Using these estimates, together with the branch input resistance estimates noted earlier for a pyramidal cell, we see that the ratio R_{SS}/R_{BI} does seem to lie in this expected range for both the distal and mid-dendritic locations, whereas the stubby spines at proximal locations would seem to lie in the flat maximum region of maximum potency without flexibility.

It should be emphasized that this agreement with prediction is based upon rough order of magnitude calculations. It is not presented as a proof that our conjecture is correct, but rather as an approximate biophysical test that suggests plausibility and indicates that this possibility cannot yet be ruled out. The design principle involved here is to sacrifice maximum power in order to gain flexibility and control. Adjustability of potency means either increase or decrease relative to other synapses. Thus we think of delicate adjustments of the relative weights (potency) of many different synapses to any given neuron. We think of these changes as

Figure 3
Summary of the effects of brief EPSP time courses based on computations by Rinzel and Rall. (unpublished)

CONCLUSIONS

THEORETICAL DEPENDENCE OF SYNAPTIC WEIGHT
UPON SPINE STEM RESISTANCE, R_{SS}, FOR SPINE LOCATION (R_{BI})

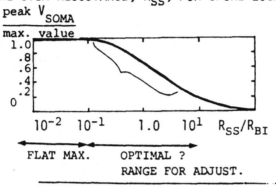

EXPERIMENTAL ESTIMATES OF R_{SS}/R_{BI}

$$\frac{R_{SS} \sim 10^8 \text{ to } 10^9 \text{ ohm}}{R_{BI} \sim 10^9 \text{ ohm}} \approx 10^{-1} \text{ to } 1.0 \quad \text{(OPTIMAL RANGE)}$$

$$\frac{R_{SS} \sim 10^7 \text{ to } 10^8 \text{ ohm}}{R_{BI} \sim 10^8 \text{ ohm}} \approx 10^{-1} \text{ to } 1.0 \quad \text{(OPTIMAL RANGE)}$$

$$\frac{R_{SS} \sim 10^5 \text{ to } 10^6 \text{ ohm}}{R_{BI} \sim R_N \sim 10^7 \text{ ohm}} \approx 10^{-2} \text{ to } 10^{-1} \quad \text{(FLAT MAX.)}$$

Figure 4
Summary of conclusions.

responsible for changes in dynamic patterns of activity in assemblies of neurons organized with convergent and divergent connective overlaps.

We do not pretend to have explained how the spine stem changes would be controlled. Also, we emphasize that other possible ways of adjusting synaptic potent should not be dismissed. Some other possibilities are: (a) the synaptic contact area could be increased or decreased, (b) the amount of chemical transmitter released could change, (c) the duration of synaptic action could be changed, (d) the caliber of the dendritic branch or its entire dendritic tree could change R_{BI}. It is noteworthy that a change in the duration would be especially valuable if the depolarization at the spine head is essentially maximal. A change in a dendritic branch or dendritic tree has some interesting properties regarding synaptic specificity (Rall, 1962) which may relate to some of Dr. Woody's earlier remarks concerning specificity. If just one spine is changed, there is only a change in the weight of that particular synapse. If the weight of the dendritic tree is changed, there is a change in the weight of *all* the synapses that end on that tree, but this is still more specific than changing the threshold of the entire neuron. One could conceive of various conditioning or plasticity situations in which either or any of the above could be most advantageous.

References

Berkley, H. J. The intra-cerebral nerve-fibre terminal apparatus and modes of transmission of nervous impulses. *Johns Hopkins Hosp. Rep.*, 6:89–93, 1897.

Chang, H. T. Cortical neurons with particular reference to the apical dendrites. *Cold Spring Harbor Symp. Quant. Biol.*, 17:189–202, 1952.

Colonnier, M. Synaptic patterns on different cell types in the different laminae of the cat visual cortex. An electron microscope study. *Brain Research*, 9:268–287, 1968.

Diamond, J., Gray, E. G., and Yasargil, G. M. The function of the dendritic spine: an hypothesis. In: *Excitatory Synaptic Mechanisms*. (P. Anderson and J. K. S. Jansen, Eds.). Oslo, Universitetsforlaget, 1970. pp. 213–222.

Gray, E. G. Axo-somatic and axo-dendritic synapses of the cerebral cortex: an electron microscopic study. *J. Anat. (Lond.)*, 93:420–433, 1959.

Jones, E. G., and Powell, T. P. S. Morphological variations in the dendritic spines of the neocortex. *J. Cell. Sci.*, 5:509–529, 1969.

Peters, A., and Kaiserman-Abramof, I. R. The small pyramidal neuron of the rat cerebral cortex. The perikaryon, dendrites and spines. *Am. J. Anat.*, 127:321–356, 1970.

Rall, W. Electrophysiology of a dendritic neuron model. *Biophys. J.*, 2:145–167, 1962.

Rall, W., and Rinzel, J. Branch input resistance and steady attenuation for input to one branch of a dendritic neuron model. *Biophys. J.*, 13:648–688, 1973.

Scheibel, M. E., and Scheibel, A. B. On the nature of dendritic spines—report of a workshop. *Comm. in Behav. Biol.* 1A:231–265, 1968.

10.3 Synaptic Amplification by Active Membrane in Dendritic Spines (1985), *Brain Res.* 325:325–330

J. P. Miller, W. Rall, and J. Rinzel

The suspected functional role of dendritic spines as loci of neuronal plasticity (possibly memory and learning) is greatly enriched when active membrane properties are assumed at the spine head. Computations with reasonable electrical and structural parameter values (corresponding to an optimal range for spine stem resistance) show that an active spine head membrane can provide very significant synaptic amplification and also strongly non-linear properties that could modulate the integration of input from many afferent sources.

Many synaptic contacts between neurons are located on dendritic spines. The possible functional significance of these spines has excited the interest of theoretical and experimental neuroscientists. Based upon the assumption that spine head membrane is passive, previous studies concluded that the efficacy of a synapse onto a spine head would be less than or equal to the efficacy of an identical synapse directly onto the 'parent' dendrite[2,4,8,12,16–21,24,32]. However, for an *active* spine head membrane, early steady state considerations suggested that a spine might act as a synaptic amplifier[8]. Here we present transient responses computed for transient synaptic conductance input. We address two questions: (1) What would be the difference in efficacy between a synapse onto a *passive* spine and onto an *active* spine? and (2) How would the efficacy of a synapse onto an active spine depend upon structural and electrical parameters of the spine? Our transient calculations demonstrate that: (1) the efficacy of a synapse onto an active spine could, indeed, be *much greater* than the efficacy of an identical synapse onto the parent dendrite or onto a passive spine; and (2) such amplification would occur only for certain ranges of spine parameters. A maximal efficacy could be attained, corresponding to a narrow optimal range of these parameters.

Calculations were performed using a commonly available program called SPICE[34] running on an IBM 370 computer. SPICE simulates the behavior of complex circuits of electrical components, and can calculate the non-linear, transient responses of circuits to time- and voltage-dependent conductance changes. The methods for modeling the structural and electrical properties of spines and dendrites, including the formulation of the action potential kinetics of active membrane[7,23], were essentially those described by Shepherd and Brayton[27]. Numerical accuracy was tested in several cases for which analytical solutions could be derived; deviations never exceeded 2%. Here, the spine head is assumed to be isopotential and the spine stem is reduced to a lumped resistance connecting the spine head to the dendrite, represented as a passive membrane cylinder of infinite length. Parameters specifying the morphology of the spine and dendrite were chosen to fall within the range of anatomical measurements reported in the literature[1,3,5,6,9,10,13,15,26,33]. The values for these parameters, as well as the electrical, synaptic and action-potential conductance parameters, are listed in Table I.

In order to compare the functional properties of an active and a passive spine, the responses of each to

TABLE I

Parameters for computations

Parameter	Value
Resting membrane resistivity	$5000\ \Omega cm^2$
Cytoplasmic resistivity	$100\ \Omega cm$
Membrane capacitance	$1\ \mu F/cm^2$
Dendrite diameter	$1\ \mu m$
Dendrite length	infinite
Spine head diameter	$0.75\ \mu m$
Spine stem resistance	0, 200, 400, 800 MΩ (see figure legends)
Synaptic conductance transient	
Time course proportional to $te^{-\alpha t/\tau}$	$\alpha = 50, \tau = 5$ ms
Peak conductance	0.25 and 0.50 nS (see figure legends)
Action potential (3 variable model)[7,23,27]	
Kinetic coefficients	$k_1 = 10^5, k_2 = 6 \times 10^4,$ $k_3 = 25, k_4 = 0.2,$ $k_5 = 1, k_6 = 0.01,$ $k_7 = 5.$
Resulting maximal inward conductance (for an isolated active spine head)	16 nS
Reversal potential for active inward current (relative to rest)	125 mV

identical synaptic inputs were computed. The results are presented graphically in Fig. 1, for two synaptic conductance amplitudes. For the smaller synaptic input the computed excitatory postsynaptic potentials (EPSPs) were all qualitatively similar and remained in the linear regime (dashed curves in all panels). For both passive and active cases, the EPSP in the dendrite (spine base) was substantially lower in amplitude than the EPSP in the spine head (note difference in voltage scales). This voltage attenuation from head to base corresponds to the I × R drop across the relatively large resistance presented by the spine stem.

When the amount of the synaptic conductance was doubled, the EPSPs shown as solid lines were obtained. In the passive case, the EPSP amplitudes are nearly doubled and the EPSP shapes are qualitatively similar to the dashed curves. However, the solid curves in the active case are qualitatively different, because the EPSP in the spine head exceeded the threshold for initiation of regenerative currents by the active spine head membrane. These regenerative

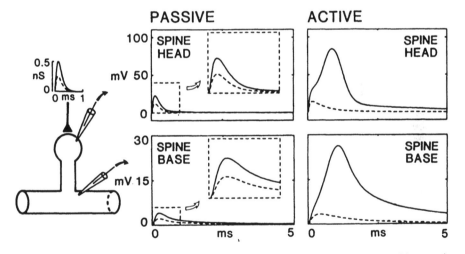

Fig. 1. Spines with active heads can greatly augment synaptic efficacy. Calculations were performed using a model representing a spine on a dendrite cylinder, shown diagramatically at the left. All model parameters are listed in Table I. Directly above the spine diagram are the time courses of the two synaptic conductances used: the dashed curve has a peak amplitude of 0.25 nS; the solid curve has peak conductance of 0.5 nS. The dashed and solid curves in the enclosed panels are the corresponding voltage transients (EPSPs) resulting from these two conductance transients, computed at two different locations (spine head or spine base) for two different types of spine head membrane (passive or active). The insets in the two left panels (passive spine membrane) are enlarged views of the areas enclosed with dashed boxes. Note that the 0.5 nS conductance transient is a suprathreshold for action potential generation in the active head (upper right panel), resulting in a substantial augmentation of the current entering the spine. This results in a much-enhanced EPSP at the base of the active spine (lower right panel).

currents have several consequences that can be described as synaptic amplification or augmentation relative to the passive case: (1) much more charge enters the spine head membrane, resulting in a spine head EPSP having a much larger amplitude and duration; and (2) the charge delivered through the spine stem into the dendrite is substantially larger, resulting in an EPSP (at the spine base) that is augmented in both amplitude and duration. The *peak amplitude* of the EPSP at the base of the active spine was 6.5 times greater than at the base of the passive spine. The *net charge* delivered to the dendrite by the active spine (proportional to the area under the EPSP at the spine base) increased 10-fold over that delivered by the passive spine (for time duration shown in Fig. 1). Thus, by either of these two criteria, synaptic efficacy was *substantially increased* by incorporation of active properties into the spine head membrane.

Previous theoretical studies have shown that changes in the structural and electrical parameters of passive spines could change synaptic efficacy[8,12,16–21,24,32]. An 'operating range' was identified within which synaptic efficacy could be increased or decreased — relative to an 'operating point' — by decreasing or increasing the spine stem resistance. (An increase in stem resistance would result, for example, from decreasing stem diameter, increasing stem length, or partially occluding the stem.) It was suggested that such changes could contribute to plasticity in central nervous systems[8,16–21,24]. Subsequently, significant activity-dependent changes in morphological parameters of spines have been reported[1,3,5,6,13]. Here we extend our study of the dependence of synaptic efficacy upon stem resistance to the case of an *active* spine head. The transient computations, illustrated by Fig. 2, show the effect of changing spine stem resistance, when the spine head and dendritic parameters remain unchanged. The amplitude and time course of the synaptic conductance (leftmost panel) was equal to the larger input (solid curve)

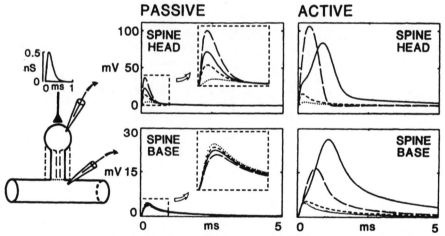

Fig. 2. There is an optimal stem resistance for maximal synaptic efficacy. The diagram at the left represents the spine model. All structural and electrical parameters of the spine and dendrite *except* spine stem resistance were as in Fig. 1. Variations in stem resistance are represented on the diagram as different spine stem diameters, although changes in length and partial occlusion could also change this resistance. Dotted curves are for the case of zero stem resistance (i.e. synapse directly on the dendrite). Resistance values of 200, 400 and 800 MΩ are represented with short-dashed, solid, and long-dashed lines, respectively (i.e. the thinner the stem, the higher the resistance). Directly above the spine diagram is the time course of the synaptic conductance used for all calculations; peak conductance was 0.5 nS. In each of the 4 enclosed panels are the voltage transient (EPSPs) corresponding to the 4 spine stem resistance values. The EPSPs were calculated at two different locations (spine head or spine base) for two different types of spine head membrane (passive or active). The insets in the two left panels (passive spine membrane) are enlarged views of the areas enclosed with dashed boxes. Note that the 400 MΩ stem results in a suprathreshold response for the *active* head (solid curve, upper right), yielding the largest EPSP at the base of the spine (solid curve, lower right). Stems of either higher or lower resistances give lower amplitude EPSPs at the base.

used in Fig. 1. The solid curves in Fig. 2 are the EPSPs calculated for a stem resistance of 400 MΩ. (These curves are identical to the solid curves of Fig. 1.) Doubling spine stem resistance yielded the curves shown as long dashes in Fig. 2; halving spine stem resistance yielded the curves shown as short dashes in Fig. 2. The dotted curves are for the limiting case of zero spine stem resistance, for which there can be no difference of potential between spine head and spine base. (The dotted curves in the upper and lower panels are identical EPSPs plotted to different voltage scales.) These dotted curves represent the reference case, corresponding to a synapse placed directly on the dendrite.

For the passive spine, comparison of the upper and lower panels of Fig. 2 shows the expected effects. For successive increases in spine stem resistance, the EPSP amplitude in the spine head (upper panel) grows successively larger than the (dotted) reference EPSP, while the EPSP amplitude at the spine base (lower panel) becomes successively smaller. The difference between these upper and lower EPSPs corresponds to the I × R drop of voltage for current flowing through the spine stem. Thus, for a passive spine, the effect of these increases in spine stem resistance is to reduce the EPSP amplitude and area at the spine base, and hence the efficacy of the synapse.

For the active spine, the computed results at the right side of Fig. 2 show more complicated (very non-linear) effects for identical increases in spine stem resistance. For an increase from 0 to 200 MΩ, the increased depolarization in the spine head does not reach the threshold for generation of an action potential; however, some regenerative response is revealed by the augmentation of both amplitude and duration of the EPSP (short dashes) at the base of the active spine, compared with the passive case. Doubling the spine stem resistance to 400 MΩ has a very dramatic effect (solid curves). In this case, the spine head depolarization exceeds threshold, resulting in a substantial regenerative augmentation of voltage amplitude and duration in the spine head, and producing a large EPSP at the spine base. Note that a further doubling of spine stem resistance to 800 MΩ causes the spine head membrane to reach threshold earlier. Even though the resulting action potential has a larger peak amplitude, its shorter latency and duration result in a smaller area under the curve.

Less charge is delivered through the spine stem to the dendrite, and the resulting EPSP at the spine base has a smaller amplitude and area. Because further increase of spine stem resistance causes further reduction of the EPSP at the spine base, it follows that the optimal (maximal) EPSP occurs for an intermediate spine stem resistance value (around 400 MΩ in this example). Because this optimum corresponds to conditions where the spine head depolarization just exceeds threshold, it is clear that these optimal conditions must correspond also to an intermediate value of synaptic conductance amplitude; that is, optimal efficacy occurs with respect to both synaptic conductance and spine stem resistance. The idea of such an optimum was briefly noted in the early steady state considerations of Jack et al.[8]; transient computations leading to similar conclusions have recently been done independently also by Perkel and Perkel[14].

An intuitive understanding of how synaptic efficacy is decreased by larger values of spine stem resistance depends upon recognizing the effect of voltage saturation in the spine head. The reversal potential sets an upper limit for the spine head EPSP amplitude and for the I × R voltage drop from spine head to spine base. Thus when R is increased while the I × R drop remains almost unchanged, the value of I, the spine stem current, must decrease almost inversely with R. This decreased current delivers less charge to the dendrite and produces a smaller EPSP there. Note that this intuitive explanation holds also for the effect of large spine stem resistance values upon a passive spine; this applies to the early steady state and transient results of Rall and Rinzel[17-21,24], and Jack et al.[8], and has also been recognized in two recent analyses of passive spines[12,32]. Negligible dependence of synaptic efficacy upon spine stem resistance results when non-linear voltage (saturation) effects in the spine head are avoided, either by treating synaptic input as a current injection[11], or by keeping synaptic conductance very small[12,32]. The small attenuation reported by Turner and Schwartzkroin[30] resulted from using a small value for the ratio of spine stem resistance to dendritic input resistance[17,18,24].

Measurements of the stem resistance in real spines have not been reported in the literature. Estimates of stem resistance based upon recently reported ranges of stem dimensions (assuming a uniform cytoplasmic resistivity) yield values at the low end of the range used in our calculations. For example, an unobstructed stem 0.1 μm in diameter and 1.0 μm in length would have a resistance of 100 MΩ. However as pointed out by Wilson et al.[33], such calculations would substantially *underestimate* the true stem resistance. A significant proportion of a spine stem may be occluded by extensive cytoskeletal structures and by large membrane-bound vesicles called the spine apparatus (SA)[28,29,31–33]. For example, occlusion of two-thirds of the volume along half the length of the above stem would double its resistance, to 200 MΩ. The resistance of this partially occluded stem would then be very sensitive to further changes in diameter of either the SA or the stem itself. For example, a 13% increase in SA diameter (or 9% decrease in stem diameter) would increase stem resistance to 400 MΩ. A further increase in SA diameter of only 5% (or a further stem diameter decrease of 5%) would increase stem resistance to 800 MΩ.

Thus, a dendritic spine could theoretically function as an EPSP amplifier, *if* the membrane in its head were active, and *if* the stem resistance and other biophysical parameters lay within the appropriate ranges. The 'gain' of the spine would be variable, and would be sensitive to small changes in stem resistance around an optimal value. Also, if such active spines were placed at distal dendritic locations, the augmentation produced by the active spine head membrane could compensate for the disadvantage of distal location. Still another kind of augmentation might take place in distal dendritic arbors. The large local depolarizations expected there would spread with negligible decrement into small branches[19,22,25] and spine heads[8,11,12,27], and those spine heads which have active membrane might thus be brought to threshold without any direct synaptic input (or they might reach threshold for a synaptic input that would be insufficient by itself). If this happens, it might be best for only some spines to have active membrane, because the distribution of active and passive spines would determine the extent to which a chain reaction of spine firings might occur, resulting in an all-or-none, and possible large, composite EPSP (for an arbor or for an entire neuron). All of these possibilities have significant functional implications for local interactions, synaptic efficacy and plasticity that merit continued attention by neurobiologists.

We thank Barry Bunow for assistance with development of computer programs, Idan Segev and Gwen Jacobs for valuable discussion. This work was supported in part by NSF Grant BNS-8202416 and a Sloan Foundation Fellowship, both awarded to J.P.M.

1 Brandon, J. G. and Coss, R. G., Rapid dendritic spine stem shortening during one trial learning: the honeybee's first orientation flight, *Brain Research*, 252 (1982) 51–61.

2 Chang, H. T., Cortical neurons with particular reference to the apical dendrites, *Cold Spring Harbor Symp. Quant. Biol.*, 17 (1952) 189–202.

3 Coss, R. G. and Globus, A., Spine stems on tectal interneurons in jewel fish are shortened by social stimulation, *Science*, 200 (1978) 787–790.

4 Diamond, J., Gray, E. G. and Yasargil, G. M., The function of the dendritic spines: a hypothesis. In P. Anderson and J. K. S. Jansen (Eds.), *Excitatory Synaptic Mechanisms*, Universitetsforlaget, Oslo, 1970, pp. 213–222.

5 Fifkova, E. and Anderson, C. L., Stimulation-induced charges in dimensions of stalks of dendritic spines in the dentate molecular layer, *Exp. Neurol.*, 74 (1981) 621–627.

6 Fifkova, E. and Van Harreveld, A., Long-lasting morphological changes in dendritic spines of dentate granule cells following stimulation of the entorhinal area, *J. Neurocytol.*, 6 (1977) 211–230.

7 Goldstein, S. S. and Rall, W., Changes of action potential shape and velocity for changing core conductor geometry, *Biophys. J.*, 14 (1974) 731–757.

8 Jack, J. J. B., Noble, D. and Tsien, R. W., *Electric Current Flow in Excitable cells*, Oxford Univ. Press, 1975, 502 pp.

9 Jacobsen, S., Dimensions of the dendritic spine in the sensorimotor cortex of the rat, cat, squirrel monkey and man, *J. comp. Neurol.*, 129 (1967) 49–58.

10 Jones, E. G. and Powell, T. P. S., Morphological variations in the dendritic spines of the neocortex, *J. Cell. Sci.*, 5 (1969) 509–529.

11 Kawato, M. and Tsukahara, N., Theoretical study on electrical properties of dendritic spines, *J. theoret. Biol.*, 103 (1983) 507–522.

12 Koch, C. and Poggio, T., A theoretical analysis of electrical properties of spines, *Proc. roy. Soc. B*, 218 (1983) 455–477.

13 Lee, K. S., Schottler, F., Oliver, M. and Lynch, G., Brief bursts of high-frequency stimulation produce two types of structural change in rat hippocampus, *J. Neurophysiol.*, 44 (1980) 247–258.

14 Perkel, D. H. and Perkel, D. J., Dendritic spines: role of active membrane in modulating synaptic efficacy, *Brain Research*, 000 (1984) 000–000.

15 Peters, A. and Kaiserman-Abramof, I. R., The small pyramidal neuron of the rat cerebral cortex. The perikaryan, dendrites and spines, *Amer. J. Anat.*, 127 (1970) 321–356.

16 Rall, W., Cable properties of dendrites and effects of synaptic location. In P. Anderson and J. K. S. Jansen (Eds.), *Excitatory Synaptic Mechanisms*, Universitetsforlaget, Oslo, 1970, pp. 175–187.

17 Rall, W., Dendritic spines, synaptic potency and neuronal plasticity. In C. D. Woody, K. A. Brown, T. J. Crow and J. D. Knispal (Eds.), *Cellular Mechanisms Subserving Changes in Neuronal Activity, Brain Inf. Serv. Rpt. no. 3,* UCLA, Los Angeles, CA, 1974, pp. 13–21.

18 Rall, W., Dendritic spines and synaptic potency. In R. Porter (Ed.), *Studies in Neurophysiology* (presented to A. K. McIntyre), Cambridge Univ. Press, Cambridge, 1978, pp. 203–209.

19 Rall, W., Functional aspects of neuronal geometry. In A. Roberts and B. M. H. Bush (Eds.), *Neurones Without Impulses,* Cambridge Univ. Press, Cambridge, 1981, pp. 223–254.

20 Rall, W. and Rinzel, J., Dendritic spines and synaptic potency explored theoretically, *Proc. I. U. P. S. (XXV Int. Congr.),* IX (1971) 466.

21 Rall, W. and Rinzel, J., Dendritic spine function and synaptic attenuation calculations, *Progr. Abstr. Soc. Neurosci. First ann. Mtg,* 1 (1971) 64.

22 Rall, W. and Rinzel, J., Branch input resistance and steady attenuation for input to one branch of a dendritic neuron model, *Biophys. J.,* 13 (1973) 648–688.

23 Rall, W. and Shepherd, G. M., Theoretical reconstruction of field potentials and dendrodendritic synaptic interactions in olfactory bulb, *J. Neurophysiol.,* 31 (1968) 884–915.

24 Rinzel, J., Neuronal plasticity (learning). In R. M. Miura (Ed.), *Some Mathematical Questions in Biology — Neurobiology, Vol. 15, Lectures on Mathematics in the Life Sciences,* Amer. Math. Soc. Providence, RI, 1982, pp. 7–25.

25 Rinzel, J. and Rall, W., Transient response in a dendritic neuron model for current injected at one branch, *Biophys. J.,* 14 (1974) 759–790.

26 Scheibel, M. E. and Scheibel, A. B., On the nature of dendritic spines — report of a workshop, *Commun. Behav. Biol.,* 14 (1968) 231–265.

27 Shepherd, G. M. and Brayton, R. K., Computer simulation of a dendrodendritic synaptic circuit for self- and lateral-inhibition in the olfactory bulb, *Brain Research,* 175 (1979) 377–382.

28 Tarrant, S. B. and Routtenberg, A., The synaptic spinule in the dendritic spine. Electron microscopic study of the hippocampal dentate gyrus, *Tissue Cell,* 9 (1977) 461–473.

29 Tarrant, S. B. and Routtenberg, A., Postsynaptic membrane and spine apparatus: proximity in dendritic spines, *Neurosci. Lett.,* 11 (1979) 289–294.

30 Turner, D. A. and Schwartzkroin, P. A., Electrical characteristics of dendritic spines in intracellularly stained CA3 and dentate hippocampal neurons, *J. Neurosci.,* 3 (1983) 2381–2394.

31 Westrum, L. E., Jones, D. H., Gray, E. G. and Barron, J., Microtubules, dendritic spines and spine apparatuses, *Cell Tissue Res.,* 208 (1980) 171–181.

32 Wilson, C. J., Passive cable properties of dendritic spines and spiny neurons, *J. Neurosci.,* 4 (1984) 281–297.

33 Wilson, C.J., Groves, P. M., Kitai, S. T. and Linder, J. C., Three dimensional structure of dendritic spines in the rat neostriatum, *J. Neurosci.,* 3 (1983) 383–398.

34 Vladimirescu, A., Newton, A. R. and Pederson, D. O., *SPICE version 26.0 User's Guide,* EECS Dept., Univ. of California, Berkeley, CA, 1980.

A   APPENDIX: MOTONEURON POPULATION MODELS FOR INPUT-OUTPUT AND VARIABILITY OF MONOSYNAPTIC REFLEX

A.1 Introduction by Julian Jack

Rall, W. (1955a). A statistical theory of monosynaptic input-output relations. *J. Cell. Comp. Physiol.* 46:373–411.

Rall, W. (1955b). Experimental monosynaptic input-output relations in the mammalian spinal cord. *J. Cell. Comp. Physiol.* 46:413–437.

Rall, W., and Hunt, C. C. (1956). Analysis of reflex variability in terms of partially correlated excitability fluctuation in a population of motoneurons. *J. Gen. Physiol.* 39:397–422.

Not long after Wil Rall decided to shift from physics into biology, he was attracted to migrate from the United States to New Zealand because John Eccles, then the leading proponent of the electrical hypotheses of synaptic excitation and inhibition (Eccles 1945; Brooks and Eccles 1947) offered him a faculty position (in response to a tentative inquiry from Wil). When Rall arrived in 1949, relative calm prevailed in the literature with respect to the ideas about synaptic mechanisms. All the leading players in the field (Lorente de Nó, Eccles, and Lloyd) agreed that synaptic excitation was a dual-component phenomenon, with a brief, spatially restricted process that secured firing of the cell and a more prolonged, general process that could lower the effective threshold for the first process. These two processes were called "detonator action" and "residual facilitation" respectively (Brooks and Eccles [1948] used the terms α and β facilitation). A representation of their respective time courses is given in figure 1, taken from a chapter by Lloyd in the sixteenth edition of *A Textbook of Physiology*, edited by J. F. Fulton (1949). The actual mechanisms envisaged were various, but one possibility was that the "detonator action" might be a very brief localized process on the nerve cell body, akin to the "local response" that had been described in peripheral nerve (Hodgkin 1938; Katz 1947), whereas "residual facilitation" simply reflected the underlying depolarization ("catelectrotonus") that spread by passive electrical propagation throughout the nerve cell membrane surface.

Although the preceding account may read rather quaintly to younger neuroscientists, the issues that were being addressed are still very alive today. The "global" hypothesis of synaptic excitation, in which depolarizing effects from all over the cell surface are "collected" at the cell body initial segment where a decision is made about firing of the cell (Eccles 1957, 1964) has been the dominant account for the motoneurone in the past 30 years; the principal evidence in favor of this account came with the advent of intracellular recording from motoneurones (Woodbury and Patton 1952; Brock, Coombs, and Eccles 1952; Coombs, Eccles, and Fatt 1955a and 1955b; Fuortes, Frank, and Becker 1957). Nevertheless, there are plenty of suggestions from the experimental literature that regenerative responses and even action potentials may sometimes be generated as a result of more restricted activity, particularly in the dendrites (Kandel and Spencer 1961; Llinas et al. 1968; etc.). The purpose of this commentary is to present an abbreviated account of the development of thinking about

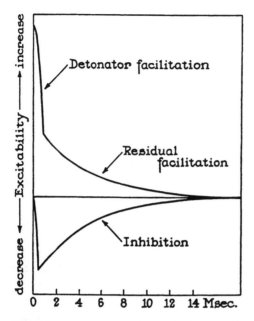

Figure 1
Schematic diagram of the presumed time course of excitability changes produced by the action of presynaptic excitatory or inhibitory volleys on spinal cord motoneurones. The illustration is based on the work of Lloyd and of Brooks and Eccles (from Lloyd 1949).

these issues in the period from 1938 to 1960 and to display the key role that Rall played in bringing quantitative clarity to some of the rather intuitive thinking that then prevailed.

Lorente de Nó (1938, 1939) argued that his evidence was incompatible with the assumption that firing threshold for oculomotor neurones could be given simply by the total number of synaptic knobs activated because he noted that a large presynaptic volley could be ineffective but a smaller volley from the same source, when combined with synaptic input from another source, also subthreshold, could evoke discharge. Similar observations and conclusions were reported by Lloyd (1945) for spinal cord motoneurones; Lloyd made this point more quantitative by considering the relationship between size of the presynaptic input volley and the magnitude of the postsynaptic output (input-output curve). In his doctoral thesis, completed in 1953 and published in 1955 (Rall 1955a, 1955b), Rall considered these arguments and pointed out that all the observations were compatible either with a simple concept of threshold in terms of total number of knobs activated or as a zonal concept in terms of a certain number of knobs being activated at a discrete zone on the neurone. "With either threshold definition, it seems sufficient to assume that the first afferent source distributes knobs fairly evenly over a large motoneurone pool, while the second afferent source distributes its knobs preferentially to a small group of motoneurones within the large pool" (Rall 1955a). The essence of Rall's point was that one could not necessarily think about the behavior of a population of neurones as if they were equivalent to a single "average" neurone. Rall went further and developed a theoretical treatment for the input-output relationship of a neurone population in which the distribution of synaptic knobs to the neurones of the pool was random in terms either of individual knobs or of knob clusters. The threshold criterion for firing of an individual neurone could be defined either in terms of total number of active knobs, irrespective of location, or as a local number of knobs active in a discrete area of the neurone. Finally, the distribution of the threshold value (on either criterion) across the pool of motoneurones was also assumed to be random and independent of active knob distribution.

With these models, Rall was able to predict the expected types of input-output curves for various values of the theoretical parameters, and in a companion experimental paper (Rall 1955b) he showed that the data for spinal cord motoneurones was equally compatible with models adopting either of the two competing threshold criteria. Thus, Rall did not claim to have disproved the zonal concept of neurone threshold, but he was able to conclude that the nature of the evidence so far offered was not adequate to establish it.

The concept of "detonator action" not only contained the idea of restricted spatial location but also of brevity: it was supposed to last about 0.5 msec (Lloyd 1949). As part of his thesis research, Rall also partly addressed this issue, by modeling the time course as well as the spatial summation properties of focal depolarizations on the membrane of a cell soma (modeled as a sphere). He was able to show that brief, focal depolarization tended to equalize around the soma on the time scale of a microsecond rather than a millisecond, so that the effect of one such input would have equalized and become uniform in its efffect over the time scale of the rising phase of a synaptic potential (Rall 1953, 1955a, p. 403). Thus, the mechanism of a brief, zonal "detonator action" could not be explained by the spatiotemporal summation characteristics of passive electrotonus, but this treatment did not exclude some form of "local response" mechanism, that is, the activation of the voltage-dependent sodium conductance in a restricted region, generating further inward, depolarizing current without necessarily securing the firing of an action potential by the cell. Indeed, this general possibility was left open by Eccles, on the basis of his intracellular studies (see Coombs, Eccles, and Fatt 1955b; Eccles 1957), although subsequently quietly forgotten.

There also still remained the experimental observations of Brooks and Eccles (1948) that there were two phases to the "facilitation" curve (see figure 2). It is interesting that Rall does not discuss this evidence explicitly in his 1955 papers, perhaps because he was skeptical about the experimental result. In the experimental paper, he does consider the problems of interpretation when two different motoneurone pools can both be contributing to the output measurement; this is certainly the situation that prevailed in the Brooks and Eccles experiment.

This was not the end of the story. Archie McIntyre had become the Professor of Physiology in Dunedin in 1952, when Eccles left to become the foundation Professor of Physiology at the Australian National University in Canberra. McIntyre had close links with Lloyd, having previously collaborated with him, and he doubtless reported to Lloyd the gist of Rall's criticisms. The obvious response for those still committed to a zonal theory of excitation was to study the behavior of individual motoneurones, rather than a population. McIntyre went on sabbatical leave to Lloyd's laboratory at the Rockefeller Institute (as Rockefeller University then was), where Carlton Hunt was also working. These three workers produced a series of five papers in volume 38 of the *Journal of General Physiology*, which occupied about 100 pages (Lloyd, Hunt, and McIntyre 1955; Lloyd and McIntyre 1955a, 1955b; Hunt 1955a, 1955b). With respect to the mechanism of firing of the motoneurone, the most detailed examination was contained in the final paper of the series (Hunt 1955b), in which it was concluded that the results "exclude the postsynaptic potential as the essential step in the normal production of discharge." By this Hunt meant that the effect he observed "could not result if transmitter potentiality resulted from a simple summation of independent knob actions. There must be an interaction between excitatory synaptic knobs." In another passage, Hunt also concluded that "transmitter potentiality must decay considerably within 0.2 to 0.3 insec." Thus, one major conclusion arising from this work was a reaffirmation of a zonal interaction of brief time course. Transmitter potentiality (the ability of synaptic input to secure firing of the cell) was concluded to have the same properties as had earlier been postulated for "detonator action."

A modern reader of these papers, not steeped in the literature of the period, would find them difficult to read and would likely dismiss them because the conclusions outlined here have not survived. This would be a mistake. These five papers, and the subsequent paper in which Rall was involved (Rall and Hunt 1956) remain important, not because they reached the aforementioned conclusions but because they were the first attempt to characterize a population of neurones in terms of the distribution of their functional responsiveness and also to give an account of the

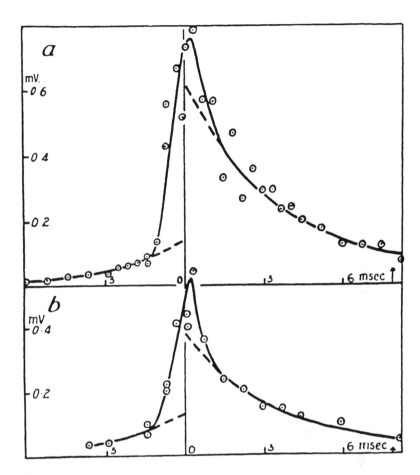

Figure 2
The time course of facilitation of monosynaptic reflex responses, recorded in the first sacral ventral root, to stimulation of the group I afferent fibres in both the medial and lateral gastrocnemius muscle nerves. When the medial gastrocnemius nerve was stimulated alone, a small reflex response was evoked, whose size is indicated by the height of the arrows to the right. Stimuli to the lateral gastrocnemius nerve alone did not evoke a reflex response. The ordinate plots the magnitude of the reflex firing when both nerves are stimulated; the abscissa gives the interval between the two stimuli, with zero being simultaneous stimulation and time intervals to the right showing how much the lateral gastrocnemius volley leads the medial gastrocnemius volley (and vice versa for intervals to the left). The upper curve (a) is for maximal group I stimuli to both nerves, and the lower curve (b) is for 30% below maximal stimuli (from Brooks and Eccles 1948).

fluctuations, about the average value, in this functional responsiveness. To my knowledge, this work has yet to be emulated for any other neuronal population, and it thus remains an exemplar for future neuroscientists who may wish to move away from models representing a single functional task by a single neurone or a population with identical properties, to the more realistic situation where a distribution of properties means the population of cells is realistically represented.

Before considering this aspect of these papers, it is best to consider why Hunt's conclusions are likely to be incorrect and, with the advantage of retrospection, to outline briefly how he came to misinterpret his data.

If the "detonator action" concept of excitation was correct for the motoneurone, then the observed neurone threshold could not be equated with a fixed level of depolarization of the soma, when initiated by different excitatory afferent inputs, for the "critical assemblage" of synaptic knobs could be activated at different levels of net generalized depolarization of the motoneurone. Subsequent to the publication of these papers, both Fatt (1957) and Eccles, Eccles, and Lundberg (unpublished observations quoted in Eccles, Eccles, and Lundberg 1957) with intracellular recording observed that there was no significant difference in the levels of depolarization required to initiate discharge from different excitatory afferent sources. That is, the neurone threshold appeared to be simply a fixed membrane potential. Additional evidence against Hunt's view came from the observation that (with group Ia afferent monosynaptic excitation) the motoneurone spike invariably arose from one part of the motoneurone (Fuortes, Frank, and Becker 1957; Fatt 1957; Coombs, Curtis, and Eccles 1957).

Relatively little experimental attention was given to Hunt's conclusion that transmitter potentiality had a rapid temporal decay. If this conclusion were correct, it would be expected that monosynaptic reflex firing of individual motoneurones should have a narrow latency range. Coombs, Eccles, and Fatt (1955a) reported that the somatic impulse arose 0.3 to 1.2 msec after the onset of the EPSP, and later Coombs, Curtis, and Eccles (1957) recorded a similar latency spread. This range, of up to one millisecond, is wider than that predicted by a transmitter potentiality that "must decay considerably within 0.2 to 0.3 msec" (Hunt 1955b, p. 823).

Thus, the various experiments indicated that Hunt's interpretations of his experimental evidence needed to be reappraised. In retrospect there were two crucial assumptions made by Hunt that are unlikely to be correct. The first was that the group Ia excitatory input was recruited linearly through the group I afferent fiber range. Rall (1955b) had already questioned this point, and subsequent experimental studies strongly suggest that it is not correct (e.g., Jack 1978). Linked to this was a problem about the measurement of input-output curves when interacting the afferent inputs from two sources. It is likely that the method used by Hunt was ineffective in separating the two pools of motoneurones that could potentially discharge; thus, his recorded input-output curve (which increased fairly linearly throughout the group I range) was a combination of a convex upward facilitation input-output curve for the conditioned motoneurone pool, and superimposed on this, a concave upward input-output curve for the effect of the conditioning volley on its motoneurone pool.

This same point is also likely to be the explanation for the time course of "facilitation" in figure 2 because the conditioning action of a volley can occur even when the conditioning volley follows the test volley into the nervous system, owing to the finite time taken to bring the motoneurones to near discharge. This effect is illustrated in figure 3 under conditions where the conditioning volley was so weak that it did not discharge its own motoneurones. By contrast, in the experiments of Brooks and Eccles illustrated in figure 2, both the "conditioning" and "testing" volleys fired

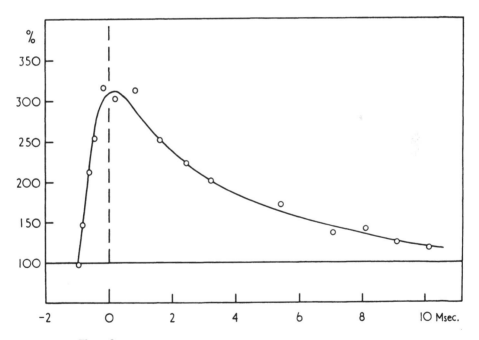

Figure 3
The effect of a weak lateral gastrocnemius-soleus afferent volley on a medial gastrocnemius test monosynaptic reflex, recorded in the first sacral ventral root. The convention for timing is that zero time represents simultaneity of the conditioning and testing volleys as they enter the spinal cord; intervals to the left of zero on the abscissa are for the testing volley leading the conditioning volley, and vice versa for intervals to the right. In this experiment care was taken to ensure that there was no discharge of the lateral gastrocnemius-soleus motoneurones, by using a very small group Ia lateral gastrocnemius-soleus conditioning volley, in contrast to the experiments shown in figure 2 (from Jack 1965).

their own motoneurones, and in the interval either side of "zero" time both volleys were acting to "condition" (i.e., facilitate) the other pool of neurones. Thus the α and β phases of facilitation ("detonator" and "residual" facilitation) do not represent two different types of facilitation; rather, facilitation has the same time course as the excitatory postsynaptic potential. β facilitation maps to the, decaying phase of the EPSP and α to the rising phase. The α phase in the left-hand half maps to the β phase in the right-hand half of the figure (and vice versa). What both Brooks and Eccles, and Lloyd, had done had been to make the attribution of both α and β phases on one side of the figure to a single conditioning volley, because they assumed that no effect could be produced before "zero" time. Once this error is realized, it is clear that "detonator action" or α facilitation could be correlated with the rising phase of the EPSP.

As already mentioned, one notable feature of the Rall and Hunt (1956) paper was to model a population of nerve cells as a distribution. The output of the pool that they analyzed was the distribution of the probabilities that individual motoneurones would fire. Lloyd and McIntyre (1955a) had already suggested that there was a uniform distribution in the average excitability of the motoneurones and a normal distribution of the fluctuation of the excitability level about the mean value. Rall and Hunt were able to define quantitatively "the extent to which excitability fluctuations of a motoneurone pool are correlated and the precise manner in which the response of the individual motoneurone is linked to the response of the population of which it is a member." They observed that for a particular motoneurone its probability of firing shows a systematic relationship to the magnitude of response of the motoneurone pool: a larger response from the pool being matched by a higher probability that the unit would fire. It is notable that Rudomin and his colleagues (Rudomin and Dutton 1969; Rudomin, Dutton, and Muñoz-Martinez 1969; Rudomin and Madrid 1972) are one of the few groups to extend and develop this pioneering population modeling by Rall and Hunt.

I would like to finish this discussion by briefly outlining how Rall and Hunt's paper inspired me to address in more detail the issue of "detonator" action of the motoneurone. Despite the observation that the motoneurone fired with a latency range of about one millisecond, it could be objected that this might have arisen as some artifact from intracellular recording; for example, that the microelectrode, as is now known, might induce a substantial electrical leak. Thus, in 1959, Lloyd and Wilson objected to the measurement of latencies of somatic spike potentials and suggested instead that the criterion should be reflex discharge of the axon.

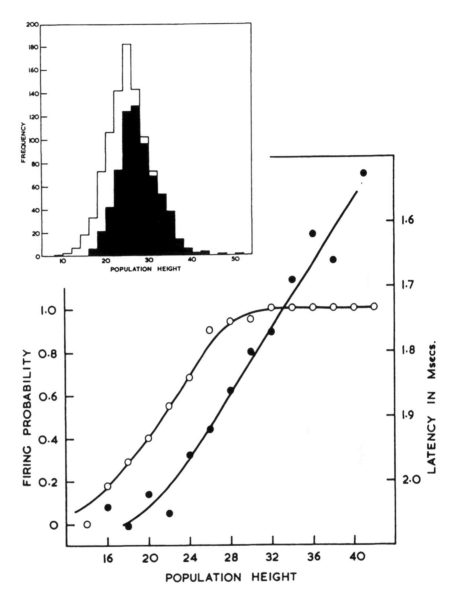

Figure 4
The abscissa plots the size (measured in arbitrary units and recorded in the first sacral ventral root) of a monosynaptic test reflex evoked by maximal group I afferent stimulation of the biceps-semitendinosus nerve. The mean amplitude was 27, with a range of reflex response sizes from 8 to 52 (see inset). In addition, the response of a single motoneurone was recorded from the seventh lumbar ventral root; this motoneurone had an average probability of firing of about 0.7. As illustrated in the inset, the single motoneurone was more likely to fire (blackened area of the histogram) when the response of the population of motoneurones was larger, indicating that the excitability of this single motoneurone was partially correlated with that of the population. In the main figure the estimated firing probability (open circles) and mean latency of firing (filled circles) for each class interval of population height is illustrated. The sigmoid shape of the firing probability curve is similar to those described by Rall and Hunt (1956). Data from Jack 1960.

As a check on the intracellular results, I recorded a single motoneurone discharge, as well as that of the population, in the ventral root. The latency range for the firing of the unit, with constant afferent stimulation, was 1.25 msec (Jack 1960), in complete accord with the intracellular data.

The data recorded included not only whether the unit fired (and, if so, at what latency) but also the size of the population response. In agreement with the results of Rall and Hunt, the probability of the unit firing was partially correlated with the size of the population response. The population response sizes were grouped, and, in addition to the firing probability associated with each size, the mean latency of unit firing was measured. As illustrated in figure 4, as the firing probability of the unit increases (with the larger population heights), the mean latency of firing decreases. Furthermore, although the firing probability curve plateaus when it reaches its maximal value, the mean unit latency continues to decrease. Associated with these changes in the mean of the unit latencies, there were characteristic changes in the distribution of the latencies about the mean, going from Gaussian for $p = 1.0$ to positively skewed for $0.5 < p < 1.0$ to Gaussian again for $p < 0.5$. It was possible, in a very informal model, to show that these latency distributions would arise if there were both correlated and uncorrelated variability between the unit and the population, with the excitatory time course being similar to that of the rising phase of an EPSP (Jack 1960). Thus, just as Rall's earlier (1955a, 1955b) papers had clarified the earlier discussion of the relationship between threshold and zonal aggregation of synapses, so did his later 1956 paper allow a further examination of this issue for the motoneurone. Doubtless the motoneurone will not prove to be typical of all cells (cf. pyramidal cells or Purkinje cells), but the vicissitudes of interpretation in the two decades from the late 1930s surely carry forward the lesson that quantitative clarity should be treasured.

References

Brock, L. G., Coombs, J. S., and Eccles, J. C. (1952) The recording of potentials from motoneurones with an intracellular electrode. *J. Physiol., London* 117:431–460.

Brooks, C. M., and Eccles, J. C. (1947) An electrical hypothesis of central inhibition. *Nature* 159:760–764.

Brooks, C. M., and Eccles, J. C. (1948) An analysis of synaptic excitatory action. *J. Neurophysiol.* 11:365–376.

Coombs, J. S., Curtis, D. R., and Eccles, J. C. (1957) The interpretation of spike potentials of motoneurones. *J. Physiol., London* 139:198–231.

Coombs, J. S., Eccles, J. C., and Fatt, P. (1955a) Tne electrical properties of the motoneurone membrane. *J. Physiol., London* 130:291–325.

Coombs, J. S., Eccles, J. C., and Fatt, P. (1955b) Excitatory synaptic action in motoneurones. *J. Physiol., London* 130:374–395.

Eccles, J. C. (1945) An electrical hypothesis of synaptic and neuromuscular transmission. *Nature* 156:680–682.

Eccles, J. C. (1957) *The Physiology of Nerve Cells.* Baltimore: John Hopkins Press.

Eccles, J. C. (1964) *The Physiology of Synapses.* Berlin: Springer.

Eccles, J. C., Eccles, R. M., and Lundberg, A. (1957) The convergence of monosynaptic excitatory afferents on to many different species of alpha motoneurones. *J. of Physiol.* 137:1.

Fatt, P. (1957) Electric potentials occurring around a neurone during its antidromic activation. *J. Neurophysiol.* 120:27–60.

Fulton, J. F. (1949). *Textbook of Physiology.* 16th Edition. Philadelphia: W. B. Saunders.

Fuortes, M. G. F., Frank, K., and Becker, M. C. (1957) Steps in the production of motoneuron spikes. *J. Gen. Physiol.* 40:735–752.

Hodgkin, A. L. (1938) The subthreshold potentials in a crustacean nerve fibre. *Proc. Roy. Soc. London Ser. B* 126:87–171.

Hunt, C. C. (1955a) Temporal fluctuation in excitability of spinal motoneurons and its influence on monosynaptic reflex response. *J. Gen. Physiol.* 38:801–811.

Hunt, C. C. (1955b) Monosynaptic reflex response of spinal motoneurons to graded afferent stimulation. *J. Gen. Physiol.* 38:813–852.

Jack, J. J. B. (1960) Inhibition and excitation in the mammalian spinal cord. Ph.D. Thesis. University of New Zealand.

Jack, J. J. B. (1965) The central latency of monosynaptic facilitation and direct inhibition of monosynaptic reflexes. *J. Physiol.* 181:52–53P.

Jack, J. J. B. (1978) Some methods of selective activation of muscle afferent fibres. In *Studies in Neurophysiology,* ed. R. Porter. Cambridge: Cambridge Univ. Press.

Kandel, E. R., and Spencer, W. A. (1961) Electrophysiology of hippocampal neurons. *J. Neurophysiol.* 24:243–259.

Katz, B. (1947) Subthreshold potentials in medullated nerve. *J. Physiol.* 106:66–79.

Llinás, R., Nicholson, C., Freeman, J. A., and Hillman, D. E. (1968) Dendritic spikes and their inhibition in alligator Purkinje cells. *Science* 160:1132–1135.

Lloyd, D. P. C. (1945) On the relation between discharge zone and subliminal fringe in a motoneuron pool supplied by a homogeneous presynaptic pathway. *Yale J. Biol. Med.* 18: 117–121.

Lloyd, D. F. C. (1949) in *A Textbook of Physiology,* ed. J. F. Fulton, 16th ed. Philadelphia: W. B. Saunders Co.

Lloyd, D. P. C., Hunt, C. C., and McIntyre, A. K. (1955) Transmission in fractionated monosynaptic spinal reflex systems. *J. Gen. Physiol.* 38:307–317.

Lloyd, D. P. C., and McIntyre, A. K. (1955a) Monosynaptic reflex responses of individual motoneurons. *J. Gen. Physiol.* 38:771–787.

Lloyd, D. P. C., and McIntyre, A. K. (1955b) Transmitter potentiality of homonymous and heteronymous monosynaptic reflex connections of individual motoneurones. *J. Gen. Physiol.* 38:789–799.

Lloyd, D. P. C., and Wilson, V. J. (1959) Functional organization in the terminal segments of the spinal cord with a consideration of central excitatory and inhibitory latencies in monosynaptic reflex systems. *J. Gen. Physiol.* 42:1219–1231.

Lorente de Nó, R. (1938) Synaptic stimulation as a local process. *J. Neurophysiol.* 1:194–206.

Lorente de Nó, R. (1939) Transmission of impulses through cranial motor nuclei. *J. Neurophysiol.* 2:402–464.

Rall, W. (1953) Electrotonic theory for a spherical neurone. *Proc. U. Otago Med. Sch.* 31:14–15.

Rall, W. (1955a) A statistical theory of monosynaptic input-output relations. *J. Cell. Comp. Physiol.* 46:373–411.

Rall, W. (1955b) Experimental monosynaptic input-output relations in the mammalian spinal cord. *J. Cell. Comp. Physiol.* 46:413–437.

Rall, W., and Hunt, C. C. (1956) Analysis of reflex variability in terms of partially correlated excitability fluctuation in a population of motoneurons. *J. Gen. Physiol.* 39:397–422.

Rudomin, P., and Dutton, H. (1969) Effects of conditioning afferent volleys on variability of monosynaptic responses of extensor motoneurons. *J. Neurophysiol.* 32:130–157.

Rudomin, P., Dutton, H., and Muñoz-Martinez, J. (1969) Changes in correlation between monosynaptic reflexes produced by conditioning afferent volleys. *J Neurophysiol.* 32:759–772.

Rudomin, P., and Madrid, J. (1972) Changes in correlation between monosynaptic responses of single motoneurons and in information transmission produced by conditioning volleys to cutaneous nerves. *J. Neurophysiol.* 35:44–64.

Woodbury, J. W., and Patton, H. D. (1952) Electrical activity of single spinal cord elements. *Cold Spring Harbor Symp. Quant. Biol.* 17:185–188.

Editorial Comment with an Excerpt from Rall (1990)

Rall, W. (1990). Perspectives on neuron modeling. In *The Segmental Motor System*, ed. M. D. Binder and L. M. Mendell. New York: Oxford University Press.

Because of space limitations, the editors have chosen not to reprint the papers of Rall that address the input-output properties of motoneuron pools involved with the segmental reflex (Rall 1955a,b; Rall and Hunt 1956). The following excerpts from Rall 1990 introduce and summarize in part the results presented in these papers.

Fractional Pool Discharge: Monosynaptic Input-Output Relation

My earliest news of Elwood Henneman came in 1954 on the day I presented my first seminar at the National Institutes of Health (NIH). Based on my Ph.D. research, this seminar included experimental results and a model for monosynaptic input-output relations in a motoneuron pool. One of the points emphasized was the need to scale the output magnitude (synchronous output volley recorded from the ventral root) relative to an elusive maximum (i.e., a complete synchronous discharge from all of the motoneurons in the pool); such scaling provides an estimate of fractional pool discharge. In the discussion following the seminar, someone mentioned that Henneman had also been concerned with estimating fractional pool discharge. It seems that both he and I had come to pursue this interest quite independently. We both explored various experimental approaches to measurement of complete pool discharge, and both recognized that posttetanic potentiation of this monosynaptic reflex (Lloyd, 1949; Eccles and Rall, 1950) provides a valuable means of demonstrating that the usual unpotentiated output represents incomplete pool discharge (Rall, 1951, 1954, 1955a, 1955b; Henneman, 1954; see also Jefferson and Benson, 1953).

My interest in this problem arose during an apprenticeship with Professors J. C. Eccles and A. K. McIntyre in Dunedin, New Zealand (1949–53). It followed from the pioneering study of the monosynaptic input-output relation that Lloyd had begun with the segmental reflex (Lloyd, 1943, 1945). On the basis of experiments by Lloyd and McIntyre in New York, and our experiments in Dunedin (Brock et al. 1951), I knew that it was important to restrict the input to a muscle nerve (triceps surae). Compared with dorsal root stimulation, this had two important advantages: (1) this restricted the input-output study to a pair of synergic motoneuron pools, in contrast to the nonfunctional combination of motoneuron pools provided by the segmental reflex (which includes antagonist and incomplete pools), and (2) the longer afferent conduction distance (from the hindlimb) helped to separate the effective portion from the ineffective portion of the input volley, because direct synapses to the motoneuron pool are made only by the group Ia afferent axons (which have the largest diameters, lowest electrical thresholds, and highest conduction velocities). Axons of group Ib and group II are also active in a maximal afferent volley, but they make no contribution to the effective input of the monosynaptic reflex because they make no direct synapses to the motoneuron pool; these ineffective axons have smaller diameters, higher electrical thresholds, and lower conduction velocities, such that their contamination of the experimental input record is greatest for large afferent volleys produced by large electrical stimuli. However, because groups Ia and Ib overlap in their threshold distributions, it was essential to determine the relation between the effective input and the experimental input record (Rall, 1955b). These points deserve emphasis because they were not recognized in another input-output study (Rosenblueth et al., 1949); consequently, those authors misinterpreted the plateau of their input-output relation as indicative of output saturation (i.e., complete discharge of their segmental pool); this error greatly complicated their effort to produce a theoretical model that could match their input-output curves.

Convincing evidence that the output plateau does not represent saturation (complete pool discharge) was provided by experiments that achieved four levels of reflex excitability in a single preparation (Rall, 1955b). These four levels were obtained by means of two depths of anesthesia, each used with and without brief tetanic conditioning. The four resulting input-output curves (see the left side of Fig. 1) all show an output plateau for experimental inputs greater than 70% of the maximum recorded afferent volley. It is important to understand that each output plateau corresponds to a different fraction of total pool discharge (approximately 37, 60, 72, and 84%). In other words, none of these curves showed output saturation; each plateau resulted from the ineffectiveness of the higher-threshold afferent axons (belonging to groups Ib and II), which contributed most of the upper 40% of the experimental input record. For small inputs, the effective component of the input volley (carried only by group Ia axons) grew linearly with the experimental input record (see the linear part of the dashed curve at the left in Fig. 1). Then, over the mid-range (from 20 to 70% of maximal experimental input), the normalized effective input curve bent and reached a maximum where the experimental input record was only 70% of its maximum. The shape of this dashed curve was verified by experiments with graded monosynaptic facilitation and with graded subthreshold synaptic potentials (of the motoneuron pool) recorded in the

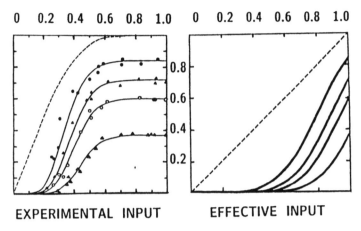

Figure 1

Output as fractional pool discharge versus two different measures of input. Each input-output curve shows an output plateau (left); transformed curves show no plateau (right). The four solid curves in the left graph were fitted to data of output versus the experimental input record (disphasic amplitude measured from intact dorsal root). The dashed line represents a normalized curve of "effective input" plotted against the experimental input record; this was based on observations of graded monosynaptic facilitation and on ventral root synaptic potentials; the linear relation for small inputs corresponds to recruitment of low-threshold group Ia fibers in the afferent muscle nerve. The ineffectiveness of increasing the experimental input volley from 60% to 100% of its maximum can be understood as resulting from the fact that the higher-threshold afferent fibers are ineffective because they belong to groups II and Ib and do not make synapses on these motoneurons. The five curves in the right panel are transformed from the five curves in the left pane; each experimental input value (abscissa, left) was replaced (in the right) by its effective input value, as defined by the ordinates on the dashed line in the left panel. This figure combines figures 2 and 6 of Rall 1955b. Straight-line fitting of the transformed data was shown in figure 4 of Rall 1955a.

ventral root. Once this dashed curve was understood, it was not surprising that the transformed input-output curves (at the right in Fig. 1) did not exhibit a plateau, because here the outputs were plotted as functions of the effective input. This transformation was the key to success in fitting the data with a relatively simple theoretical model (Rall, 1955a, 1955b).

In this model, it was assumed that the distribution of activated synaptic knobs could be treated as random over the motoneuron population. Suppose that each neuron has the same number, N, of potential synaptic sites (e.g., $N = 5000$) and that each site has the same probability, γ, of being occupied by a synapse belonging to the monosynaptic pathway (e.g., $\gamma = 0.02$); then the average number of relevant synapses per motoneuron is γN (e.g., $\gamma N = 100$). The effective input, β, ranges from 0 to 1, and for any particular value of β, we assume that $\beta\gamma$ defines the probability that a synaptic site receives an activated synapse (belonging to this pathway); thus, the average number of such activated synapses per motoneuron is $n = \beta\gamma N$ (e.g., n equals 100, 75, and 50 for β values of 1, 0.75, and 0.5, respectively). Because these probabilities were assumed to be independent,

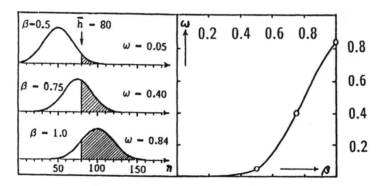

Figure 2
Schematic illustration of a mathematical model that gives output (ω) as fractional pool discharge versus effective input (β). At the left, the three input values, $\beta = 0.5$, 0.75, and 1.0, result in three normal distributions of the motoneuron population with respect to the number (n) of synapses activated on a motoneuron; these normal distributions are centered about mean values of 50, 75, and 100, with a standard deviation of 20; the mean threshold value is shown as 80, for the number of activated synapses needed to fire a motoneuron spike. The fractional pool discharge is shown as the shaded area under each normal distribution curve; this is the fraction of the motoneuron population for which the number of activated synapses exceeds threshold. These fractions are shown as $\omega = 0.84$ for $\beta = 1$, $\omega = 0.40$ for $\beta = 0.75$, and $\omega = 0.05$ for $\beta = 0.5$ at the left, and by the open circles on the input-output curve at the right. (Figure 1 in Rall 1955a.)

the result is a binomial (nearly Poisson) distribution of the motoneuron population with respect to the number, n, of activated synapses that each receives; the variance of this distribution is very close to n (e.g., var(n) $\approx$ 100 when $\beta = 1$).

A motoneuron was assumed to fire an impulse when the number of its simultaneously activated synapses, n, exceeded some threshold number, h. The value of h was assumed to have a variability that could result both from inherent variability of motoneuron excitability and from background synaptic activity in other synapses. Because this variability in h was assumed to be independent of the variability in n, it was reasonable to approximate the combined variability of the motoneurons, with respect to their $n - h$ values, as a normal distribution with a variance, var($n - h$) = var(n) + var(h). In this case, good results were obtained for a normal distribution with a standard deviation very close to $\sigma = \gamma N/5$, (e.g., $\sigma = 20$).

The normal distributions in Fig. 2 are shown with $\sigma = 20$, but to simplify the diagram, these distributions are shown as though all of the combined variability were in the value of n (the number of synapses activated on an individual motoneuron). This permitted the threshold to be shown as though it were fixed at its average value, $\bar{h}$. The diagrams at the left illustrate how this normal distribution becomes shifted (relative to $\bar{h}$) for different values of effective input ($\beta = 0.5$, 0.75, and 1.0). In each case, the shaded area of the distribution corresponds to the output, ω, as fractional pool discharge ($\omega = 0.05, 0.40$, and 0.84, respectively). The resulting input-output curve is shown at the right in Fig. 2.

This model has basically two theoretical parameters; both are scaled to the number γN, the average number of (direct group Ia) synapses per motoneuron (e.g., $\gamma N = 100$). One of these two parameters is the standard deviation, $\sigma/\gamma N$, of the motoneuron population with respect to the difference variable, $n - h$ (i.e., the difference between the number, n, of synapses activated on a particular motoneuron and the threshold number, h, required to fire that neuron). The other basic parameter is the average threshold value, $\bar{h}/\gamma N$. It was satisfying to find that one of these parameters had the same value for all four of the input-output curves shown in Fig. 1; i.e., $\sigma/\gamma N = 1/5$. Because of this, each input curve could be obtained by resetting the value of other parameter, $\bar{h}/\gamma N$; four values, very close to 0.80, 0.88, 0.95, and 1.07, yielded the four input-output curves of Fig. 1.

The agreement found between theory and experiment thus implied that the shift to a deeper level of anesthesia (in the experiment) was matched by an increase in the value of a single model parameter (the average threshold, $\bar{h}$, the motoneuron population) without a significant change in the variance or standard deviation of the population with respect to $n - h$. In addition, the effect of brief tetanic conditioning was matched by a decrease in the effective value of that same model parameter (or by an increase in the effective value of n). It may be noted that complications, such as possible departures from a normal distribution, and the possible role of higher densities of activated synapses in local zones of the soma surface were addressed in the original paper (Rall, 1955a) and found to result in similar input-output curves.

Because this model also predicted how the factor of output potentiation should depend on the level of fractional pool discharge (Fig. 5 of Rall, 1955a), it was pointed out that this could be developed into a method of estimating fractional pool discharge. Further, an extension of the model to include distinctions between homonymous and heteronymous synapses was shown to yield agreement with "cross-facilitation" of one motor pool by input from heteronymous afferents, in contrast to little or no mono-synaptic "cross- discharge" in the absence of homonymous input (Figs. 6 and 7 of Rall, 1955a). A related modeling effort (Rall and Hunt, 1956) was able to account for experimental observations of the firing indices of individual motoneurons, in relation to motoneuron pool discharge, during repeated trials, for several different levels of reflex excitability.

Looking back about 33 years, it seems fair to say that these early efforts did succeed in providing explicit models that correspond reasonably well with the general concept of spatial summation in motoneuron pools, originally introduced by Denny-Brown and Sherrington (1928) and discussed by Lloyd (1945) in terms of an "excited zone," a "discharge zone," and a "subliminal fringe." The discharge zone corresponds to the shaded area in Fig. 2, while the subliminal fringe is composed of motoneurons in a band just to the left of the vertical threshold line; the excited zone probably includes the entire population for effective inputs greater than 50% of maximum.

One result of this study was to show that the shape of the input-output curve does not require spatial summation to be the very local process envisaged by Lorente de Nó (1938) and by Lloyd (1945). Moreover, another theoretical model, for passive electrotonic spread over a spherical soma, led to the conclusion that the membrane depolarization becomes essentially uniform over the closed soma surface by the time the synaptic potential reaches its maximum amplitude (Rall, 1953, 1955a, 1959); this result weighed against the validity of very local spatial summation on the motoneuron soma surface. It is interesting that the concept of local synaptic interactions has recently returned in a different context, namely, for synapses on excitable dendritic spines at distal dendritic locations (Rall and Segev, 1987, 1988).

In concluding this section on motoneuron populations, it is important to point out several limitations of these early models. No distinction was then made between motoneurons of different size or functional type; these important distinctions have been explored by Henneman and by other contributors to this volume. The assumption of random synaptic distributions was a convenience that was justified by ignorance of actual synaptic distributions. In addition, no distinction was made between different sequences of afferent fiber recruitment, and no consideration was given to distinguishing between synapses at different (proximal to distal) dendritic locations in the motoneuron population. The task of incorporating such considerations into a more comprehensive model of a motoneuron pool provides an interesting challenge for future modeling.

References

Brock, L. G., Eccles, J. C., and Rall, W. (1951). Experimental investigations on the afferent fibres in muscle nerves. *Proc. R. Soc. (Biol.)*, 138:453–475.

Denny-Brown, D. E., and Sherrington, C. S. (1928). Subliminal fringe in spinal flexion. *J. Physiol. (Lond.)* 66:175–180.

Eccles, J. C., and Rall, W. (1950). Post-tetanic potentiation of responses of motoneurones. *Nature* 166:465.

Henneman, E. (1954). Maximal discharge of a motoneuron pool during potentiation. *Fed. Proc.* 13:69.

Jefferson, A., and Benson, A. (1953). Some effects of post-tetanic potentiation of monosynaptic responses of spinal cord of cat. *J. Neurophysiol.* 16:381–396.

Lloyd, D. P. C. (1943). Reflex action in relation to pattern and peripheral source of afferent stimulation. *J. Neurophysiol.* 6:111–120.

Lloyd, D. P. C. (1945). On the relation between discharge zone and subliminal fringe in a motoneuron pool supplied by a homogenous presynaptic pathway. *Yale J. Biol Med.* 18: 117–121.

Lloyd, D. P. C. (1949). Post-tetanic potentiation of response in monosynaptic reflex pathways of the spinal cord. *J. Gen. Physiol.* 33:147–170.

Lorente de Nó, R. (1938). Synaptic stimulation as a local process. *J. Neurophysiol.* 1:194–207.

Rall, W. (1951). Input-output relation of a monosynaptic reflex. *Proc. Univ. Otago Med. Sch.* 29:17–18.

Rall, W. (1953). Electrotonic theory for a spherical neurone. *Proc. Univ. Otago Med. Sch.* 31: 14–15.

Rall, W. (1954). Monosynaptic reflex input-output analysis. *J. Physiol. (Lond.)* 125:30–31.

Rall, W. (1955a). A statistical theory of monosynaptic input-output relations. *J. Cell. Comp. Physiol.* 46:373–412.

Rall, W. (1955b). Experimental monosynaptic input-output relations in the mammalian spinal cord. *J. Cell Comp. Physiol.* 46:413–438.

Rall, W. (1959). Branching dendritic trees and motoneuron membrane resistivity. *Expt. Neurol.* 2:503–532.

Rall, W. (1990). Perspectives on neuron modeling. In *The Segmental Motor System*, ed. M. D. Binder and L. M. Mendell. New York: Oxford University Press.

Rall, W., and Hunt, C. C. (1956). Analysis of reflex variability in terms of partially correlated excitability fluctuations in a population of motoneurons. *J. Gen. Physiol.* 39:397–422.

Rall, W. and Segev, I. (1987). Functional possibilities for synapses on dendrites and on dendritic spines. In *Synaptic Function* (ed. G. M. Edelman, W. E. Gall, and W. M. Cowan). Wiley, New York, pp. 605–636.

Rall, W. and Segev, I. (1988). Synaptic integration and excitable dendritic spine clusters: Structure/function. In *Intrinsic Determinants of Neuronal Form and Function* (ed. R. J. Lasek and M. M. Black) New York: Alan R. Liss, pp. 263–282.

Rosenblueth, A., Wiener, N., Pitts, W., and Garcia-Ramos, J. (1949). A statistical analysis of synaptic excitation. *J. Cell. Comp. Physiol.* 34:173–205.

Complete Bibliography of Wilfrid Rall

(A): abstract, (B): book review, (C): book chapter, (J): journal article, (R): report, (T): thesis.

1944–1946 (R) Nine classified research reports for the Manhattan Project (at the Metallurgical Laboratory, University of Chicago); some of these reports overlap the next three items.

1946 (A) Rall, W. Mass assignments of some radioactive isotopes of Pd and Ir. *Phys. Rev.* 70:112.

1947 (J) Shaw, A. E., and W. Rall. An a.c. operated mass spectrograph of the Mattauch type. *Rev. Sci. Insts.* 18:278–288.

1948a (A) Rall, W. The packing fraction of Zirconium. *Phys. Rev.* 73:1222.

1948b (T) Rall, W. The field of biophysics. Univ. of Chicago M.S. Thesis.

1950 (J) Eccles, J. C., and W. Rall. Post-tetanic potentiation of responses of motoneurones. *Nature* 166:465.

1951a (J) Eccles, J. C., and W. Rall. Effects induced in a monosynaptic reflex path by its activation. *J. Neurophysiol.* 14:353–376.

1951b (J) Brock, L. G., J. C. Eccles, and W. Rall. Experimental investigations on the afferent fibres in muscle nerves. *Proc. Roy. Soc. Lond. Ser. B* 138:453–475.

1951c (J) Eccles, J. C., and W. Rall. Repetitive monosynaptic activation of motoneurones. *Proc. Roy. Soc. Lond. Ser. B* 138:475–498.

1951d (A) Rall, W. Input-output relation of a monosynaptic reflex. *Proc. U. Otago Med. Sch.* 29:17.

1953a (T) Rall, W. Spatial summation and monosynaptic input-output relations in the mammalian spinal cord. Univ. of New Zealand, Ph. D. Thesis; Univ. of Otago, Dunedin, New Zealand.

1953b (A) Rall, W. Electrotonic theory for a spherical neurone. *Proc. U. Otago Med. Sch.* 31:14–15.

1954 (A) Rall, W. Monosynaptic reflex input-output analysis. *J. Physiol. London* 125:30–31 P.

1955a (J) Rall, W. A statistical theory of monosynaptic input-output relations. *J. Cell. Comp. Physiol.* 46:373–411.

1955b (J) Rall, W. Experimental monosynaptic input-output relations in the mammalian spinal cord. *J. Cell. Comp. Physiol.* 46:413–437.

1956 (J) Rall, W, and C. C. Hunt. Analysis of reflex variability in terms of partially correlated excitability fluctuation in a population of motoneurons. *J. Gen. Physiol.* 39:397–422.

1957a (J) Rall, W. Membrane time constant of motoneurons. *Science* 126:454.

1957b (A) Rall, W. Theory of electrotonus and synaptic potentials on a spherical nerve model. *Abstracts of First National Biophysics Conference*, Columbus, Ohio, p. 58.

1958a (A) Freygang, W. H., K. Frank, W. Rall, and A. McAlister. Evidence for electrical inexcitability of soma-dendritic membrane in motoneurones. *Abstracts of Biophysical Society*, p. 23.

1958b (A) Rall, W. Mathematical solutions for passive electrotonic spread between a neuron soma and its dendrites. *Fed. Proc.* 17:127.

1958c (B) Rall, W. Book review of "An Introduction to Cybernetics," by W. Ross Ashby. London: Chapman and Hall, 1956. In *Archives Italiennes de Biologie*, 96:113–114.

1959a (R) Rall, W. Dendritic current distribution and whole neuron properties. Naval Medical Research Institute Research Report, NM 0105 00.01.02, pp. 479–525.

1959b (J) Rall, W. Branching dendritic trees and motoneuron membrane resistivity. *Exptl. Neurol.* 1:491–527.

1960a (J) Rall, W. Membrane potential transients and membrane time constant of motoneurons. *Exptl. Neurol.* 2:503–532.

1960b (A) Nelson, P. G., K. Frank, and W. Rall. Single spinal motoneuron extracellular potential fields. *Fed. Proc.* 19:1–5.

1960c (B) Rall, W. Book review of "Conduction of Heat in Solids," by H. S. Carslaw and J. C. Jaeger. Oxford University Press, London, 1959. In *Archives Italiennes de Biologie*, 98:118–119.

1961a (R) Rall, W. Mathematical model of dendritic neuron electrophysiology. In *Proceedings of the 3rd IBM Medical Symposium*, Endicott NY pp. 443–489.

1961b (A) Frank, K., P. G. Nelson, and W. Rall. Extracellular action potential fields of single motoneurons, and theoretical extracellular action potentials. *Abstracts of First International Biophysics Congress*, Stockholm, p. 244.

1962a (J) Rall, W. Theory of physiological properties of dendrites. *Ann. N.Y. Acad. Sci.* 96:1071–1092.

1962b (J) Rall, W. Electrophysiology of a dendritic neuron model. *Biophys. J.* 2: (No. 2, part 2) 145–167.

1964 (C) Rall, W. Theoretical significance of dendritic trees for neuronal input-output relations. In *Neural Theory and Modeling*, ed. R. F. Reiss. Stanford Univ. Press.

1965 (C) Rall, W. Dendritic synaptic patterns: Experiments with a mathematical model. In *Studies in Physiology*, presented to John C. Eccles, ed. D. R. Curtis and A. K. McIntyre. New York: Springer-Verlag.

1966 (J) Rall, W., G. M. Shepherd, T. S. Reese, and M. W. Brightman. Dendro-dendritic synaptic pathway for inhibition in the olfactory bulb. *Exptl. Neurol.* 14:44–56.

1967a (J) Rall, W. Distinguishing theoretical synaptic potentials computed for different soma-dendritic distributions of synaptic input. *J. Neurophysiol.* 30:1138–1168.

1967b (J) Rall, W., R. E. Burke, T. R. Smith, P. G. Nelson, and K. Frank. Dendritic location of synapses and possible mechanisms for the monosynaptic EPSP in motoneurons. *J. Neurophysiol.* 30:1169–1193.

1968a (J) Rall, W., and G. M. Shepherd. Theoretical reconstruction of field potentials and dendrodendritic synaptic interactions in olfactory bulb. *J. Neurophysiol.* 31:884–915.

1968b (C) Rall, W. Synaptic activity at dendritic locations: Theory and experiment. In *Neural Networks*, ed. E. R. Caianiello. New York: Springer-Verlag.

1969a (J) Rall, W. Time constants and electrotonic length of membrane cylinders and neurons. *Biophys. J.* 9:1483–1508.

1969b (J) Rall, W. Distributions of potential in cylindrical coordinates and time constants for a membrane cylinder. *Biophys. J.* 9:1509–1541.

1970a (C) Rall, W. Dendritic neuron theory and dendrodendritic synapses in a simple cortical system. In *The Neurosciences: Second Study Program*, ed. F. O. Schmidt. New York: Rockefeller Univ. Press.

1970b (C) Rall, W. Cable properties of dendrites and effects of synaptic location. In *Excitatory Synaptic Mechanisms*, ed. P. Andersen and J. K. S. Jansen. Oslo: Universitetsforlaget.

1971a (A) Rall, W., and J. Rinzel. Dendritic spines and synaptic potency explored theoretically. *Proc. I.U.P.S.* (XXV Intl. Congress) IX:466.

1971b (A) Rall, W., and J. Rinzel. Dendritic spine function and synaptic attenuation calculations. *Program and Abstracts Soc. Neurosci. First Annual Mtg.* p. 64.

1973 (J) Rall, W., and J. Rinzel. Branch input resistance and steady attenuation for input to one branch of a dendritic neuron model. *Biophys. J.* 13:648–688.

1974a (J) Rinzel, J., and W. Rall. Transient response in a dendritic neuron model for current injected at one branch. *Biophys. J.* 14:759–790.

1974b (J) Goldstein, S. S., and W. Rall. Changes of action potential shape and velocity for changing core conductor geometry. *Biophys J.* 14:731–757.

1974c (R) Rall, W. Dendritic spines, synaptic potency and neuronal plasticity. In *Cellular Mechanisms Subserving Changes in Neuronal Activity*, ed. C. D. Woody, K. A. Brown, T. J. Crow, and J. D. Knispel. Brain Information Service Research Report No. 3, U.C.L.A, Los Angeles, pp. 13–21.

1977a (C) Rall, W. Core conductor theory and cable properties of neurons. In *The Handbook of Physiology, The Nervous System, Vol. 1, Cellular Biology of Neurons*, ed. E. R. Kandel, J. M. Brookhart, and V. B. Mountcastle. Bethesda, MD: American Physiological Society.

1977b (J) Klee, M., and W. Rall. Computed potentials of cortically arranged populations of neurons. *J. Neurophysiol.* 40:647–666.

1978 (C) Rall, W. Dendritic spines and synaptic potency. In *Studies in Neurophysiology, presented to A. K. McIntyre*, ed. R. Porter. Cambridge: Cambridge Univ. Press.

1981 (C) Rall, W. Functional aspects of neuronal geometry. In *Neurones without Impulses*, ed. B. M. H. Bush and A. Roberts. Cambridge: Cambridge Univ. Press.

1982a (A) Rall, W. Theoretical models which increase R_m with dendritic distance help fit lower value of C_m. *Soc. Neurosci. Abst.* 8:115.11.

1982b (A) Miller, J. P., and W. Rall. Effect of dendritic length upon synaptic efficacy. *Soc. Neurosci. Abst.* 8:115.10.

1983a (J) Lev-Tov, A., J. P. Miller, R. E. Burke, and W. Rall. Factors that control amplitude of EPSPs in dendritic neurons. *J. Neurophysiol.* 50:399–412.

1983b (A) Segev, I., and W. Rall. Theoretical analysis of neuron models with dendrites of unequal electrical lengths. *Soc. Neurosci. Abst.* 9:102.20.

1983c (A) Rall, W. Introduction to passive cable properties of neurons. *Proc. IUPS XXIX Intl. Congress*, Sydney, Australia.

1984 (A) Segev, I., and W. Rall. EPSP shape indices when dendritic trees have unequal length. *Soc. Neurosci. Abst.* 10:215.12.

1985a (C) Rall, W., and I. Segev. Space clamp problems when voltage clamping branched neurons with intracellular microelectrodes. In *Voltage and Patch Clamping with Microelectrodes*, ed. T. G. Smith, H. Lecar, S. J. Redman, and P. Gage. Bethesda, MD: American Physiological Society.

1985b (J) Miller, J. P., W. Rall, and J. Rinzel. Synaptic amplification by active membrane in dendritic spines. *Brain Res.* 325:325–330.

1985c (J) Shepherd, G. M., R. K. Brayton, J. P. Miller, I. Segev, J. Rinzel, and W. Rall. Signal enhancement in distal cortical dendrites by means of interaction between active dendritic spines. *Proc. Nat. Acad. Sci.* 82:2192–2195.

1986 (A) Segev, I., and W. Rall. Excitable dendritic spine clusters: Nonlinear synaptic processing. *Soc. Neurosci. Abst.* 12:196.6

1987a (C) Rall, W., and I. Segev. Functional possibilities for synapses on dendrites and dendritic spines. In *Synpatic Function*, ed. G. M. Edleman, W. E. Gall, and W. M. Cowan. New York: Wiley.

1987b (C) Rall, W. Neuron, Cable Properties. In *Encyclopedia of Neuroscience*, ed. G. Adelman. Boston: Birkhauser.

1987c (A) Holmes, W. R., and W. Rall. Estimating the electrotonic structure of neurons which cannot be approximated as equivalent cylinders. *Soc. Neurosci. Abst.* 13:422.7.

1988a (C) Rall, W., and I. Segev. Synaptic integration and excitable dendritic spine clusters: Structure/function. In *Intrinsic Determinants of Neuronal Form and Function*, ed. R. J. Lasek and M. M. Black. New York: Alan R. Liss.

1988b (C) Rall, W., and I. Segev. Dendritic spine synapses, excitable spine clusters and plasticity. In *Cellular Mechanisms of Conditioning and Behavioral Plasticity*, ed. C. D. Woody, D. L. Alkon, and J. L. McGaugh. New York: Plenum Press.

1988c (C) Rall, W., and I. Segev. Excitable dendritic spine clusters: Nonlinear synaptic processing. In *Computer Simulation in Brain Science*, ed. R. M. J. Cotterill. Cambridge: Cambridge Univ. Press.

1988d (J) Segev, I., and W. Rall. Computational study of an excitable dendritic spine. *J. Neurophysiol.* 60:499–523.

1989 (C) Rall, W. Cable theory for dendritic neurons. In *Methods in Neural Modeling; from Synapses to Networks*, ed. C. Koch and I. Segev. Cambridge, MA: The MIT Press.

1990a (C) Rall, W., and I. Segev. Dendritic branches, spines, synapses and excitable spine clusters. In *Computational Neuroscience*, ed. E. Schwartz. Cambridge, MA: The MIT Press.

1990b (C) Rall, W. Some historical notes. In *Computational Neuroscience*, ed. E. Schwartz. Cambridge, MA: The MIT Press.

1990c (C) Rall, W. Perspectives on neuron modeling. In *The Segmental Motor System*, ed. M. D. Binder and L. M. Mendell. Oxford: Oxford Univ. Press.

1991 (A) Segev, I., and W. Rall. Computer models of dendritic excitability. *Soc. Neurosci. Abst.* 17:605.5.

1992a (C) Rall, W. Functional insights about synaptic inputs to dendrites. In *Analysis and Modeling of Neural Systems*, ed. F. H. Eeckman. Boston: Kluwer Academic Publishers. pp. 63–68.

1992b (C) Holmes, W. R., and W. Rall. Electrotonic models of neuronal dendrites and single neuron computation. In *Single Neuron Computation*, ed. T. McKenna, J. Davis, and S. F. Zornetzer. Boston: Academic Press.

1992c (C) Rall, W. Path to biophysical insights about dendrites and synaptic function. In *The Neurosciences: Paths of Discovery II*, ed. F. Samson and G. Adelman. Boston: Birkhauser.

1992d (J) Rall, W., R. E. Burke, W. R. Holmes, J. J. B. Jack, S. J. Redman, and I. Segev. Matching dendritic neuron models to experimental data. *Physiol. Rev.* 72:S159–S186.

1992e (J) Holmes, W. R., I. Segev, and W. Rall. Interpretation of time constant and electrotonic length estimates of multi-cylinder or branched neuronal structures. *J. Neurophysiol.* 68:1401–1420.

1992f (J) Holmes, W. R., and W. Rall. Electrotonic length estimates in neurons with dendritic tapering or somatic shunt. *J. Neurophysiol.* 68:1421–1437.

1992g (J) Holmes, W. R., and W. Rall. Estimating the electrotonic structure of neurons with compartmental models. *J. Neurophysiol.* 68:1438–1452.

1993 (J) Rall, W. Transients in neuron with arbitrary dendritic branching and shunted soma: A commentary for "New and Notable." *Biophys. J.* 65:15–16.

Index